Fourth Edition

Cara and MacRae's

Psychosocial Occupational Therapy

An Evolving Practice

Fourth Edition

Cara and MacRae's
Psychosocial Occupational Therapy
An Evolving Practice

Anne MacRae, PhD, OTR/L, BCMH, FAOTA

Professor Emerita
San Jose State University
San Jose, California

Previously edited by Elizabeth Cara & Anne MacRae

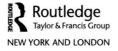

Routledge
Taylor & Francis Group

NEW YORK AND LONDON

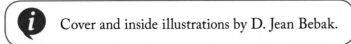
Cover and inside illustrations by D. Jean Bebak.

Cara and MacRae's Psychosocial Occupational Therapy: An Evolving Practice, Fourth Edition includes ancillary materials specifically available for faculty use. Included are supporting charts, learning activities, and reproducible forms. Please visit http://www.routledge.com/9781630914776 to obtain access.

First published 2019 by SLACK Incorporated

Published 2024 by Routledge
605 Third Avenue, New York, NY 10158

and by Routledge
4 Park Square, Milton Park, Abingdon, Oxon OX14 4RN

Routledge is an imprint of the Taylor & Francis Group, an informa business

Library of Congress Cataloging-in-Publication Data

Names: MacRae, Anne, author. | Preceded by (work): Cara, Elizabeth.
   Psychosocial occupational therapy.
Title: Cara and MacRae's psychosocial occupational therapy : an evolving
   practice / Anne MacRae.
Other titles: Psychosocial occupational therapy
Description: Fourth edition. | Thorofare, NJ : Slack Incorporated, 2019. |
   Preceded by Psychosocial occupational therapy : an evolving practice /
   Elizabeth Cara, Anne MacRae. 3rd ed. c2013. | Includes bibliographical
   references and index.
Identifiers: LCCN 2019004953 (print) | ISBN 9781630914776 (hardback)
Subjects: | MESH: Occupational Therapy--methods | Mental
   Disorders--rehabilitation
Classification: LCC RC487 (print) | NLM WM 450.5.O2 | DDC
   616.89/165--dc23
LC record available at https://lccn.loc.gov/2019004953

ISBN: 9781630914776 (hbk)
ISBN: 9781003522805 (ebk)

DOI: 10.4324/9781003522805

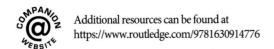
Additional resources can be found at
https://www.routledge.com/9781630914776

Dedication

This book is dedicated to the memory of my late husband, Joseph Hemm. My career would not have been the same without his constant support and encouragement. He was my best friend and helped me keep my priorities straight and maintain some balance in my life! We also shared in the upbringing of our two wonderful children, Nora and Malcolm Hemm. It is a comfort and delight to see them blossom into thoughtful, talented, and kind adults who pursue their life interests with passion.

My deepest appreciation and thanks also go to the many colleagues, students, service users, families, and friends who have graced my life. They have greatly enriched my knowledge and understanding and, in turn, I do my best to share what I have learned with others.

CONTENTS

Cara and MacRae's Psychosocial Occupational Therapy: An Evolving Practice, Fourth Edition includes ancillary materials specifically available for faculty use. Included are supporting charts, learning activities, and reproducible forms. Please visit http://www.routledge.com/9781630914776 to obtain access.

ABOUT THE EDITOR

Anne MacRae, PhD, OTR/L, BCMH, FAOTA received her bachelor's degree in education from Antioch College, Yellow Springs, Ohio, and her master's degree in occupational therapy from San Jose State University (SJSU) in California. She also has a doctorate in human science from Saybrook Institute, San Francisco, California. She is now retired after over 30 years on the faculty at SJSU and was granted the status of Professor Emerita. Anne remains active in occupational therapy as a frequent guest lecturer and consultant, both nationally and internationally. In addition to teaching and consulting, Anne actively engaged in practice throughout her career. She supervised the SJSU campus-based psychosocial occupational therapy clinic for 20 years, provided direct service and developed programs in rural areas, practiced in an urban psychiatric hospital and a partial hospitalization program, and occasionally still sees clients through private practice.

CONTRIBUTING AUTHORS

Tiffany (Debra) Boggis, MBA, OTR/L (Chapter 8)
Associate Professor, School of Occupational Therapy
Pacific University, College of Health Professions
Hillsboro, Oregon

Elizabeth Cara, PhD, OTR/L, MFT (Chapter 9)
Professor Emerita
San Jose State University
San Jose, California

Elizabeth Carley, OTD, OTR/L (Chapter 11)
Occupational Therapist
Northwest Center
Seattle, Washington

Bernadette Hattjar, DrOT, MEd, OTR/L, CWCE (Chapter 12)
Gannon University
Erie, Pennsylvania

William L. Lambert, MS, OTR/L (Chapters 10, 11)
Faculty Specialist
The University of Scranton
Department of Occupational Therapy
Scranton, Pennsylvania

Karen McCarthy, OTD, OTR/L (Chapter 12)
Dominican University of California
San Rafael, California

Jerilyn (Gigi) Smith, PhD, OTR/L, FAOTA (Chapters 3, 14)
Associate Professor
Graduate and Undergraduate Coordinator/Advisor
Occupational Therapy Program
San Jose State University
San Jose, California

INTRODUCTION

The mental health arena is in some ways undergoing rapid change, but in other ways, needed change is excruciatingly slow. Philosophical principles of recovery, justice, and trauma-informed care are certainly driving changing attitudes, but the practical methods used to incorporate these principles need further exploration and clarity. In order to address this need, the *Fourth Edition* of *Cara and MacRae's Psychosocial Occupational Therapy* is completely revised and reorganized.

Providing timely and significant new material creates a dilemma of how to edit material from earlier editions to produce a streamlined and affordable resource. Salient information from previous editions, including history, theory, assessments, techniques, diagnoses, specialized programs, and research are woven throughout this edition.

Keeping current with the significant shifts in thinking and practice can be challenging, but also extremely rewarding. This text is designed to meet practice challenges as the occupational therapy profession continues to evolve to meet the current needs of our communities.

Section I addresses practice settings and service delivery, with an emphasis on describing the entire continuum of health, social service, and community settings and how psychosocial occupational therapy is valuable in all settings. The chapters in this part of the book are all new but do incorporate relevant information from chapters published in previous editions. New to this book is the exploration of models of integrated primary care and the emergence of an occupational therapy presence in primary care, especially suited for occupational therapists because of our generalist background.

Chapter 1: Philosophical Worldviews of Mental Health. The differences in practice settings and service delivery are philosophical as well as practical, and these differences are highlighted in the opening chapter. Understanding the medical, rehabilitative, and social approaches to health, wellness, and recovery helps occupational therapists craft our practice to meet the needs of specific populations, communities, and practice settings.

Chapter 2: Psychiatric Institutions and Hospitals. This chapter provides a historical perspective of mental health care and also describes the current status of the hospital system. Also presented is the case that inpatient hospitals are an integral part of the continuum of service provision and that occupational therapists have a vital role in this service.

Chapter 3: Community Behavioral Health Services. Integrated primary care, especially with a focus on behavioral health concerns and healthy communities, includes several different models in various levels of development and implementation. This chapter describes the current status of integrated primary care and advocates for a strong occupational therapy presence. This chapter also discusses community behavioral health services, elements of healthy communities, and community partnerships. The future of occupational therapy practice is contingent on retaining and expanding our role in community behavioral health services, and suggestions to meet this goal are provided.

Chapter 4: Direct Service Provision. In order for occupational therapy to maintain its identity and credibility, direct service must remain the backbone of the profession. This chapter includes many examples and suggestions while describing the occupational therapy process. This process is changing as we move away from a medical model, so the chapter addresses up-to-date concepts of referrals, goals, assessment, intervention, and discontinuation of services. Core values and interpersonal strategies as well as documentation are also discussed.

Chapter 5: Consultation and Program Development. Although occupational therapists must maintain our roles in direct service, other roles that are responsive to the changing needs of service users and providers must also be expanded. There are a number of potential roles, but keeping with the practice orientation of this book, consultation and program development are discussed.

Section II provides a greater emphasis on understanding the person in multiple contexts. The cultural and environmental content found in previous editions is expanded into two chapters, and there is a new chapter discussing personal and social identity. This new chapter explores the personal and social interrelatedness of stigma and dimensions of identity. Although trauma awareness and trauma-informed care are discussed throughout this book, it is in this chapter that the trauma-related issues of poverty, violence, and human displacement are discussed, as well as the role of occupational therapy in all issues presented.

Section III maintains a much-heralded section of the previous editions—*Mental Health Across the Lifespan*—now expanded to include new chapters on the mental health of emerging adults and mid-life adults. The expansion of this part of the book is designed to allow a more thorough examination of lifespan issues. However, readers are urged to keep in mind that defining lifespan stages is a somewhat arbitrary concept based on chronology alone. Lifespan stages can significantly overlap depending on developmental age, emotional maturity, cultural and societal norms, and personal experiences.

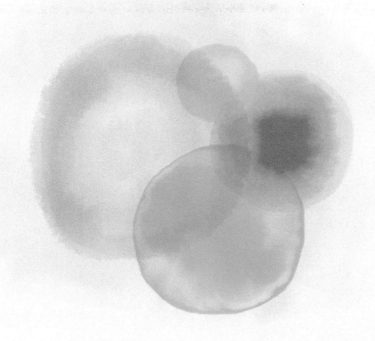

SECTION I
Practice Settings and Service Delivery

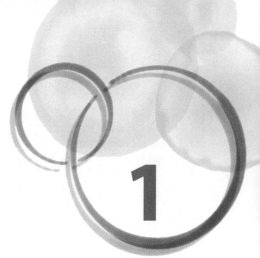

Philosophical Worldviews
of Mental Health

Anne MacRae, PhD, OTR/L, BCMH, FAOTA

Psychological health care literature, as well as academic training, focuses on well-established theoretical frameworks. These include the humanistic, biological, psychodynamic, behavioral, and cognitive perspectives. However, most discussions of these theories pertain to the etiology of mental illness and theoretically consistent interventions. This chapter focuses on the overarching philosophical worldviews that address not only interventions and outcomes, but also the broad belief systems that acknowledge emerging trends and paradigm shifts and, therefore, influence service delivery. It is important to recognize that although there is some relationship between traditional theoretical frameworks and the philosophical worldviews discussed in this chapter, it is not an automatic transference or a simple change in terminology. Readers are encouraged to immerse themselves in the scholarly literature, engage in self-reflection, and collaborate with organizational stakeholders to craft the most effective occupational therapy approaches for identified service users and practice settings.

Figure 1-1 shows a simple three-legged stool representing the three pillars of comprehensive mental health service. These pillars are often identified in the literature as *models*, but for the reasons previously discussed, it is perhaps more accurate to identify them as *philosophical worldviews*. These worldviews, compared in Table 1-1, are the medical model, rehabilitation model, and social model. Although there is some overlap between these models, there are also significant philosophical differences. For example, all three of these worldviews now acknowledge a wellness/recovery perspective and consider recovery to be the desirable outcome. However, as outlined in Table 1-1, each model defines recovery in very different ways. It is the position of this author that all three approaches should be incorporated, or at least considered, for comprehensive and effective service delivery. However, the priorities and emphasis can and should change with the needs of the service users and the practice setting. It does appear that there is movement toward the delivery of comprehensive services. One indicator is that the preferred term for services is now *behavioral health* rather than *mental health*. Behavioral health encompasses all aspects of mental/emotional well-being and actions that affect wellness. Problems include alcohol and drug addiction, serious psychological distress and mental disorders. In addition to standard interventions, behavioral health is also concerned with prevention and health promotion, as well as other recovery support. Although many agencies in the United States, particularly public community services, have now adopted the behavioral health title, it remains to be seen how the three pillars of comprehensive services will incorporate the concepts of behavioral health. Perhaps more critically, it is not clear that this broadened definition will affect the narrow parameters for reimbursement by public and private insurance. For the purposes of this chapter, and indeed the entire book, the terms *mental health* and *behavioral health* are both used, depending on context.

MacRae, A. (Ed.). *Cara and MacRae's Psychosocial Occupational Therapy: An Evolving Practice, Fourth Edition* (pp 3-17).
© 2019 Taylor & Francis Group.

TABLE 1-1. COMPARISON OF MENTAL HEALTH WORLDVIEWS

ATTRIBUTE	MEDICAL MODEL	REHABILITATION MODEL	SOCIAL MODEL
Power	Hierarchical	Collaborative partnership	Individual (service user)
Focus	Illness and symptoms	Function	Wellness, hope, and justice
Knowledge base	Pathology	Pathology and strengths; context	Lived experience, context
Techniques	Component based	Skill development in vivo	Support, inclusion
Outcomes	Clinical recovery (remission and management)	Functional recovery (adaptation)	Personal recovery (acceptance)

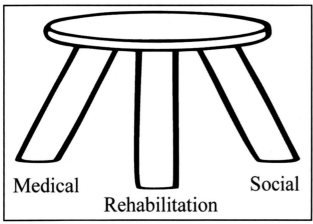

Figure 1-1. The three pillars of comprehensive mental health care.

MEDICAL MODEL

As is outlined in Table 1-1, the medical model is focused on illness and symptoms, necessitating a strong knowledge base in pathology. Therefore, the process of intervention is to determine a diagnosis and then consider the appropriate interventions. Practitioners most closely aligned with the medical model are physicians, nurses, pharmacists, and psychologists. Also, clinicians or counselors who use clinical approaches are essentially medical in nature because of their defined scope of practice and reimbursement schemas that focus on diagnostic assessment with the desired outcome to manage the related symptoms. Despite the obvious medical orientation in these practitioners' training and scope of practice, it should also be acknowledged that many medical clinicians actively collaborate with rehabilitative and socially oriented colleagues and embrace their values.

Diagnoses and Symptoms

The determination of a clinical diagnosis in psychiatry is, at best, an inexact process based on both deductive and inductive reasoning, and it often lacks precise data on psychiatric illness. Although knowledge of the structure and chemistry of the brain is growing, it is rare that measurable or visible objective data, such as X-rays and blood tests, as are used in physical diagnosis, can be used in psychiatry. Glackin (2010) suggests that diagnoses may be viewed as a destructive force that serves only to inappropriately label and dehumanize individuals. This sentiment is echoed by many mental health service users. Box 1-1 contains quotes from clients who participated in a focus group that describe their ambivalence regarding psychiatric diagnosis. Case Illustration 1-1 describes Brian's diagnostic history and highlights some of the limitations of psychiatric diagnosis.

Still another significant concern about diagnosis is cultural bias—specifically, a White, male, Judeo-Christian orientation. This issue is beginning to be addressed, but it remains essential that clinicians be aware of the inherent ethnocentrism found in the current diagnostic system (van de Water, Suliman, & Seedat, 2016). According to Alarcón et al. (2009):

> Careful attention to the sociocultural dimensions of mental illness serves both a scientific and social justice agenda. For example, when assessment fails to attend to sociocultural factors, it risks misdiagnosis and the perpetuation of clinical stereotypes based on race, ethnicity, gender, religion, or sexual orientation, among other factors, which can lead to mental healthcare disparities. (p. 559)

It has also been suggested that not taking into account all contextual factors has caused an increase in false positive diagnoses in community-based treatment (Wakefield, 2010). Given these limitations, why are diagnoses used at all? Shortly after the first publication of the *Diagnostic and Statistical Manual of Mental Disorders* (DSM) in 1952, justifications for using a diagnostic taxonomy were published, and the reasoning has been generally accepted for decades. As stated by Zigler and Phillips (1961), "a classificatory system in psychiatry serves the same essential purpose as

Box 1-1. Service User Attitudes About Diagnosis

- It's sort of weird, like a label stuck on my forehead.
- My diagnosis of bipolar disorder seems to make me think that's all of me. It isn't, though. There is so much more to me than my diagnosis of a mental illness.
- I guess there have to be different diagnoses. It gives the doctors something to work on and hopefully prescribe the right medication.
- The diagnosis of a mental illness is not so different than a medical diagnosis. It helps everyone understand his or her disease or problem.
- If only the "normies" could understand that the diagnosis of a mental illness is only a way to figure out how to help the client, just like with a medical diagnosis, then it wouldn't be such a bad thing.
- My diagnosis of schizophrenia has followed me around my entire adult life. It is like a plague. I hate it. It's like being called a wart and having a wart sitting right in the middle of my forehead!
- There are so many different diagnoses. I always wonder how the doctors come up with the right one, or if maybe they just guess.

CASE ILLUSTRATION 1-1: BRIAN'S MANY DIAGNOSES

Brian is a 58-year-old man who was first diagnosed with depression in his senior year of high school after fracturing his neck. With the physical pain, he remembers that the emotional pain that had been hidden suddenly rushed to the surface and he could no longer control it. His diagnosis of depression was only the first of many more diagnoses to come. Over the years, he recalls being diagnosed with bipolar disorder, borderline personality disorder, schizophrenia, schizoaffective disorder, posttraumatic stress disorder, and others. He isn't sure if any of those diagnoses were correct. Brian has symptoms that fit into just about all of those diagnoses at one time or another, but the diagnoses seemed to change with new psychiatrists and therapists. He now wonders if the different medications prescribed for his various diagnoses were possibly the wrong ones. He'll never know, but he still thinks about what would have happened if he had one psychiatrist, one therapist, and one (correct) diagnosis.

Discussion

There are many reasons why a diagnosis may change, including the differing theoretical perspectives of the primary clinician. However, diagnoses may also change because of the adopting of new criteria and diagnostic procedures by the psychiatric establishment, changing environmental stressors of the client, the development of new symptoms, or even new information coming to light within the therapeutic relationship. Regardless of the reasons for changing a client's diagnosis, this story demonstrates the need for caution against over-reliance or interpretation based on diagnosis alone.

taxonomy in science in general, and that a simple, coherent, and meaningful system of classification based on behavioral correlates of psychiatric syndromes is possible" (p. 607). Despite legitimate controversy, the diagnostic process helps facilitate interdisciplinary communication and fosters research, both of which are essential for high-quality mental health care. It is hoped that as research continues, the process of diagnosing will become increasingly objective, culturally sensitive, and accurate.

The most commonly used instrument to record diagnoses, disorders, and symptoms is the World Health Organization's (WHO's) *International Classification of Diseases*, currently in its 11th edition (ICD-11; WHO, 2018). WHO also publishes a companion document known as the *International Classification of Functioning, Disability and Health* (ICF), which not only covers the diagnostic concerns of body structure and functions but also includes ratings of activities and participation and contextual factors such as the influence of personal causation and environment (WHO, 2001).

The ICD and the ICF are not limited to mental illness and do not contain the diagnostic specificity found in the American Psychiatric Association's (APA's) DSM, which is currently in its fifth edition (APA, 2013).

This manual is a significant part of the academic curricula of mental health professionals, especially in the United States. Furthermore, according to Hebebrand and Buitelaar (2011):

TABLE 1-2. CATEGORIES OF PSYCHOPATHOLOGY AND DESCRIPTION OF TYPICAL SYMPTOMS

CATEGORY	SYMPTOMS
Thought	*Executive dysfunction:* Difficulty in planning, organizing, and strategizing *Concrete thinking:* Thought processes focused on immediate experiences and specific objects or events, as well as an inability to think metaphorically or abstractly *Delusions:* Deep-seated beliefs not based in reality, including delusions of grandeur as well as self-deprecating and paranoid delusions; these are typically not an exaggeration of real experiences but rather an essentially inaccurate, though powerful, belief *Obsessions:* Specific and repetitive thoughts that are typically unwanted and cannot be eliminated by reason
Language	*Concreteness:* Extremely literal verbal responses due to concrete thinking patterns; the speaker does not recognize the nuances of language, including abstractions or metaphors *Loosening of associations:* Ideas shift from one subject to another that is completely unrelated; the speaker does not show any awareness that the topics are unconnected *Perseveration:* Repetition of the same word, phrase, or idea; also, an inability to shift from one task to another *Circumstantiality and tangentiality:* The person digresses, giving unnecessary, irrelevant information; when speech is circumstantial, there is difficulty getting to the point of the conversation, yet in the person's mind, the answers are related; in tangential speech, the person starts answering a question but then rapidly digresses *Echolalia:* Repetition (echo) of the words and phrases of others; this speech is repetitive and persistent *Clanging:* The sound or rhyme of the words takes precedence over the meaning or content of the replies *Neologism:* An invented word that may closely resemble an existing word or may be known only to the individual

(continued)

[the] DSM not only influences how mental health specialists diagnose and treat their patients but also sways how US insurance companies decide which disorders to cover, how pharmaceutical companies design clinical trials and how funding agencies decide which research to fund. (p. 57)

With such widespread influence, it is sometimes difficult to keep in mind that the information being presented is not clear-cut, concrete, or complete. It is important to analyze the data critically and be aware of their limitations. Furthermore, the process of assessment and treatment planning is far more comprehensive than can be covered in a manual such as the DSM, and each particular discipline has something unique and specific to offer. It is important to be familiar with the information in the DSM; however, it should not be assumed that this knowledge is all that is required for practice, as it barely constitutes a beginning.

Inherent in the diagnostic process is the recognition of specific symptoms of mental illness. Although the trend in mental health practice is toward minimizing the focus on

symptoms alone and avoiding overpathologizing behavior, appropriate and effective treatment planning is dependent on identifying and understanding the symptoms of mental illness and the various ways they can interfere with a person's recovery. Symptoms of mental illness may present in a wide variety of combinations, and there are various schemas for organizing the information. Table 1-2 outlines the categories of psychopathology and descriptions of typical symptoms.

Psychopharmacology

By far the most common medical intervention for mental illness is the prescribing of psychotropic medications. Table 1-3 lists the types of psychopharmaceuticals, along with some examples of medicines that are in common use. However, this table is not meant to be a comprehensive source, and practitioners and students are encouraged to keep up with the rapid advances in this field by using related websites with up-to-date information. (See Suggested Resources at the end of this chapter.)

TABLE 1-2 (CONTINUED). CATEGORIES OF PSYCHOPATHOLOGY AND DESCRIPTION OF TYPICAL SYMPTOMS	
CATEGORY	**SYMPTOMS**
Perception and sensation	*Sensory-processing deficits*: Dysfunction is in the delivery or integration of the sensory message such as oversensitivity, avoidance, or low registration; deficits include distorted time sense and spatial awareness, poor visual perception, poor body scheme, and hyper- or hyposensitivity to stimuli *Hallucinations*: Perceptual images experienced as sensations but not based on actual stimulation from the external environment; can involve any of the senses: visual (seeing images), auditory (hearing voices or sounds), tactile (feeling sensations on the skin surface), gustatory (taste), olfactory (smell), and somatic (feeling sensations within the body) *Illusions*: A form of perceptual distortion in which the outside object causing the stimuli is real but the person misinterprets the object; like hallucinations, illusions may involve any of the senses, but auditory and visual illusions are most common
Affect	*Flat affect*: A lack of observable emotion *Anxiety/hostility*: Only considered pathologic if the emotional state is either inappropriate or out of proportion to the environmental stimuli *Depression*: Significant decrease of interest or pleasure in most daily activities, commonly identified as a sense of hopelessness; it may be seen with many psychiatric diagnoses *Mania*: A condition in which the individual responds in an eager, exuberant, and even joyful manner, regardless of the environmental reality; the dysfunction resulting from the manic state is usually caused by the associated features of poor judgment and impulsivity *Lability*: A state of unstable emotions not necessarily related to external stimuli; may present as incontrollable laughter or tears
Orientation and memory	*Orientation*: A person's awareness and appropriate identification of time, place, and person *Procedural memory*: An automatic sequence of behavior such as conditioned responses *Declarative memory*: Memory specific to consciously learned facts such as school subjects *Semantic memory*: The knowledge of the meaning of words and the ability to classify information or ideas *Episodic memory*: The knowledge of personal experiences *Prospective memory*: The capacity to remember to carry out actions in the future; in essence, "to remember to remember"
Energy and motoric response	*Lethargy and agitation*: Very commonly found in a wide variety of psychiatric disorders; considered pathologic when responses interfere with daily function *Disruption of the sleep–wake cycle*: Either excessive or insufficient sleep can contribute to poor overall functioning and to worsening of other symptoms *Catatonia*: Rigidity or immobility most likely observed during an acute and severe psychotic episode rather than as a persistent state *Stereotypy*: The repetition of apparently senseless actions *Tics*: Muscular spasms or twitching *Compulsions*: Repetitive, irrational behaviors acted out in response to an overwhelming urge

Despite widespread use, psychopharmacology is not without controversy, and pharmaceuticals rarely work in isolation to control all of the symptoms and deficits found in persons with mental illness. Drug therapy should be viewed as one possible facet of comprehensive, interdisciplinary treatment. Compliance with prescribed medication regimes is often the primary goal and the focus of medically oriented intervention. Prescribing clinicians walk a fine line between respecting the rights of the service user to choose a course of treatment and ensuring that the

TABLE 1-3. OVERVIEW OF PSYCHOTROPIC MEDICATIONS

CLASSES/TYPES	SUBTYPES	GENERIC EXAMPLES (SAMPLE BRAND NAME)
Antidepressants	Selective serotonin reuptake inhibitors	Fluoxetine (Prozac); sertraline (Zoloft); paroxetine (Paxil)
	Serotonin norepinephrine reuptake inhibitors	Venlafaxine (Effexor XR); duloxetine (Cymbalta); desvenlafaxine (Pristiq)
	Atypical	Bupropion (Wellbutrin); mirtazapine (Remeron); trazodone (Desyrel)
Antipsychotics	First generation (typical)	Chlorpromazine (Thorazine); haloperidol (Haldol); pimozide (Orap)
	Second generation (atypical)	Aripiprazole (Abilify); quetiapine (Seroquel); risperidone (Risperdal)
Mood stabilizers		Divalproex (Depakote); carbamazepine (Tegretol); lithium (Eskalith)
Antianxiety agents		Diazapam (Valium); lorazepam (Ativan); buspirone (Buspar)
Stimulants		Amphetamine (Adderall); methylphenidate (Ritalin); dextroamphetamine (Dexedrine)

person has access to information and understands all of the positive and negative consequences of taking or not taking prescribed medication. In an effort to improve communication regarding medication choices, the process of shared decision making is now highly recommended and considered to be essential for meaningful recovery (Paudel, Sharma, Joshi, & Randall, 2018). A decision team may consist of several stakeholders, including staff, service users, family, and peers (Bradley & Green, 2018).

Although occupational therapists do not prescribe medication, the occupational therapy focus on function (doing) provides an ideal perspective from which to observe the effectiveness of the medication regimen and work with both the team and the service user to establish an individualized and optimum plan of treatment. "Occupational therapists analyze and formulate tailored solutions to problems associated with the performance of medication management activities. Occupational therapy practitioners implement interventions that reduce barriers and promote routine, effective medication management" (American Occupational Therapy Association, 2017, p. 6).

Table 1-4 lists commonly cited reasons for refusal or inability to take medication and some techniques that the occupational therapist or other team members may use to help the individual adhere to prescribed treatment. However, the ultimate choice remains the service user's, and that must be respected.

REHABILITATION MODEL

Although the rehabilitation model is well understood and accepted in physical medicine, it is not as broadly understood or consistently applied in mental health services. Even the terminology can vary depending on geographic location, as well as history of use and preference in practice settings. For example, the term *psychosocial rehabilitation* is often used interchangeably with *psychiatric rehabilitation*. In practice, the more colloquial term *psych rehab* is common and is the term of choice for this chapter.

Psych rehab is the process of restoring community functioning and well-being of an individual who has a psychiatric disability. The categories of service and examples of interventions that comprise the psych rehab scope of practice are delineated in Table 1-5. Rehabilitation practitioners seek to effect changes in a person's environment and in a person's ability to deal with his or her environment in order to facilitate improvement in symptoms, full community integration, and improved quality of life. The key concepts of psych rehab service delivery are as follows:

- Psych rehab is contextual, requiring knowledge of home and community as well as individual life events, influences, and experiences.
- Psych rehab is skill based; therefore, it requires practice.
- Psych rehab is action oriented and may be provided individually, in groups, or through consultation.
- Psych rehab has immediate application to daily living.

TABLE 1-4. INTERVENTIONS FOR MEDICATION MANAGEMENT

REASON	DESCRIPTION	INTERVENTIONS
Delusions or beliefs of potential harm	Paranoid delusions may include fears of poisoning or other physical damage. However, clients also may refuse medication based on nonpathological belief systems grounded in their sociocultural and religious upbringing.	*Trust building*: Clients who have a solid therapeutic relationship with someone in the system are less likely to think they will come to harm. *Correcting misinformation*: Erroneous beliefs such as an individual's fear of becoming a "drug addict" can be addressed through education.
Admission of illness	Denial is a common reaction to the onset of severe illness. With psychiatric disorders, there are the added problems of dealing with social stigma and the possible presence of thought disorder.	*Create an accepting environment*: Rather than attempting to "convince" someone of his or her illness, it is important to convey that individuals are accepted for who they are. *Peer counseling*: Often, clients can benefit from hearing about the personal experience of others. *Education*: The realities of the illness may not be as frightening as the assumptions. It is important for service users to know that many people are able to live satisfying and productive lives with the presence of a mental illness.
Side effects	Individual reaction to psychotropic medication is extremely variable. Many side effects disappear or decrease with time. However, others may be ongoing and difficult to tolerate or manage.	*Medical interventions*: This may include switching medications or reducing dosages, as well as adding additional medications. *Educational techniques (individual or group) for medication management*: This may include instruction in nutrition (increasing fluid and fiber, decreasing caffeine), avoidance of direct sunlight (sunscreen, outing schedule, hats), regulation of sleep and exercise, and relaxation techniques.
Cognitive deficits	Deficits may include poor memory, confusion, poor time orientation, concrete thinking, and poor organizational skills.	*Medical intervention*: Simplify regime by decreasing dosages per day and using long-acting agents. *Supervision*: This includes health care staff or appropriately instructed caregivers. *Memory and orientation strategies*: This includes reminder notes, pill organizers, and schedules.
Perceived loss of freedom	Complaints are of restrictive monitoring and dislike of precautions, including recommendations to avoid caffeine or alcohol and the necessity of remaining on a schedule and reporting to the clinic for follow-up lab work.	*Education*: Clients are more likely to adhere to recommendations if they understand the consequences of avoiding advice. *Change of medication*: The choice may be for a medication with limited side effects or precautions, even if it is considered less effective than alternatives. *Adaptation of daily living*: Help clients switch to decaffeinated, nonalcoholic beverages and using a calendar, day planner, and/or clock and visual reminders.

From the definition provided and the key concepts, it is obvious that occupational therapists are psych rehab practitioners, and examples of rehab-oriented occupational therapy assessments and interventions are discussed throughout this text. Other psych rehab practitioners may include case managers and social workers, as well as peer specialists operating in a behavioral health arena. Further discussion of peer specialists can be found in the subsequent section

TABLE 1-5. PSYCHIATRIC REHABILITATION SERVICES AND INTERVENTIONS

CATEGORY OF SERVICE	EXAMPLES OF INTERVENTIONS
Symptom management	Relaxation techniques and coping skills, techniques to manage medication side effects, memory strategies and anger management
Social relationships	Friendship encouragement and identification of support persons, communication and social skill development
Community integration	Social outings, stigma reduction and advocacy, linkage with community social groups
Vocational and educational skills	Work readiness program, volunteer opportunities, General Equivalency Diploma prep course, linkage with community college, referrals to Department of Rehabilitation and Employment Development
Basic living skills	Group and individual interventions for self-care such as hygiene and grooming, meal preparation
Financial management	Budget and shopping skills, assistance with entitlement applications and management (e.g., Social Security, disability insurance)
Community and legal resources	Collaboration with the faith-based community, linkage with agencies to provide health and human service support as needed (e.g., Medicaid, food stamps), linkage with affordable or pro bono attorneys and legal clinics for specialized services such as immigration issues and criminal record expungement
Health maintenance	Accompanying peers to medical and dental appointments, groups focused on prevention and wellness such as nutrition and exercise
Housing	Linkage with governmental housing services such as Housing and Urban Development), services provided at homeless shelters as needed, home management skill development, home visits as needed

on the social model but is included here because some peer specialists, particularly those with recognized certification, can work in traditional settings, and the services are reimbursable (Daniels, Ashenden, Goodale, & Stevens, 2016; Walsh, McMillan, Stewart, & Wheeler, 2018).

It is important to recognize that, unlike the traditional medical model, there is no assumption in the rehab worldview that the underlying causes of dysfunction are directly or solely due to the psychiatric illness. Rather, myriad issues may be contributing factors to the diagnosis that initiated services. In addition, it is often the case that obstacles to recovery concurrently exist that should inform the course of intervention. Case Illustration 1-2 highlights these complex issues.

Habilitation and Prevention

Another complication in understanding rehab terminology is differentiating between *habilitation* and *rehabilitation*. Rehabilitation focuses on regaining skills and abilities that have been lost or diminished because of a disability or

illness. Habilitation focuses on attaining skills of daily living that may have never been developed or refined due to a number of circumstances not limited to new diagnoses. Physical medicine is almost exclusively focused on rehabilitation, whereas in pediatric or school-based settings, habilitation has recently gained more attention (Hooper, 2017). However, in psych rehab, it is often difficult to determine previous levels of function due to poor reporting and limited access to accurate records. Therefore, it is up to the practitioner to determine an accurate baseline of knowledge and skills. Although addressing habilitation for mental health service users requires different interventions than might be used in rehabilitation, all interventions are typically under the umbrella of rehab or are not addressed at all because of preexisting organizational structures. For example, having to learn new skills may not be seen by insurance companies as being a result of the diagnosis that triggered treatment authorization. Therefore, the services will not be reimbursed unless the issue is framed as rehabilitation (connected to diagnoses) rather than habilitation. In some cases, depending on the interpretation of protocols

CASE ILLUSTRATION 1-2: REBECCA'S MULTIFACETED TREATMENT

Rebecca sought services at the county (public) behavioral health agency at the insistence of her sister. She was subsequently diagnosed with major depression and was prescribed Zoloft. It was also recommended that she participate in the psych rehab groups offered at the center. Through informal interviews and observation, it became apparent that Rebecca had a difficult childhood with abusive parents and persistent poverty. To escape her past, Rebecca dropped out of school at age 16 and moved in with her boyfriend. It is unclear if there was a pattern of intimate partner abuse because Rebecca refused to discuss this. She was very dependent on the boyfriend because he financially supported her for 3 years prior to being arrested and sent to prison for dealing drugs. Because she could not afford the rent for the apartment they had shared, she returned to her parents' house, where her sister observed her lethargy, poor eating, and lack of affect or interaction. Her sister also noticed that her prescription pain medicine was missing and feared that Rebecca had taken them, potentially for a suicide attempt.

Discussion

It is likely that the diagnosis of major depression is accurate and that medication may reduce the symptoms of depression. Rebecca can also benefit from psychotherapy to address suicidal ideation and dysfunctional relationships. However, she will have great difficulty in improving her quality of life, sustaining health, and promoting her own recovery without intensive psych rehab. Rehabilitation would address a wide range of independent living skills, including educational and vocational preparedness, financial management, communication skills, and healthy living strategies. In addition to direct services, the rehab specialist or team would likely refer Rebecca to several community resources, including a trauma support group, government agencies for entitlement benefits (food, shelter, health care), and a vocational training agency.

and rules, habilitation can only be addressed through non-medical services such as may be provided in recovery and wellness centers (see the section on the social model).

A related concept to habilitation that is much discussed in the literature but unfortunately not adequately funded is prevention. In the psych rehab arena, this specifically refers to the development of coping and management skills but also addresses the likelihood of psychological distress or psychiatric illness manifesting if preventative techniques are not provided. For example, children or adolescents who have "missed out" on typical skill development due to deprived environments or who are transitioning to independence, such as aging out of the foster care system, are at high risk of a variety of mental health challenges, including depression and posttraumatic stress disorder (Rapaport, 2015).

The Importance of Rehabilitation in Behavioral Health Care

In many ways, rehabilitation is the bridge between the social and medical models, having elements of both. Psych rehab specialists are generally well trained in psychopathology, understand the diagnostic system, and are versed in addressing symptom management. However, psych rehab also recognizes the necessity of identifying a service user's strengths and using such strengths in all interventions.

Psych rehab specialists, especially occupational therapists, are equally versed in the personal, social, cultural, and environmental issues that may represent strengths or cause significant distress and dysfunction, and they are trained to address all of these areas simultaneously. These areas are sufficiently complex to warrant separate chapters in Section II of this text.

Unfortunately, it is common for people with either a medical and social perspective to attempt to provide and even claim reimbursement for psych rehab without a complete understanding of the focus or parameters. Many organizations, including policy makers and public/private funders, have poorly defined rehab goals, limited staff trained in the philosophy of psych rehab, and a poor understanding of the competencies needed to provide authentic rehabilitative services. Readers are encouraged to not only expand their knowledge of psych rehab but also to develop strategies for educating stakeholders about its value and to become active advocates for psych rehab inclusion in all services. Organizations such as the Psychiatric Rehabilitation Association provide a wealth of resources for such purposes. (See Suggested Resources for the website.)

In conclusion, a robust, well-defined psych rehab service can be the bridge between the clashing paradigms of the medical and social models and can fill the gaps in consumer services. It is an essential leg of the three-pronged approach to comprehensive mental health care. Furthermore, occupational therapists, because of our unique skill set, should be at the forefront of the advocacy and education efforts.

Figure 1-2. History of the recovery/
wellness movement.

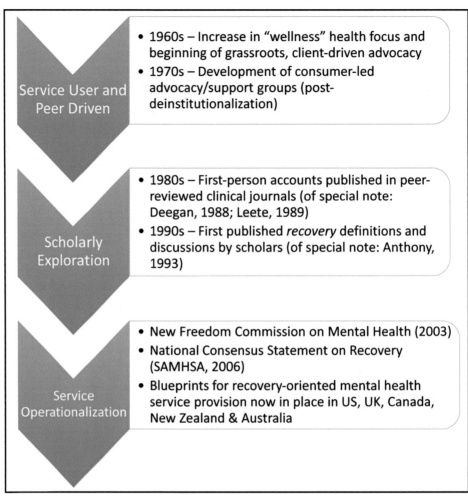

Service User and Peer Driven

- 1960s – Increase in "wellness" health focus and beginning of grassroots, client-driven advocacy
- 1970s – Development of consumer-led advocacy/support groups (post-deinstitutionalization)

Scholarly Exploration

- 1980s – First-person accounts published in peer-reviewed clinical journals (of special note: Deegan, 1988; Leete, 1989)
- 1990s – First published *recovery* definitions and discussions by scholars (of special note: Anthony, 1993)

Service Operationalization

- New Freedom Commission on Mental Health (2003)
- National Consensus Statement on Recovery (SAMHSA, 2006)
- Blueprints for recovery-oriented mental health service provision now in place in US, UK, Canada, New Zealand & Australia

SOCIAL MODEL

The social model is the driving force in the establishment of peer-driven support groups and wellness centers, as well as advocacy and outreach organizations. As described in Table 1-1, the focus of the social model is on wellness, hope, and justice. The worldview of the social model is that mental health challenges are primarily, but not exclusively, determined by external factors of the environment and other contexts, as well as social factors such as stigma, exclusion, marginalization, and oppression. In order to understand how the social model can benefit people with mental illness or psychosocial distress, it is necessary to leave the comfort zone of conventional Western health care and explore the knowledge bases of social justice, politics, advocacy, and policy.

Recovery and Wellness

The hallmark of the social model is the advent of the recovery movement, which recognizes personal or lived experience as the most authentic source of knowledge. As discussed in previous sections, recovery is now considered the ultimate outcome for all mental health services, and there can be considerable overlap in the beliefs of mental health practitioners, regardless of their initial professional training. Nevertheless, it would be disingenuous to not acknowledge that the recovery movement started as a grassroots effort by former and current service users. It was only after people with lived experience began to speak out and organize that serious scholarly exploration and governmental policy development occurred. Key events in the history the recovery movement are shown in Figure 1-2.

One of the first scholars to write about recovery with mental illness was Professor William (Bill) Anthony of Boston University. Although there are many scholarly interpretations and critiques of recovery, Anthony's early definition captures the key elements of the principle of recovery as it is used today:

> Recovery is described as a deeply personal, unique process of changing one's attitudes, values, feelings, goals, skills, and/or roles. It is a way of living a satisfying, hopeful, and contributing life even with limitations caused by illness. Recovery involves the development of new meaning and purpose in one's life as one grows beyond the catastrophic effects of mental illness. (1993, p. 11)

By the turn of the century, policy statements to operationalize recovery principles were being discussed and eventually published. For example, the Substance Abuse and Mental Health Services Administration (SAMHSA), together with other federal agencies, developed a National Consensus Statement, which states:

> Mental health recovery is a journey of healing and transformation enabling a person with a mental health problem to live a meaningful life in a community of his or her choice while striving to achieve his or her full potential. (2006)

In addition to this definition, SAMHSA added 10 components of recovery, which are depicted in Figure 1-3.

Inherent in the social model is a focus on wellness. In 2006, Swarbrick, an occupational therapist, developed a pictorial representation of "the eight dimensions of wellness" that has been extensively used by SAMHSA as well as other agencies to explain the holistic nature of wellness. The dimensions include the following:

1. Emotional
2. Financial
3. Social
4. Spiritual
5. Occupational
6. Physical
7. Intellectual
8. Environmental

Peer Leaders

A key to sustaining the recovery movement as a positive force is the emergence of leaders who have the lived experience of mental illness and are willing to talk about their past. These leaders have not only been successful with their own recovery but are also inspirational to others in the recovery process by being positive role models. They also play a major role in educating the community and influencing the political process related to mental health services.

Because the social model is predicated on the idea that lived experience (of mental illness) is the primary source of knowledge, it stands to reason that peer leaders or specialists should have a major role in providing services in any program that identifies as a recovery or wellness center. Case Illustration 1-3 describes Chanlina's horrific life events and psychological distress and highlights the unique gifts and special bond that a peer leader can offer. Although many people in the recovery process use and value professional mental health services, intervention within the recovery perspective is not limited to clinical treatment. Peer support, self-help groups, information sharing, peer teaching, and role modeling, as well as community and family support, are all important components of recovery.

Successful recovery, which includes regaining meaningful roles and social participation, is also dependent

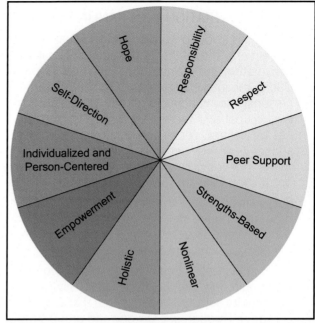

Figure 1-3. Components of recovery. (Adapted from Substance Abuse and Mental Health Services Administration. [2006]. *National consensus statement on mental health recovery* [Publication SMA-05-4129]. Rockville, MD: Author.)

on support from all aspects of the community. The most immediate community is often family members, who can be a valuable social support for the person with mental illness. Empathy from family members can be overwhelmingly comforting and often makes the difference between stability and relapse. It can be a far more difficult road for individuals with mental illness who are estranged or isolated from family. For these individuals, peer leaders can help develop surrogate family with healthy friendships and meaningful roles in the community. Behavioral health drop-in or wellness centers often provide the environment for developing such surrogate families through peer support, opportunities for socialization and activities, shared meals, and group celebrations of cultural and community events.

Peer teaching takes many forms, from one-on-one instruction and providing informational literature to running groups. One particular intervention, the Wellness Recovery Action Plan (WRAP), is an exemplary intervention that can be led by peer specialists but ultimately directed by peer participants. WRAP is a system that was developed by and for people who want to be active participants in gaining and retaining their personal health. It has also been studied as a means of supporting recovery after a crisis (Ashman, Halliday, & Cunnane, 2017). A facilitator who has completed the certification course in WRAP facilitation guides the process. According to Copeland (2002):

> The Wellness Recovery Action Program is a structured system for monitoring uncomfortable and distressing symptoms, and, through planned responses, reducing, modifying, or eliminating

CASE ILLUSTRATION 1-3: CHANLINA—PEER-PROVIDED RECOVERY SERVICES

Chanlina is a young woman being seen at an outpatient behavioral health agency for an intake assessment. The referral to this agency was initiated as she was released from the hospital for acute dehydration and malnutrition after she was found wandering the streets with no shoes or coat. During the intake assessment, Chanlina became highly agitated when asked to fill out forms with personal information and refused to sign a consent to treatment form. She was about to leave when the occupational therapist, who headed the rehab team, asked Chanlina's permission to contact the nearby wellness center and arrange to have a peer specialist meet her. She explained that the wellness agency peer provider could help Chanlina negotiate available services and provide support. She agreed to the meeting only on the condition that she would not need to share any personal information. The occupational therapist waited with Chanlina in the lobby until Rose, the peer specialist, arrived.

Rose walked Chanlina over to the wellness center to show her the facility and explain the many programs offered. Because it was clear that English was not Chanlina's first language, Rose offered to find her a translator. However, Chanlina not only refused translation services, she also would not disclose her primary language.

Although Chanlina began to attend the center regularly, she only stayed through the provided lunch and would only talk with Rose. Eventually, Chanlina became a regular participant in groups and community activities and reported that the wellness center was the only place that she felt safe and accepted. Through one-on-one and group support, Chanlina's traumatic past was slowly revealed to Rose. She was taken from her home in Cambodia at the age of 14 as part of a human trafficking operation and brought to the United States. She was forced into prostitution, regularly beaten, and often denied food. After she escaped from her confines, she did not know how to get help, including food or shelter, which resulted in her hospitalization. Rose was able to provide emotional support by sharing her own story of being a survivor of intimate partner violence and being estranged from her family. She also shared her history of being treated for posttraumatic stress disorder and depression. Chanlina admitted to having many of the same symptoms that Rose described but was not yet willing to seek clinical help.

Chanlina wanted to continue practicing her English, but it was sometimes difficult. Rose found a Khmer (Cambodian) language app that helped them communicate. She also arranged for Chanlina to attend an English as a second language course at the local community college. As Chanlina's history came to light, it became clear to Rose that there were services needed beyond what the wellness center could provide. She referred Chanlina to an additional outside support group specializing in the trauma of sex slavery and human trafficking. She also referred her to a refugee and immigrant assistance program that offered many services, including pro bono legal help and specialized clinical services.

Discussion

Without the consistent and dedicated support of the peer specialist, coupled with the welcoming and noninvasive atmosphere of the wellness center, it is likely that Chanlina's path to recovery would have been thwarted and service would have simply fallen between the cracks. The peer specialist provided Chanlina with empathetic and nonjudgmental support while providing linkage with many needed community services.

those symptoms. It also included plans for responses from others when your symptoms have made it impossible for you to continue to make decisions, take care of yourself, and keep yourself safe. (p. 3)

The Role of Professional Mental Health Providers in the Social Model

Given that diagnoses and symptoms may or may not be a focus of service, professional mental health care providers often struggle to find their place within the social model. However, mental health professionals, especially occupational therapists, can provide meaningful contributions to social model programs. These contributions sometimes occur through direct services but more often through mentoring and consultation. Examples of these services are highlighted in Chapter 5.

Psych rehab practitioners may be better able to assimilate into the social model than medical practitioners because of their multiple frames of reference involving social justice and environmental dimensions. For example, occupational therapy has extensive grounding in occupational justice, as well as conceptual models that explore the interrelatedness between a person and the environment (society), including the Model of Human Occupation, the Canadian Model of Occupational Performance and Engagement, and all of the ecological frameworks.

Some emphasis has been placed on social issues in the occupational therapy literature for a long time. An argument could be made that the founders were at least implicitly aware of issues of justice. Schwartz (2009) pointed out in her Eleanor Clark Slagle Lecture:

> [T]he reformers of the early 20th century had strong views about democracy and social justice, and a firm belief in the power of science to influence proposed social, educational and medical reforms. In particular, the reform movements involving arts and crafts, moral treatment, scientific management, and women's suffrage would have a significant and direct influence on the founders of the profession of occupational therapy.… The founders displayed confidence, courage, hard work, creativity and a willingness to take risks. These characteristics are what we need to cultivate if we are going to lead our profession in implementing the Centennial Vision.

Obstacles to Professional Involvement in Socially Oriented Programs

Programs designed on a complete social model (rather than as a hybrid with medical and rehabilitative services) present unique challenges for professionals who want to work in such settings. The first challenge is that the practitioner must gain the trust of the service users and be willing to give up control of the situation and follow the lead of the service users, providing their unique expertise only as requested. However, even practitioners prepared for this power shift face other challenges. By far the largest obstacle relates to reimbursement for services. In the United States, payment, from either public or private insurance, is entirely based first on medical principles and second on rehabilitation principles, and then only if interventions are related to current diagnoses and the reduction of symptoms. Even in the systems of other countries that have varying degrees of socialized health care, there are still parameters for qualified services that tend to be medical in nature. Therefore, the most effective method of employing health care practitioners in social model programs is to use multiple funding streams. These funding sources often include public and private grants but may also be generated from partnering with nonmedical service organizations from the community, the education sector, social services, or criminal justice agencies. Such designs are becoming more common in the United States but can also be found in many other places in the world, especially in high-need areas.

An excellent example is Grandmothers Against Poverty and AIDS (GAPA), which started in South Africa but has been replicated in multiple African countries. This organization was founded by a small group of grandmothers with the assistance of an occupational therapist in 2001 to provide education and psychosocial support. The original funding was derived from research grants and ongoing program needs, and funding continued through a wide variety of sources, including several branches of the South African government, corporate donations, universities, religious institutions, and benevolent societies. (See Suggested Resources for GAPA website.) They have also devised some self-income generation schemas based on selling crafts and garden products (GAPA, 2015). The mission and programs of GAPA are consistent with the philosophy of occupational therapy, and occupational therapists remain very involved in the activities of GAPA. However, it must always be recognized that it is the grandmothers who are the leaders of this organization, and indeed the entire movement. It is hoped that occupational therapists around the world can follow the lead of GAPA and similar organizations to partner with others in developing much-needed services in their home countries.

RECOMMENDATIONS AND SUMMARY

The delivery of mental and behavioral health services is going through a period of rapid transformation in which occupational therapists, as all practitioners, must align their practice with new trends. This includes understanding the dissidence between worldviews but also exploring ways in which the best elements of all perspectives can be honored and merged for best practice. A key feature of these changes will be the further development of collaborative models of service, together with people with the lived experience of mental illness. An area of particular urgency is establishing a research agenda and approach that is consistent with the worldviews described in this chapter. Currently, all health care fields hold the medical-scientific research agenda as the gold standard to develop evidence-based practice. This type of research is extremely difficult to conduct in small, community-based mental and behavioral health settings, so there is a perceived paucity of evidence-based practices. However, reversing the priority to be practice-based evidence is certainly possible and much desired. In other words, rather than focusing on large-scale, highly controlled studies of specific interventions, the focus on data collection and analysis of the actual services provided can identify meaningful interventions, document successful outcomes, and improve practice protocols. The obstacle to the practice-based evidence approach is primarily the perception that such data are somehow inferior, which results in difficulty publishing or otherwise sharing practice-based results.

Furthermore, it stands to reason that if behavioral health professionals are going to study recovery outcomes, it must be done in collaboration with people in recovery. Collaborative and participatory research are typically qualitative or mixed-method designs that, like practice generated data, often do not meet the hierarchical and empirical criteria that many scholarly journals require for publication. There is debate within the social and recovery framework about the value of measuring generalized outcomes because they are seen by some recovery advocates as dehumanizing and impersonal (Browne, 2006). Inherent in the recovery perspective is the concept that desired outcomes are determined by the service user, but conventional outcome measures used in research are meant to be applied with all people identified within a particular population (Dickens, 2009). Although there are certainly ways to individualize outcome measures, large-scale, population-based outcome studies are the most professionally valued and hence most frequently published. Clearly, a rethinking of both research priorities and valued methodologies is in order. "If we are to embrace outcome measures, let's measure things that are relevant to the new culture" (Browne, 2006, p. 153).

ACKNOWLEDGEMENT

Material for the diagnostic case illustration and the service user quotes found in the figures were gathered in focus groups conducted by Carol Underwood. She also contributed to some of the writing regarding recovery and wellness.

REFERENCES

Alarcón, R. D., Becker, A. E., Lewis-Fernández, R., Like, R. C., Desai, P., Foulks, E., … Cultural Psychiatry Committee of the Group for the Advancement of Psychiatry. (2009). Issues for DSM-V: The role of culture in psychiatric diagnosis. *Journal of Nervous and Mental Disease, 197,* 559-660.

American Occupational Therapy Association (2017). Occupational therapy's role in medication management. *American Journal of Occupational Therapy, 71*(Suppl 2), 7112410025. doi:10.5014/ajot.716S02

American Psychiatric Association. (2013). *Diagnostic and statistical manual of mental disorders* (5th ed.). Washington, DC: Author.

Anthony, W. (1993). Recovery from mental illness: The guiding vision of the mental health service system in the 1990s. *Psychosocial Rehabilitation Journal, 16*(4), 11-13.

Ashman, M., Halliday, V., & Cunnane, J. G. (2017). Qualitative investigation of the Wellness Recovery Action Plan in a UK NHS crisis care setting. *Issues in Mental Health Nursing, 38*(7), 570-577.

Bradley, E., & Green, D. (2018). Involved, inputting or informing: "Shared" decision making in adult mental health care. *Health Expectations, 21,* 192-200.

Browne, G. (2006). Outcome measures: Do they fit with a recovery model? *International Journal of Mental Health Nursing, 15,* 153–154.

Copeland, M. E. (2002). *Wellness Recovery Action Plan.* West Dummerston, VT: Peach Press.

Daniels, A. S., Ashenden, P., Goodale, L., & Stevens, T. (2016). *National Survey of Compensation Among Peer Support Specialists.* Albuquerque, NM: The College for Behavioral Health Leadership. Retrieved from www.leaders4health.org

Deegan, P. (1988). Recovery: The lived experience of rehabilitation. *Psychiatric Rehabilitation Journal, 11,* 11-19.

Dickens, D. (2009). Mental health outcome measures in the age of recovery-based services. *British Journal of Nursing, 18*(15), 940-943.

Glackin, S. (2010). Tolerance and illness: The politics of medical and psychiatric classification. *Journal of Medicine and Philosophy, 35,* 449-465.

Grandmothers Against Poverty and Aids. (2015). GAPA annual report: Together we are stronger. Retrieved from http://www.gapa.org.za/

Hebebrand, J., & Buitelaar, J. K. (2011). On the way to DSM-V. *European Child & Adolescent Psychiatry, 20,* 57-60.

Hooper, L. (2017). Associations press for continued HHS support for rehabilitation and habilitation. *OT Practice, 22*(6), 6.

Leete, E. (1989). How I perceive and manage my illness. *Schizophrenia Bulletin, 15*(2), 197-200.

New Freedom Commission on Mental Health. (2003). *Achieving the promise: Transforming mental health care in America.* Washington, DC: Author.

Paudel, S., Sharma, N., Joshi, A., & Randall, M. (2018). Development of a shared decision making model in a community mental health center. *Community Mental Health Journal, 54,* 1-6.

Rapaport, L. (2015, October 22). Teens leaving foster system may lack needed mental health care. *Reuters Health News.* Retrieved from https://www.reuters.com/article/us-health-fostercare-teens/teens-leaving-foster-system-may-lack-needed-mental-health-care-idUSKCN0SG2OX20151022

Schwartz, K. B. (2009). Reclaiming our heritage: Connecting the founding vision to the centennial vision (Eleanor Clarke Slagle lecture). *American Journal of Occupational Therapy, 63,* 681-690.

Substance Abuse and Mental Health Services Administration. (2006). *National consensus statement on mental health recovery* (Publication SMA-05-4129). Rockville, MD: Author.

Swarbrick, M. (2006). A wellness approach. *Psychiatric Rehabilitation Journal, 29*(4), 311–314.

van de Water, T., Suliman, S., & Seedat, S. (2016). Gender and cultural issues in psychiatric nosological classification systems. *CNS Spectrums: The International Journal of Neuropsychiatric Medicine, 21*(4), 334-340.

Wakefield, J. C. (2010). Misdiagnosing normality: Psychiatry's failure to address the problem of false positive diagnosis of mental disorder in a changing professional environment. *Journal of Mental Health, 19*(4), 337-351.

Walsh, P. E., McMillan, S. S., Stewart, V., & Wheeler, A. J. (2018). Understanding paid peer support in mental health. *Disability & Society, 33*(4), 579-597.

World Health Organization. (2001). *International classification of functioning, disability and health.* Geneva, Switzerland: Author.

World Health Organization. (2018). *International classification of diseases* (11th ed.). Geneva, Switzerland: Author.

Zigler, E., & Phillips, L. (1961). Psychiatric diagnosis: A critique. *The Journal of Abnormal and Social Psychology, 63*(3), 607-618.

Suggested Resources

American Psychiatric Association: www.psychiatry.org

Boston University Center for Psychiatric Rehabilitation: www.bu.edu/cpr

Grandmothers Against Poverty and Aids (GAPA): www.gapa.org.za

National Library of Medicine MedlinePlus: www.medlineplus.gov

Mental Health America: www.mentalhealthamerica.net

Mental Health Recovery (and WRAP): www.mentalhealthrecovery.com

National Alliance on Mental Illness (NAMI): www.nami.org

Prescribers' Digital Reference: www.pdr.net

Psychiatric Rehabilitation Association: www.psychrehabassociation.org

Substance Abuse and Mental Health Services Administration: www.samhsa.gov

World Health Organization *International Classification of Diseases* (ICD): www.who.int/classifications/icd/en

World Health Organization *International Classification of Functioning, Disability and Health* (ICF): www.who.int/classifications/icf/en

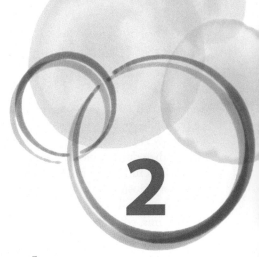

Psychiatric Institutions and Hospitals

Anne MacRae, PhD, OTR/L, BCMH, FAOTA

Psychiatric hospitals have been experiencing steady and significant downsizing for decades, and although behavioral health services in the community are preferred to hospitalization, the closure of many facilities has led to a situation where hospital beds are not available when needed.

Although there is no argument that occupational therapy is a good match for community services, this chapter advocates for occupational therapy to preserve and even expand our role in acute psychiatric services. The role of occupational therapy in acute psychiatry is often misunderstood and has sometimes been considered nonproductive, overtly difficult, and frightening. Actually, it is quite the opposite. The occupational therapist in these settings has the opportunity for a deeply satisfying and enjoyable work experience while providing authentic and effective occupational therapy.

THE RISE AND FALL OF PSYCHIATRIC INSTITUTIONS

In order to understand the current situation regarding psychiatric hospitalization, it is helpful to provide a brief history of the treatment of people with mental illness. Throughout the ages, what are now commonly thought of as symptoms of mental illness were seen as spiritual phenomena, and in some parts of the world, in certain cultures, and in some religious groups, these beliefs can still be found. In some cases, the person is revered as having "special knowledge" and is considered a shaman (or cultural equivalent). People so designated are protected and cared for if needed. However, much more frequently, the differences in behavior are interpreted as demonic, leading to harsh, sometimes brutal treatment. Even without the spiritual interpretation of "abnormal" behavior, people with symptoms of mental illness have often been ostracized from society. For example, writings from the Civil War era in the United States provided the following description:

> If the insane person is peaceful, people generally let him run loose. But if he becomes raging or troublesome, he's chained down in a corner of the stable or an isolated room, where his food is brought to him daily. (Caradec, 1860, as quoted in Shorter, 1997, p. 11)

In England, if people were not kept at home they might be sent to workhouses or poorhouses, and the situation in the United States was similar to that in Europe. In rural Massachusetts in 1840, social reformer Dorothea Dix noted finding a woman in a cage in Lincoln, a man chained in a stall in Medford, and four women in animal pens in Barnstable (Dix, 1843). In an almshouse she visited, she came upon a woman beating on the bars of a cage, "the unwashed frame invested with fragments of unclean garments, the air so extremely offensive, though ventilation

MacRae, A. (Ed.). *Cara and MacRae's Psychosocial Occupational Therapy: An Evolving Practice, Fourth Edition* (pp 19-31). © 2019 Taylor & Francis Group.

was afforded to all sides save one, that it was not possible to remain beyond a few moments" (p. 6). Before 1800, there were only two hospitals in the United States that admitted people then designated as "insane": Pennsylvania Hospital, established in 1752 by the Religious Society of Friends, and New York Hospital, which had a separate psychiatric building that was called the *Lunatic Asylum.*

Asylums, which had existed in Europe since the Middle Ages, were frequently referred to as *madhouses* and, for obvious reasons, were regarded as places to be avoided. That began to change with the introduction of a new approach in the 19th century that became known as *moral treatment.* Phillipe Pinel of France is commonly recognized as its initiator, although efforts were underway in all of Europe and England to create new asylums based on the moral treatment philosophy. Moral treatment was humanitarian and therapeutic. Pinel's philosophy was a humanistic one characterized by kindness and respect, in which individuals would be treated with dignity and optimism in place of the previous view of persons with mental illness as dangerous and incurable. The asylums for moral treatment were designed around the belief that orderly routines and occupations would have a therapeutic effect. Pinel (1809) advocated a carefully planned treatment approach based on the use of "occupational activities of different kinds according to individual taste; physical exercise, beautiful scenery, and from time to time soft and melodious music" (p. 260).

What began in Europe ultimately came to the United States, where several private institutions were created under the moral treatment philosophy. They included McLean Asylum in Massachusetts, Hartford Retreat in Connecticut, Friends Hospital in Pennsylvania, and Sheppard Enoch Pratt Asylum in Maryland. Public asylums using the moral treatment approach were also established, with one of the most prominent founded in Worcester, Massachusetts. These facilities were impressively equipped with a variety of craft rooms, gardens, and recreational areas designed to provide residents with an active schedule of productive, creative, and recreational occupations. Another such program, Gardner State Colony in Massachusetts, also provides a typical example of the rich occupation base of treatment: the residents were largely responsible for the development of 1500 acres of productive farmlands that yielded 142,526 quarts of milk and 2000 dozen eggs (Hall, 1914, p. 302). Inside the facility there was a carpenter shop, furniture factory, machine shop, shoemaking department, and rug weaving department (p. 304).

> But it is not all work at Gardner. The patients have a good time … [with] tennis, golf … reading and entertainment. They have their orchestra and have musicals frequently. They have an excellent library, bowling and billiard rooms, and on the whole it is not such a terrible thing to be insane if one can be sure of the happy, even passage of one's life at a place like Gardner. (Hall, 1914, p. 305)

In a way, the success of the asylums based on moral treatment ultimately led to their demise. Once asylums gained a good reputation, people were willing to be admitted to them. After a while, there were more people than could be accommodated with the available resources. Ultimately, the asylums did not have the funding to support the increasing numbers of individuals needing care. This resulted in overcrowded conditions and understaffing (Rothman, 1971). Moreover, by the beginning of the 20th century, there was a shift in the view of mental illness away from the beliefs of moral treatment that centered on the importance of the therapeutic environment to the view that the science of brain pathology would provide the information that would ultimately lead to a cure.

The 20th century was a time of great experimentation in the treatment of mental illness. Because no one had discovered a "cure," any and all theories, modalities, and approaches that might work were tried. Unfortunately, these interventions included intense sessions of electroconvulsive therapy; psychosurgery such as lobotomies (excision of part of the frontal lobe of the brain); high doses of sedating medicines, including morphine, phenobarbital, or chloral hydrate; and long periods of forced hydrotherapy (hot or cold baths). When all these techniques failed, physical restraints were used, including straightjackets and chains.

During this time, there were attempts to revive the ideas of moral treatment with the introduction of the concept of a therapeutic community called *milieu therapy.* This approach added a new dimension in advocating that participants should have autonomy and a voice in determining how the therapeutic community would be run. The idea of the therapeutic community became so popular in the United States that, by 1960, almost all mental health facilities claimed to use this approach. Unfortunately, the necessary resources to make it successful were never provided, and it was not fully embraced by psychiatrists.

The dire situation in the care of people with mental illness began to change in 1954 when chlorpromazine was introduced in the United States. Clinical trials revealed that this drug calmed agitation and ameliorated the severe behaviors associated with psychosis (Rollin, 1990). Thus began the era of psychopharmacology, which has since seen the development of a wide range of highly marketed medications. There is little doubt that the introduction of these drugs represented a significant step forward for many people who otherwise might have been lifelong inmates in institutions. The drugs, however, did come at a price. One problem was the side effects, particularly of the early drugs. (See Chapter 1 for further discussion of side effects). Also, the false hope that medications would provide a cure, or at least an effective method of controlling all symptoms, was one factor in the deinstitutionalization movement that started in the United States in the late 1950s and continued through the following decades. The closing of psychiatric hospitals also occurred in many other countries in the world. For example, in Great Britain, the number of psychiatric hospital beds steadily declined from 1962 to the mid-1980s (Craig & Timms, 1992). In India, the trend took hold in the 1970s and continues to the present day (Sheth, 2009). Many countries did not experience the same degree of profound negative effects found in the United States, partly because the transitions to the community were conducted over a longer period of time, better planned, and, in some cases, more appropriately funded than in the United States.

Although there is no doubt that the advent of psychopharmaceutical treatments contributed to the deinstitutionalization movement, there were other factors. The social movement favoring community-based, rather than institutional, care took hold concurrently with the advent of psychopharmacology. Also, the beginnings of a self-advocacy movement and the increase in legal protections could be seen as both causes and effects of hospital closures. Still another oft-cited contributor to the deinstitutionalization movement was short-sighted cost cutting. Whether the experiment in deinstitutionalization was a failure or success remains controversial. In theory, treatment provided in the least restrictive environment is an agreed-upon aim. Community-based services have helped many individuals improve quality of life and social inclusion. Nevertheless, it is generally accepted that the closure of psychiatric hospitals is linked to an increase in homelessness and a vast number of people with mental illness incarcerated in the criminal justice system. In fact, prisoners with mental illness outnumber the people with mental illness in state hospitals (Torrey et al., 1992). The issues of homelessness and criminal justice as they relate to mental illness are covered in several other chapters of this text, but the role of psychiatric hospitals in our overall health care service needs to be discussed and clarified throughout many sectors of society. Some scholars, expressing concern of failing systems and overwhelming mental health crises, go so far as to propose the return of the asylum system (Sisti, Segal, & Emanuel, 2015). Although most experts disagree with that approach, clearly there is a need to rethink the community, housing, and service needs of people with serious and persistent mental illness.

THE NEED FOR COMPREHENSIVE BEHAVIORAL HEALTH SERVICES

As described in Chapter 1, behavioral health disorders include both substance abuse and mental illness, which until recently were considered separate concerns with different treatment protocols, payment for services, data collection, and policies. Because there can be significant overlap between substance abuse and some mental illnesses or being at risk for mental illness, gathering data and developing treatments that can be used in many situations is an efficient means of addressing multiple issues. According

to the Substance Abuse and Mental Health Services Administration (SAMHSA), substance use disorders "occur when the recurrent use of alcohol or other drugs (or both) causes clinically significant impairment, including health problems, disability, and failure to meet major responsibilities at work, school, or home" (2015a). Of the more than 20 million adults with a substance use disorder, almost 8 million (at least 39%) have a co-occurring mental illness (SAMHSA, 2015a). Although substance use disorders, as well as mental illness, can and often should be treated in the community, there is no doubt that people with severe and/or multiple comorbidities may be in dire need of hospitalization in order to eventually thrive or even survive in the community. "It is known that in cases of substance use disorder with psychiatric comorbidity, clinical presentation and symptoms are more severe than in patients diagnosed with either substance abuse disorder or another psychiatric disorder only" (Darcin, Nurmedov, Noyan, Yilmaz, & Dilbaz, 2015, p. 197). Therefore, the likelihood of a needed hospitalization increases with dual diagnoses. Although inpatient treatment for drug and alcohol rehabilitation is available for people able to pay out of pocket, many of these private programs do not accept people with mental illness, particularly if the condition requires medication management. Public or low-cost options are scarce for both substances abuse or dual diagnoses and often have long waiting lists for admission. Particularly because the opioid crisis is now at an epidemic stage, it is hoped that more inpatient facilities will be funded.

According to the National Institute of Mental Health (2017), one in six adults (44.7 million people) in the United States lives with a mental illness, and according to the National Alliance on Mental Illness "approximately 1 in 25 adults in the United States—9.8 million, or 4.0%—experiences a serious mental illness in a given year that substantially interferes with or limits one or more major life activities" (n.d.). These statistics are roughly similar to worldwide statistics; however, recording strategies vary widely. What is not debated is the dire need for services worldwide. According to the World Health Organization:

> … the gap between the need for treatment and its provision is wide all over the world. In low- and middle-income countries, between 76% and 85% of people with mental disorders receive no treatment for their disorder. In high-income countries, between 35% and 50% of people with mental disorders are in the same situation. (2017)

Having a meaningful, productive life while being socially included in the community is the ultimate aspiration of people in recovery. However, there are times that individuals need higher levels of structure and care than can be provided in the community. In an ideal model of service delivery, there are many levels of care that are matched to the needs at the time. A system that allows for the continuity of care, from acute short-term hospitalizations to

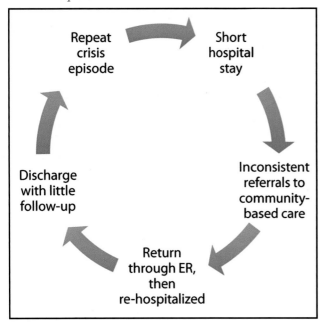

Figure 2-1. The revolving door syndrome. Abbreviation: ER, emergency room.

intermediate or long-term care facilities to various levels of assistance and support in the community, is ideal but is woefully lacking.

Violence and Behavioral Health Disorders

Contrary to the persistent and highly damaging myth largely fostered by the media, people with mental illness are generally not dangerous and violent. Statistically, people who have a mental illness who live in the community are no more likely to commit a serious crime than are people in the general population. However, most of the available data are derived from treatment facilities and therefore do not include people who have never received services or been diagnosed with a mental illness. (The need for prevention and early intervention is further discussed in the following chapter on community services.)

Another confounding factor in determining the potential for violence is the high incidence of substance use disorders with or without a dual diagnosis with mental illness. Alcohol and street drugs decrease judgment and reasoning and increase impulsivity, thereby reducing awareness of consequences of actions. Hence, it is possible that intoxicated individuals act on behavior that would otherwise be controlled. The other link to violence is the potential for being involved with a wide range of illegal activities, especially when the substance being used is illegal.

People who are actively psychotic, particularly if they are paranoid, sometimes do become very violent, which is most often self-afflicting violence, but they may also present a danger to others. These are two criteria that can initiate an involuntary hospitalization.

PSYCHIATRIC HOSPITALIZATION

One of the major differences between the goals of current psychiatric hospitalization and the historic institutions described earlier in this chapter is the expected length of time and resultant outcome of the service. As Swarbrick (2009) described, there was little expectation in the past that institutional residents would ever return to the community, and their conditions were viewed as life-long afflictions. In modern-day psychiatric hospitals, the goal is to release people back into the community in as short a time as possible. Although philosophically this is consistent with the principles of recovery, it is also driven by economic decisions that have nothing to do with the medical needs of patients or sustainable recovery in the community. The number of available psychiatric hospital beds has been steadily dwindling for decades. Based on 2015 data, it is estimated that there is one "psych bed" for every 5,006 people in the United States; however, there should be a minimum of one psych bed for every 2,000 people (California Hospital Association, 2018). The shortage of available beds sometimes forces hospitals to release people before they are stabilized or have a plan for community integration. This phenomenon triggers what is known as the *revolving door syndrome*, which is graphically displayed in Figure 2-1. This destructive pattern not only contributes to painful setbacks in the recovery process, but it is also fiscally irresponsible due to the high cost of emergency rooms and repeated potentially nonproductive hospitalizations.

Another factor that contributes to short-stay hospitalization is the limited, sometimes unrealistic, payment schemas for services. This is especially problematic in the United States with its privatized and fragmented health care system. Even people with private insurance are subject to stringent limitations in reimbursement and access to services. Unless someone has substantial personal wealth, hospitalization will be limited in length, if possible at all. For those without the means to pay for psychiatric hospitalization, there are mandated public psychiatric hospitals that are meant to provide acute short- and long-term care in every state in the United States (Mental Health America [MHA], n.d.-a). However, length of stay in acute care hospitals is extremely limited, some only accept patients placed on legal involuntary holds for admission, and the geographic availability of hospitals varies tremendously state to state and region to region. The situation is even more problematic in public long-term facilities. The waiting list for an available bed is often months long, and the options are very limited. Should a person who is no longer in need of acute care continue to occupy an expensive hospital bed? Or should that same person, who has significant functional limitations, be released to the streets even if there are no available supports? The issues raised by such scenarios go beyond the need for further health care reform. Rather, they are complex phenomena involving societal values, legal rulings, and the allocation of resources throughout the entire

CASE ILLUSTRATION 2-1: DANGER TO SELF—INVOLUNTARY PSYCHIATRIC HOSPITAL ADMISSION

Elise is a 25-year-old graduate student who tends to procrastinate and then pull all-nighters to complete assignments. Her behavior deteriorated over the semester and started to alarm her housemates. One night, they found Elise on the floor of the bathroom, crying uncontrollably and holding a razor blade to her wrists. Elise's housemates tried to get her to drop the blade, but she kept screaming that there was "no use in even trying." One housemate called 911, and when the police arrived, she attempted to strike an officer but then sank to the floor, shaking and crying. An ambulance arrived, and the emergency medical technicians transported Elise to an emergency room (ER), where she was eventually transferred to the locked psychiatric unit on a 72-hour involuntary hold.

Discussion

Elise meets the criteria for involuntary admission based on the observation that she is an immediate danger to herself. She appears to be struggling with a mood disorder, but the precise diagnoses are yet to be determined (differential diagnosis: bipolar disorder or major depression). The number of entities (housemates, police, emergency medical technicians, ER, hospitalization) involved in this process is not unusual, and the process was in fact relatively smooth. Errors can occur at every step along the way. The housemates could have ignored the behavior, the police could have arrested Elise and taken her to jail, or she could have been immediately released from the ER without psychiatric care.

spectrum of medical, social, and educational services. Although some of these issues are discussed throughout this book, for the purposes of this chapter, the focus is on acute care hospitalization.

Many people have distorted ideas about psychiatric hospitalization. Some have a very negative view, partially because of a history of neglectful and abusive treatment, but also because of prolonged media misrepresentation. Others have an extremely positive view, thinking that once someone is sent to the hospital, the individual will be "cured," or at least managed, and thereby the community will be safer. Neither of these conflicting views is entirely fair or accurate. The purpose of psychiatric hospitalization is primarily to stabilize the person sufficiently to be able to return to the community or to move on to a less restrictive environment, such as an intermediate-level or long-term facility. Although this role is minimal compared with the role of psychiatric institutions in the past, it is still a daunting mission given the extreme time limitations, intermittent or minimal community services, and lack of coordination throughout the spectrum of mental health services. In order to have a better understanding of the value and limitations of psychiatric hospitalization, it is helpful to discuss what actually happens in an acute care psychiatric setting.

Admission

Hospital admission is typically a very stressful event for anyone, but for someone who might be confused, psychotic, and/or involuntarily admitted, it can be especially frightening. The process of involuntary admission varies from state to state and country to country, but typically the individual must show a present and immediate danger to self or others and/or be "gravely disabled." "Danger to self"

is the most common reason for psychiatric admission and is described in Case Illustration 2-1. "Danger to others" is a needed caveat for involuntary admission, but, as previously discussed, it is probably overplayed in the media. The qualification *gravely disabled* is the most nebulous and, therefore, open to interpretation. However, in most jurisdictions, it is reserved for people who are incapacitated to the point of being unable to perform even the most basic survival skills. Case Illustration 2-2 provides an example of a gravely disabled man brought into the hospital on an involuntary commitment hold.

Given the severity of symptoms and behaviors found in people eligible for an involuntary admission, it is not unusual for the police to be involved. Unfortunately, sometimes seriously mental ill people are brought directly to jail. However, if the local police are well trained and there are relevant protocols as well as available services, the police will initiate the involuntary commitment process, generally starting in an emergency room before follow-up transport to a locked psychiatric unit.

The ideal situation is that the newly admitted patient has a psychiatric advanced directive in place and can, in some form, relay contact information for people who have permission to share such documentation. A psychiatric advance directive lists medical treatment preferences as well as other instructions. It is created when a person is stable but can "grant legal decision-making authority to another person who will serve as [an] advocate and health care agent until the mental health crisis is over" (MHA, n.d.-b). One such directive, the Wellness Recovery Action Plan, was discussed in Chapter 1, but there are other formats for advanced directives. For example, MHA provides thorough information regarding the content and legal issues involved when preparing an advanced directive.

CASE ILLUSTRATION 2-2: GRAVELY DISABLED—INVOLUNTARY PSYCHIATRIC HOSPITAL ADMISSION

The police respond to a storekeeper's complaint of a "homeless guy" who was huddled in his doorway and refused to leave. Upon finding the man, the police attempted to assess his status, initially assuming that he was drunk, but several clues suggested that there may be multiple issues. His speech was mostly incoherent, with some evidence of paranoid delusions. Also, he appeared to be significantly underweight and could not remember when he last ate. In addition, he was possibly dehydrated. When the police attempted to forcibly move him from the shop's doorway, he collapsed. The police called the paramedics to transport the nameless man to the ER, which they did with him in restraints. Blood for lab analysis was drawn at the ER, which somewhat surprisingly showed a blood alcohol level well below the legal level of intoxication. The ER treated him with intravenous fluids, but his mental state did not significantly clear. Considering that there was no apparent physical illness or injury to account for his behavior, he was transferred to the psych unit under a 72-hour involuntary hold for observation.

Discussion

This man meets the criteria for gravely disabled because he is not able to meet his basic survival needs. The staff in the psych unit has no information on this man, so other than continuing to care for his physical needs, observation will be the first form of assessment and intervention. It may be that his mental status will clear with no further intervention, but even if it does, the psychiatric service will attempt to discern the underlying cause of his grave disability. It is somewhat of a misnomer to call these admissions "involuntary" because, in many cases, particularly with those who are gravely disabled, the individual is unable to give an informed consent for treatment.

Trauma-Informed Care in Hospital

Trauma-informed care (TIC) must be adapted to the meet the demands of a particular environment. (TIC is more thoroughly discussed in Chapter 7.) Given the events that usually lead to a psychiatric hospitalization, it is to be expected that the person is traumatized. Moreover, people in this population are highly likely to have experienced past trauma and are at risk of retraumatization. Therefore, initial contact must be brief and calming. Muskett (2014) advocates for the use of specific trauma-informed approaches for inpatient mental health settings precisely because of significant evidence of the high incidence of trauma in the backgrounds of people with mental illness. Beckett, Holmes, Phipps, Patton, and Molloy (2017) support this position and further state that trauma-informed practice can have a positive effect on reducing seclusion and restraints and improving therapeutic engagement. According to SAMHSA (2015b), survivors of trauma "need to be respected, informed, connected, and hopeful regarding their own recovery." Although a trauma-informed approach is especially critical during the admission process and initial contact, the principles should be combined with other principles of recovery and therapeutic techniques throughout the entire hospitalization.

It is not uncommon for newly admitted patients to refuse to disclose their names, let alone any details about their lives. Therefore, unless the person has been previously hospitalized in the same location and is remembered, the team needs to start from the beginning, building a profile that includes all diagnoses, medication history, precautions,

cultural and religious beliefs, prior living arrangements, and social support—all while respecting that verbal exchanges are extremely difficult when in an acute crisis. Consistent with a trauma-informed approach, staff must convey information regarding patient's rights and recovery-oriented approaches while in hospital; however, it is not realistic to expect prolonged verbal exchanges typical of most interview formats. Upon admission and during the first few days of hospitalization, observation may provide more detailed and accurate information than an interview. Patients who are at risk for harm to self or others may be additionally placed on a continued observation protocol, meaning that the patient must be within eyesight of a staff member at all times. The lack of privacy can be uncomfortable, but some patients report feeling safe because of the continued observation (Barnicot et al., 2017).

Medical Care

The primary medical function of psychiatric hospitalization is to determine a course of psychotropic medication. Some medications are only used short-term to address immediate safety concerns. Although these medications deescalate a potentially dangerous situation, they delay engagement and active pursuance of recovery due to their sedating nature. The more common types of psychotropic prescriptions are antipsychotic medications to control florid symptoms such as hallucinations, delusions, or bizarre behavior. Antidepressants and mood stabilizers are also frequently prescribed depending on the presentation of symptoms. (See Chapter 1 for further discussion of psychopharmaceuticals.) People are rarely in hospital long enough to observe the full effects of medication, so the goal is to have people sufficiently stable to safely return to the community with medical follow-up. This follow-up is to promote medication compliance, adjust dosages or change medication as needed, and assist in managing side effects. Unfortunately, this follow-up does not always happen for a variety of reasons, leading to the revolving door syndrome previously discussed.

In addition to the psychiatric crisis that brings an individual to the hospital, it is common for admitted patients to also have a whole array of physical maladies. Therefore, staff in psychiatric hospitals must be prepared to deliver a complete range of health services. Among the most prevalent physical health issues are drug and alcohol withdrawal, infectious diseases, and health neglect.

Drug and Alcohol Withdrawal

One of the most common presenting physical concerns involves individuals who are in the process of withdrawal and detoxification from various substances. Alcohol, opioids, and tranquilizers have the most dangerous physical symptoms of withdrawal, including the risk of cardiovascular incidents (e.g., heart attack, stroke, palpitations), seizures, delirium tremens or other tremors, and gastrointestinal disorders (Addictions and Recovery, 2018). Even substances that are not as physically addictive can present with an array of physical, emotional, and cognitive symptoms during the withdrawal process.

Some street drugs can also cause psychosis, which is difficult to differentiate from psychosis attributed to a mental illness. The psychosis may dissipate once the drug is out of one's system. However, some drugs, particularly habitual use of crystal methamphetamine, can cause a psychosis that may last months or longer. If the methamphetamine user also has a mental illness with psychotic features, the psychosis may be resistant to treatment.

Infectious Diseases

People admitted to psychiatric hospitals have an increased likelihood of having engaged in a variety of high-risk behaviors, including drug and alcohol abuse and unprotected sexual encounters. This population is also more likely to have come from high-risk environments, including living on the street (homeless) or in shelters or other overcrowded conditions. It is also possible that a transient lifestyle without access to health care (either by choice, economic necessity, or immigration status) may contribute to the spread of infectious diseases. Piri, Greer, Weissgarber, Liverant, and Safren (2005) found that state psychiatric hospital patients had a significantly higher incidence of tuberculosis as well as hepatitis B and C than the general population. Unfortunately, many of these diseases require a period of time in quarantine or isolation, which may be contrary to the psychiatric needs of patients. Even

when quarantine is not required, all staff must be cognizant of infection control procedures with all patients.

Health Neglect

People in emotional crisis tend not to take care of their personal health needs because of either disinterest in maintaining health (including suicidality), poor environmental conditions (e.g., homelessness), limited access to daily life necessities (e.g., food, water, hygiene supplies), or poor health status awareness (e.g., risk factors of diabetes, heart disease). Skin issues such as decubiti ulcers, infections, parasitic infestations, and insect bites from lice and bedbugs are common.

Individuals who reside in less-than-optimal living conditions have significant challenges in monitoring and managing any chronic illness, but some are more difficult than others. For example, diabetes, which is a known complication of alcoholism, may lead to blindness and amputation if not carefully managed. Therefore, isolation, increased daily life stressors, decreased accessibility, and inability to maintain independent living can all lead to a decompensation of mental status. The challenge during a psychiatric hospitalization is not limited to immediate medical care of complications; it also requires significant education on health management and sensitive and appropriate discharge planning to find placements to help the individual manage chronic health conditions.

THE STRUCTURE OF ACUTE PSYCHIATRIC PROGRAMMING

Consistent with recovery principles, inpatient hospitalization offers a variety of group and individual interventions, and every attempt is made to do so in a calm, warm environment that promotes healing and social interaction. In order to accomplish this, a highly coordinated team approach is needed, which is sometimes challenging with the very limited amount of time of hospital stays and the subsequent rapid rate of patient turnover. Table 2-1 presents a sample weekly schedule that includes team preparation, education, and coordination, as well as group and individual interventions. In the table, there are 6 hours of time dedicated to direct service provision, which takes priority. However, due to the unpredictability of behavior, tolerance, scheduling conflicts, and variable census, it is not possible to predict accurate time use. As a general rule, short individual sessions (20 minutes or less) are optimal for at least the first few days of hospitalization, and not every person will be seen daily (frequency is often decided based on team recommendations). Flexible scheduling with rotating staff may allow for evening and/or Saturday groups. The following is an expanded explanation of some of the items in this table.

TABLE 2-1. SAMPLE WEEKLY SCHEDULE IN AN ACUTE PSYCHIATRIC HOSPITAL

TIME	MONDAY	TUESDAY	WEDNESDAY	THURSDAY	FRIDAY
8:00 to 8:15 AM	Change of shift; brief report for patient updates and immediate concerns				
8:15 to 9:00 AM	Individual visits by occupational therapist to patient rooms for daily orientation and hygiene cart; individual nursing visits for check-in				
9:00 to 10:00 AM	Community meeting	Team meeting	Community meeting	Team meeting	Community meeting
10:00 to 11:00 AM	Living skills group (occupational therapy)	Thematic group	Living skills group (occupational therapy)	Thematic group	Goal-setting group
11:00 AM to 12:00 PM	Individual assessment and intervention/documentation				
LUNCH	*Patients are encouraged to have all meals in communal dining area*				
1:00 to 3:00 PM	Occupational therapy workshop OR other structured group offering				
3:00 to 4:00 PM	Individual assessment and intervention/documentation				
4:00 to 5:00 PM	Continued direct service provision if needed; opportunity to address a variety of administrative and organizational tasks such as documentation and preparation, committee meetings, supply ordering, supervision; end-of-shift patient check-in and staff report				

Morning Check-In

This applies to the brief sharing of information among staff, usually at change of shift, to make sure that urgent situations are addressed and any new patient information is relayed. More extensive team meetings are usually scheduled a couple of times per week to thoroughly review cases. Check-ins also apply to morning rounds to patient rooms by a variety of professionals. Coordination is needed to prevent the all-too-common situation where multiple staff are visiting the patient simultaneously or in rapid succession, causing the patient to become overwhelmed. The occupational therapist may use the morning check-in to provide occupation-based, continuous assessment and intervention. For example, in the weekly schedule outlined in Table 2-1, the occupational therapist uses a cart of hygiene supplies to orient the individual to occupational therapy and begin the occupational engagement process.

Community Meetings

A critical part of a mental health milieu is to have a mechanism for all patients to have social interaction, express concerns, ask questions, and provide information to the staff regarding their needs and interests. All patients are strongly encouraged to attend community meetings unless their behavior would be disruptive to the group process. It is not uncommon for people to remain passive and quiet during meetings, so it is sometimes up to the group leader(s) to broach new topics and to facilitate further engagement. Group leaders are typically part of the professional staff (e.g., nurses, social workers, occupational therapists) but could also be peer specialists or patient rights advocates.

Groups

People in acute crisis and/or displaying severe symptoms usually cannot tolerate group attendance for a full hour or more (even in a passive way). Mechanisms should be allowed for brief visits to observe group without being disruptive. (The room can be arranged with space near the door for pacing or sitting outside of the group.) Ideally, these people would have a one-on-one support person to gently coax them into greater involvement or accompany them to another room if necessary. Sometimes, this person would be the assigned nurse, but more often, the support person would be an occupational therapy assistant, psych tech, intern/student, or peer specialist.

CASE ILLUSTRATION 2-3: GOAL CONFLICT WITH DISCHARGE PLANS

Diamond has a long history of repetitive decompensations while living in the community. During her most recent hospitalization, the team recommended that she be placed in a residential care facility to help monitor her symptoms and medication. Diamond strongly objected, stating that she liked living alone in an apartment and that her goal was to return to independent living. After repeated discussions with the team, Diamond reluctantly agreed to the placement. Two weeks later, Diamond walked out of the facility and has not gotten in touch with her therapist or case manager in the ensuing month.

Discussion

This scenario might have been avoided if more effort had been made to understand the meaning of Diamond's goals. Although a residential care facility may be a safer alternative than independent living, it cannot be a feasible alternative without the individual's cooperation. Negotiation about follow-up care in the community, including day treatment and case management options, might have addressed the team's legitimate concerns while allowing Diamond to remain in an independent living situation.

As part of the overall goal of stabilization, expectations are graded/increased as tolerated. Examples include minimizing disruptive behavior, staying in the room for a full session, participating in an activity, and participating in socialization. Specific occupational therapy groups that could be used in hospital settings are discussed elsewhere in this text, but groups in psychiatric units can be run by any number of staff, and it is not uncommon for groups to be co-led with an interdisciplinary focus.

Thematic groups have rotating themes that address current issues/events, including seasonal celebrations or political involvement such as engagement in a letter-writing campaign on issues related to mental health. Thematic groups may also be the designated time for specialized interventions such as Wellness Recovery Action Plan, TIC, or sensory processing.

Goal-setting groups can also have an interdisciplinary structure. The occupational therapist may use this group to conduct assessment activities such as completion of the Kawa or the Canadian Occupational Performance Measure (COPM; Law et al., 2015). (See Chapter 4 for further discussion.) Depending on the group's needs, it can be the setting where initial (collaborative) discharge planning takes place because, through self-awareness, individuals can best determine their future needs for support and placement. Although goal setting is an evolving process throughout hospitalization, it tends to be more realistic toward the end of hospitalization when patients are getting ready for the next step. Cooperative goal setting can be hampered by the individual's pathology. People with delusions, poor insight, concrete thinking, or avolition may initially be incapable of healthy and realistic goal setting. Nevertheless, within the person's capabilities, every effort should be made to seek out and honor his or her expressed interests and desires, even if they sometimes conflict with the team's opinion. Case Illustration 2-3 shows the negative consequences of unresolved conflict regarding goals and discharge planning.

THE ROLE OF OCCUPATIONAL THERAPY IN ACUTE PSYCHIATRY

As discussed in the previous section, service in acute psychiatric hospitalization is highly dependent on a well-coordinated team approach. Although occupational therapy is often part of that team, there are unique aspects of occupational therapy service delivery that should be clarified and communicated.

Given that the primary role of acute psychiatric hospitalization is stabilization of the patient, that also needs to be the focus of acute psychiatric occupational therapy. Although this particular concept has not been discussed in recent scholarly literature, stabilization as a goal was well documented in earlier literature and is part of the profession's collective belief system. For example, it is universally accepted in occupational therapy that daily structure and activity are healing and stabilizing. According to Hutcheson, Ferguson, Nish, and Gill (2010), there is a well-known and recognized problem of patient inactivity on acute psychiatric wards. This point alone makes the case that occupational therapy should retain and expand a significant role in psychiatric hospitalization. Furthermore, stabilization is also dependent on addressing basic self-care such as grooming and hygiene, sleep, healthy eating, and adequate hydration. Although medically oriented staff take care of deficits in these areas, the skill development necessary for increased independence in these basic activities of daily living is best achieved through occupational therapy. Skill development in occupations is the core of occupational therapy practice across all settings. It is not realistic to assume that achieving functional goals and mastering skills can be accomplished in a short-stay hospitalization. However, occupational therapy can play a significant role in providing the beginnings of rehabilitation with skill development, helping patients develop and refine realistic goals, and helping with referrals to the community where

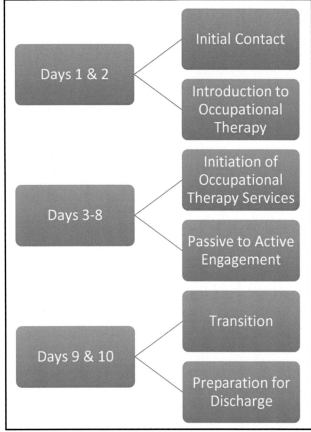

Figure 2-2. Occupational therapy progression in acute psychiatric hospitalization.

goal attainment is possible. Furthermore, in acute psychiatry, the pace and methods need to be adjusted to meet the needs of the patient. In order to have a better understanding of occupational therapy on acute units, Figure 2-2 shows the typical progression of occupational therapy services in a 10-day hospitalization, and Table 2-2 expands on that progression. The table gives a day-by-day account of the story of Elise, which was presented in Case Illustration 2-1.

A review conducted by Lloyd and Williams (2010) included the following findings:

> There was found to be a paucity of current literature relating to occupational therapy practice in acute mental health. From the literature that was available, four core elements of occupational therapy practice in acute mental health were identified: individual assessment, individual treatment, therapeutic groups, and discharge planning. (p. 483)

These elements are shared with many mental health professionals, but there are specific processes in these elements that are unique to occupational therapy. These processes have been discussed in this chapter as well as others throughout this text. Although these elements are enormously important and well within the occupational therapy scope of practice, there is another element that it

is equally important: the role of occupational therapy in environmental adaptation.

Occupational Therapy in the Institutional Environment

One of the principles of milieu therapy is the importance of creating a healing environment. The need for a calming environment is also of paramount importance in the application of trauma-informed principles (Huckshorn & LeBel, 2013). Occupational therapists are under-recognized as environmental experts and should be playing a major role in the arrangement and modification of any treatment setting. These skills are perhaps especially important in acute care psychiatry precisely because there is a strong desire to create a healing and calming environment that is part of recovery and TIC. However, the reality is that the settings are first and foremost hospitals with significant safety concerns. Therefore, there are great limitations on what can be environmentally altered. Even if an occupational therapist cannot have a role in the adaptation of an entire facility, each therapist working in acute care psychiatry should advocate for a separate clinic or designated space to be a therapeutic healing environment in which to conduct occupational therapy. The psychosocial health benefits of a structured and organized environment have been recognized in occupational therapy since the early writings of the profession. In 1954, Wade and Franciscus stated the following:

> An orderly, well-kept, attractive unit is good mental hygiene in itself and is important for the morale of patient and therapist alike. It gives to the patient a feeling of order and direction rather than one of chaos and indirection. All supplies and equipment should have a given place in which to be kept when not in use, and the therapist must assume the responsibility of seeing that each item is returned to its proper place, not merely pushed aside in a heap on a shelf until it is impossible to locate desired items as they are needed. In addition, a working area need not be drab and depressing, for with ingenuity, some inexpensive material and paint, any room can be made inviting and attractive, and many patients would enjoy working on a project, taking pride in the end result. These latter considerations are an important part of the therapist's responsibility in creating a therapeutic atmosphere. (p. 83)

Sometimes, the environmental changes can be very simple, but with thoughtful design and proper supplies, the space can provide a safe and comfortable place to enhance recovery goals and to offer a range of opportunities for increasing self-efficacy, responsibility, and socialization. These concepts are highlighted in Case Illustration 2-4. As shown in this case, patients may be asked to volunteer for a

TABLE 2-2. OCCUPATIONAL THERAPY FOR ELISE

DAY 1	The morning after Elise is admitted to hospital, Cathleen, the occupational therapist, stops by her room. However, Elise is sleeping, so Cathleen decides to check back later in the day. She stops by several times, but each time Elise has the sheet over her head and is apparently sleeping. Before the end of the shift, Cathleen tries one more time, but again finds Elise in bed with the sheet over her head. However, she suspects that Elise is probably awake and is using the sheet to isolate herself. Although she does not expect a response, Cathleen introduces herself and informs Elise that she will be back in the morning.
DAY 2	Cathleen stops by Elise's room to find her still in bed but apparently awake. Elise pulls the sheet over her head again to avoid interaction. Cathleen offers Elise supplies from the hygiene cart, which triggers a response. Elise shouts, "The damn nurses forced me into the shower!" Cathleen responds that when she is ready to perform her daily hygiene independently, she would be happy to help her with supplies because she visits all patients every morning with the hygiene cart. At that point, Elise rolled over and faced the wall with the sheet completely covering her. Cathleen lets her know that she will visit again later. By that afternoon, Elise is awake and appears calm. However, she refuses to get out of bed and does not have any eye contact. Cathleen briefly explains occupational therapy and shares the calendar of groups. Although Elise initially refuses to attend any groups, she does provide monosyllabic answers regarding her daily routines and hesitantly agrees that she is struggling with taking care of herself.
DAY 3	Elise accepts a toothbrush, toothpaste, a washcloth, and "nice" body wash from the hygiene cart and is coaxed to the bathroom with Cathleen to perform very basic hygiene. Then Elise states that she is "really tired" and wants to go back to bed. The occupational therapy session is interrupted by the arrival of the psychiatrist, so plans are made for an afternoon visit, when Cathleen manages to coax Elise out of her room. She agrees to walk down the hall and peek into the occupational therapy clinic, but then she starts to panic and returns to her room.

Hospital commitment extended to a maximum of 14 days because Elise is still considered a danger to self and is not yet stabilized on optimum medication regime.

DAYS 4 TO 8	Cathleen continues to visit Elise every morning to provide hygiene supplies and observes a steadily increasing ability for self-care. There is also individual occupational therapy time as tolerated to complete brief assessments in functional (occupational) performance, cognition, and environmental stressors. However, verbal communication tends to be both exhausting and challenging for Elise, so assessment is also conducted via observation during groups. For example, the Kawa model, which requires minimal verbal exchange, can be done as a group assessment activity. By day 5, Elise is attending all groups but initially does not participate at all. Eventually, Elise advances from passive observation to active but isolated involvement, and finally engages in some social interaction with other participants.
DAYS 9 TO 10	Additional one-on-one meetings are scheduled to discuss referrals for after discharge. The COPM is administered for the purpose of goal setting, and permission is sought to share results of the COPM with the occupational therapist in the recommended follow-up outpatient group, which uses a wellness/recovery and support model.

CASE ILLUSTRATION 2-4 : THE SAFETY AND COMFORT OF THE OCCUPATIONAL THERAPY CLINIC

Mrs. Vigar is a 57-year-old housewife with a long history of schizophrenia who recently stopped taking her medication and subsequently decompensated. She was brought to the psychiatric hospital because of escalating threatening behavior and paranoid delusions. Initially, Mrs. Vigar refused to leave her room, even though she was quite agitated by the noise of her roommate and the proximity to the nurses' station. The occupational therapist was able to coax her out of her room for a short visit to the occupational therapy clinic for a cup of tea. The following day, the therapist once again escorted Mrs. Vigar to the clinic, invited her to look at the artwork on the walls, and engaged her in the task of watering the plants. Mrs. Vigar attended clinic regularly thereafter, sometimes engaging in clinic activity, other times simply observing. However, she never missed a session, and the nursing staff reported that she was less agitated during and after occupational therapy.

Discussion

The occupational therapy clinic environment was arranged to provide a sense of comfort, familiarity, and safety, as well as a balance of sensory stimulation. This had a direct impact on Mrs. Vigar's sense of control and symptom reduction.

---

variety of tasks, including feeding the fish in an aquarium, watering the potted plants, setting up the tea cart, helping set up or put away activity supplies, and cleaning tables. However, these responsibilities should be presented as part of the recovery process and a means of group ownership/inclusion rather than as chores that may be seen as punishment.

An occupational therapy room should be a warm, inviting, and safe place. The visual representations found in an occupational therapy room are ideally pleasant and calming, but most important, they should have some personal meaning for the service users. All aspects of the individual service user's humanity should be recognized and acknowledged. What may seem like trivial details on the surface can greatly affect the overall feel of the treatment area. For example, it is optimum if fresh water is available at all times in the room. This is a gesture of courtesy and a reflection of the desire to have service users in occupational therapy feel comfortable. It is also an acknowledgment of the problems of dehydration and dry mouth commonly found in people on medication. It is, therefore, a tool to educate service users about symptom and side effect management, as well as role-modeling healthy nutritional habits.

Determining the level of sensory stimulation in the clinic can be difficult, especially regarding auditory stimulation. People have very different thresholds of tolerance to sound. For some individuals, it is necessary to have a quiet room for them to engage in any task. It is especially important for the therapist to provide a quiet place for some people to retreat to if others are engaging in a particularly noisy activity. On the other hand, sound (as in music), if used judiciously, can enhance the therapeutic effect of an activity and the clinic environment. "Music can facilitate mood changes, alter states of awareness, modify one's consciousness and increase affective response. Music can be effectively used to shift a person's attention, soothe agitation and as an aid with visualization techniques" (MacRae, 1992, p. 275).

SUMMARY

The trend away from hospitalization has occurred over several decades and has had both positive and negative effects. However, it is possible that a point has now been reached where further hospital closures are not realistic and, in fact, a reactionary and cyclical process may be beginning, calling for an increase in psychiatric in patient services. It is hoped that all changes in the delivery of mental health services are thoughtfully coordinated to make sure that people in need of service do not fall through the cracks, but also that service settings are a good match for the needs of service users.

Although occupational therapy services in mental health are appropriately focused on the community, this chapter advocates for the preservation of occupational therapy's role in acute care psychiatry. Occupational therapists have unique skills that are invaluable in acute settings. Furthermore, it is in the best interest of the profession to stay involved in all areas of service delivery, ensuring the continuity of care.

ACKNOWLEDGEMENT

Information on the history of institutions was provided by Kathleen Schwartz, EdD, OTR (Ret.), FAOTA.

REFERENCES

Addictions and Recovery. (2018). Retrieved from https://www.addictionsandrecovery.org

Barnicot, K., Insua-Summerhayes, B., Plummer, E., Hart, A., Barker, C., & Priebe, S. (2017). Staff and patient experiences of decision-making about continuous observation in psychiatric hospitals. *Social Psychiatry and Psychiatric Epidemiology, 52,* 473-483.

Beckett, P., Holmes, D., Phipps, M., Patton, D., & Molloy, L. (2017). Trauma-informed care and practice: Practice improvement strategies in an inpatient mental health ward. *Journal of Psychosocial Nursing and Mental Health Services, 55*(10), 34-38.

California Hospital Association. (2018). *California psychiatric bed annual report.* Retrieved from https://www.calhospital.org/sites/main/files/file-attachments/cha_whitepaper_psychbeds.pdf

Craig, T., & Timms, P. (1992). Out of the wards and onto the streets? Deinstitutionalization and homelessness in Britain. *Journal of Mental Health, I,* 365-327.

Darcin, A. E., Nurmedov, S., Noyan, C. O., Yilmaz, O., & Dilbaz, N. (2015). Psychiatric comorbidity among inpatients in an addiction clinic and its association with the process of addiction. *The Journal of Psychiatry and Neurological Sciences, 28,* 196-203.

Dix, D. (1843). *Memorial to the Legislature of Massachusetts.* Boston, MA: Munroe & Francis.

Hall, H. J. (1914). Occupational treatment of patients in state hospitals. *Modern Hospital, 2*(4), 302-305.

Huckshorn, K., & LeBel, J. (2013). Trauma-informed care. In K. Yeager, D. Cutler, & G. Sills (Eds.), *Modern community mental health: An interdisciplinary approach* (pp. 62-83). New York, NY: Oxford University Press.

Hutcheson, C., Ferguson, H., Nish, G., & Gill, L. (2010). Promoting mental wellbeing through activity in a mental health hospital. *British Journal of Occupational Therapy, 73*(3), 121-128.

Law, M., Baptiste, S., Carswell, A., McColl, M. A., Polatajko, H., & Pollock, N. (2015). *Canadian Occupational Performance Measure (COPM)* (5th ed.). Toronto, Canada: Canadian Association of Occupational Therapists.

Lloyd, C., & Williams, L. (2010). Occupational therapy in the modern adult acute mental health setting: A review of current practice. *International Journal of Therapy and Rehabilitation, 17*(9), 483-493.

MacRae, A. (1992). The issue is: Should music be used therapeutically by occupational therapists? *American Journal of Occupational Therapy, 46,* 275-277.

Mental Health America. (n.d.-a). *Hospitalization.* Retrieved from http://www.mentalhealthamerica.net/hospitalization

Mental Health America. (n.d.-b). *Psychiatric advance directives: Taking charge of your care.* Retrieved from http://www.mentalhealthamerica.net/psychiatric-advance-directives-taking-charge-your-care

Muskett, C. (2014). Trauma-informed care in inpatient mental health settings: A review of the literature. *International Journal of Mental Health Nursing, 23,* 51-59.

National Alliance on Mental Illness. (n.d.). *Mental health by the numbers.* Retrieved from https://www.nami.org/learn-more/mental-health-by-the-numbers

National Institute of Mental Health. (2017). *Mental illness.* Retrieved from https://www.nimh.nih.gov/health/statistics/mental-illness.shtml

Pinel, P. (1809). *Traite medico-philosophique sur l'alientation mentale* (2nd ed.). Paris, France: J. A. Brosson.

Piri, W., Greer, J., Weissgarber, C., Liverant, G., & Safren, S. (2005). Screening for infectious diseases among patients in a state psychiatric hospital. *Psychiatric Services, 56*(12), 1614-1616.

Rollin, H. R. (1990). The dark before the dawn. *Journal of Psychopharmacology, 4,* 109-114.

Rothman, D. J. (1971). *The discovery of the asylum.* Boston, MA: Little, Brown.

Sheth, H. C. (2009). Deinstitutionalization or disowning responsibility. *International Journal of Psychosocial Rehabilitation, 13*(2), 11-20.

Shorter, E. (1997). *A history of psychiatry.* New York, NY: Wiley.

Sisti, D., Segal, A., & Emanuel, E. (2015). Improving long-term psychiatric care: Bring back the asylum. *Journal of the American Medical Association, 313*(3), 243-244.

Substance Abuse and Mental Health Services Administration. (2015a). *Behavioral health trends in the United States: Results from the 2014 National Survey on Drug Use and Health.* U.S. Department of Health and Human Services (Publication No. SMA4927). Rockville, MD: Author.

Substance Abuse and Mental Health Services Administration. (2015b). *Trauma-informed approach.* Retrieved from https://www.samhsa.gov/nctic/trauma-interventions

Swarbrick, M. (2009). Historical perspective: From institution to community. *Occupational Therapy in Mental Health, 25,* 201-223.

Torrey E. F., Stieber, J., Ezekial, J., Wolfe, S. M., Sharfstein, J., Noble, J. H., & Flynn, L. M. (1992). *Criminalizing the seriously mentally ill: The abuse of jails as psychiatric hospitals.* Washington, DC: Public Citizen's Health Research Group.

Wade, B., & Franciscus, M. L. (1954). Occupational therapy for the mentally ill. In H. Willard & C. Spackman (Eds.), *Principles of occupational therapy* (2nd ed.). Philadelphia, PA: Lippincott.

World Health Organization. (2017). *Mental disorders.* Retrieved from http://www.who.int/mediacentredg/factsheets/fs396/en

Community Behavioral Health Services

Anne MacRae, PhD, OTR/L, BCMH, FAOTA
and Jerilyn (Gigi) Smith, PhD, OTR/L, FAOTA

Since its inception in the 1960s, the provision of community behavioral health services in the United States has vacillated between spurts of creative proposals and hopeful energy to profound discouragement with the lack of cohesive planning and support. The implementation of the Patient Protection and Affordable Care Act (ACA) of 2010 (better known as *Obamacare*) brought to the forefront the mandate to health care systems to improve health care value, quality, and efficiency. The ACA spurred the development of new models of service delivery, some of which enhance existing services and some of which demonstrate a major rethinking of how services could be provided. This has led to a plethora of new terms for actualized and proposed models, which are highlighted in Figure 3-1. Unfortunately, the political climate in the United States has changed drastically since the passing of the ACA, resulting in considerable concern and confusion about the status of health care funding and the commitment, or lack thereof, to solidifying and expanding services in the community. Although it is not clear what the future may hold, it is imperative that we continue to protect the services currently being offered as well as advocate for improvements and expansion to meet the needs of all community members. Most importantly, all providers, including occupational therapists, must keep up to date on the ever-changing landscape of service delivery and be prepared to step up to create opportunities and address needs, particularly in the behavioral health arena.

To that end, this chapter discusses integrated primary care and behavioral health centers.

Furthermore, the premise of this chapter is that community services for behavioral health should extend far beyond specific settings, and the community must be understood as an interactive system that can either support or inhibit mental health and recovery. Therefore, this chapter also discusses qualities of healthy communities as well as the importance of developing community partners.

Prior to discussing professional behavioral health services, it is important to acknowledge that peer-provided services are essential for supporting recovery and wellness. However, they are not the focus of this chapter because, by definition, professionals are only peripherally involved, if at all. For example, 12-step programs such as Alcoholics Anonymous are found in communities throughout the country, and other forms of support groups can be found internationally. They are primarily operated on a volunteer basis and do not have professional staff. Therefore, the only role for a behavioral health service provider is as a referral source. Other models of peer support, such as consumer-operated services, are gaining in popularity and recognition. The Substance Abuse and Mental Health Service Administration (SAMHSA) defines consumer-operated services as "peer-run service programs that are owned, administratively controlled, and operated by mental health consumers and emphasize self-help as their operational

MacRae, A. (Ed.). *Cara and MacRae's Psychosocial Occupational Therapy:*
An Evolving Practice, Fourth Edition (pp 33-48).
© 2019 Taylor & Francis Group.

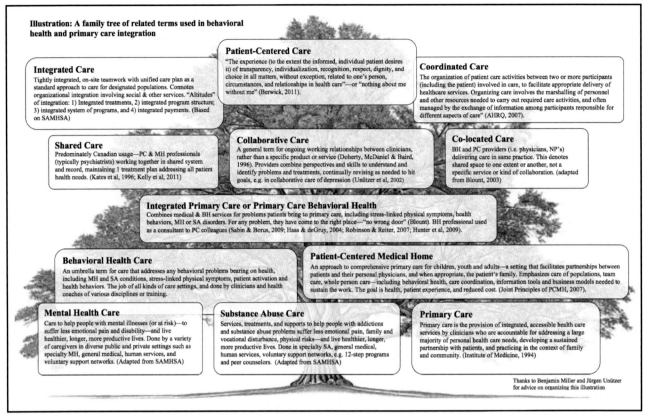

Figure 3-1. Related terms used in behavioral health and primary care integration. (Reprinted from Peek, C. J., & the National Integration Academy Council. [2013]. *Lexicon for behavioral health and primary care integration* [AHRQ Publication No.13-IP001-EF]. Rockville, MD: Agency for Healthcare Research and Quality. Retrieved from http://integrationacademy.ahrq.gov/sites/default/files/Lexicon.pdf)

approach" (2011, p. 1). Nevertheless, SAMHSA suggests that such centers can sometimes benefit from outside training and technical support. Therefore, there is a potential role for a behavioral health service provider as a consultant. (See Chapter 5 for further discussion of consultation.)

INTEGRATED PRIMARY CARE

For the purpose of this chapter, primary care is defined as "the provision of integrated, accessible health care services by clinicians who are accountable for addressing a large majority of personal health care needs, developing a sustained partnership with patients, and practicing in the context of family and community" (Institute of Medicine, 1994, p. 1). Reimbursement systems heavily influence the model of service provision, and as these systems change, they create opportunities as well as challenges for both the recipients of the services and for health care providers.

The emergence of alternative payment models that give added incentive payments to encourage the provision of high-quality, cost-efficient care related to client outcomes has provided important opportunities for occupational therapy to have a key role in primary care (Halle, Mroz, Fogelberg, & Leland, 2018).

Although the term *primary care* has been used since the early 1960s, interest in the primary care model, especially as it relates to behavioral health needs, was renewed with the implementation of the ACA because primary health care was specifically identified as a key avenue of service delivery. This model of health care provision is designed around the concept of providing integrated care from a team of professionals that addresses health care needs in collaboration with the client in the context of their family and community. Outcomes emphasize prevention, wellness, and the empowerment of individuals to manage their conditions (Dahl-Popolizio, Manson, Muir, & Rogers, 2016). The ACA provides financial incentives to health care providers and support for the development of innovative models of service delivery of care that emphasize improving health care outcomes and client experiences.

Primary Care and Behavioral Health

Individuals with serious mental illness are at a significantly higher risk for morbidity and mortality than the general population (Bahorik, Satre, Kline-Simon, Weisner, & Campbell, 2017). Failure to recognize and appropriately treat behavioral health conditions has a negative impact on health outcomes and quality of life and significantly increases the overall cost of health care. Individuals with untreated behavioral and mental health conditions, especially those who also have chronic medical conditions, use more medical resources and are associated with persistent medical illness (Kathol, Patel, Sacks, Sargent, & Melek, 2015). Behavioral health intervention delivered under the primary care model is ideally suited to provide integrated services to this population to improve health and cost outcomes. In primary care, the interprofessional team is responsible for the coordinated treatment of acute conditions, management of chronic illness, prevention of disease, facilitation of wellness, and management of mental and behavioral health issues (Dahl-Popolizio et al., 2016).

Multi-morbidity (the presence of two or more chronic conditions) creates an additional challenge in managing the medical care of individuals, particularly for older adults. As life expectancy increases, so do the number of people with multiple long-term conditions, which includes both physical and mental conditions. Individuals with multi-morbidity have the highest risk of safety incidents for many reasons, including more vulnerability due to poor overall health, complications due to difficulties with medication management, cognitive impairment, limited health literacy, and comorbidity of depression and/or anxiety (World Health Organization [WHO], 2018).

Having behavioral health care services available within primary care is crucial. Providing specialized mental health support for those who have mixed physical and mental health issues, as well as those struggling with addiction or those who have developed behavioral health needs as a result of a chronic physical condition, will improve the knowledge and capacity of the other primary care professionals in the practice and result in better health outcomes.

The primary care interprofessional team is responsible for the assessment and treatment of acute conditions, management of chronic conditions, promotion of wellness, and management of mental and behavioral health issues. Behavioral health domains include health behaviors, mental health and substance abuse, life stressors and crises, stress-related physical symptoms, and ineffective patterns of health care utilization. Primary care providers are often the first line of care for individuals with mental health problems. It is estimated that approximately 70% of primary care visits for older adults involve underlying mental health or behavioral health issues (e.g., panic, generalized anxiety, major depression, somatization, stress, adjustment disorders) and behaviors that lead to increased risk of chronic illness (American Psychological Association, n.d.).

Primary Care Models

There are many different models of service delivery that fall under the umbrella of primary care, all having the common theme of providing integrated, team-based, accessible health care services with the goal of promoting and maintaining health and preventing illness and disability. Table 3-1 describes the most commonly cited models.

The patient-centered medical home is a model that is currently envisioned as one of the preferred models of primary care service delivery, at least from a medical perspective. The term *home* does not refer to a place but to a model of care in which the physician is a member of a team who will offer comprehensive care under one roof (Tello, 2017). The physician receives one flat payment from insurance to cover most of the care provided. Services such as therapies, nutrition education, and behavioral health are located within the same building. The goal is to have a centralized setting that fosters partnerships between the client, physician, and clinical care team, where the client can get the care he or she needs and wants in a culturally and linguistically appropriate manner. The physician sees the client and is able to immediately send him or her to the appropriate service to address his or her needs. The goal is to provide better coordinated, more comprehensive and personalized care, improved access to medical care and services, and improved health outcomes, especially for those with chronic conditions.

Federally qualified health centers deliver services from a more social perspective, fitting in better with the recovery and wellness paradigm that is dominant in current behavioral health services. These centers primarily provide social services as well as medical services to low income, homeless, or otherwise designated vulnerable populations, but may also be open to the general population. One such center, the Integrated Care Center, operated by Healthright 360, was opened in San Francisco in 2017 and provides a wide range of services (Box 3-1).

Occupational Therapy in Primary Care Services

Occupational therapy has much to contribute to the team to facilitate positive client outcomes. Interprofessional collaborative practice to improve health and manage chronic conditions (including mental illness), improve access to services, and increase client satisfaction is at the heart of the primary health care model (Fong, 2008; WHO, 2008). A collaborative, client-centered approach that addresses these areas of concern is at the heart of occupational therapy practice and makes for a natural fit between occupational therapy and primary health care.

Since the passage of the ACA in 2010, various models of primary care service delivery have emerged to innovatively meet the need to provide integrated, comprehensive care. Occupational therapy has been actively involved in defining the role of the occupational therapist on the primary care team and has been working to ensure that occupational therapy is included in state and federal policies that dictate the provision of care.

Having professionals on the team who have experience in behavioral health is necessary to address these needs. Occupational therapy education and clinical training

TABLE 3-1. PRIMARY CARE SERVICE DELIVERY MODELS

COMPREHENSIVE PRIMARY CARE PLUS	NEXT-GENERATION ACCOUNTABLE CARE ORGANIZATIONS
• 5-year multi-payer initiative (began January 2017) • Regionally based multi-payer payment reform and delivery care transformation program • Offers incentives based on quality and utilization metrics • Targets 20 U.S. geographic regions • Involves 20,000 doctors and practitioners • Provides practices with learning systems, patient cost, and utilization data feedback to guide their decision making (Patient-Centered Primary Care Collaborative, 2018)	• Groups of doctors, hospitals, and other health care providers and suppliers who come together voluntarily • Provide coordinated care to Medicare patients • Offer Medicare beneficiaries better control over their health care • Provide opportunities for shared savings to create increased incentives (Centers for Medicare & Medicaid Services, 2018b)
FEDERALLY QUALIFIED HEALTH CENTER	**PATIENT-CENTERED MEDICAL HOME**
• Reimbursement designation from Centers for Medicare & Medicaid Services for safety net providers who provide comprehensive services to medically underserved populations or areas • Have ongoing quality assurance programs (Centers for Medicare & Medicaid Services, 2018a)	• A model for the organization and delivery of primary health care • Focused on reducing costs by providing care that is comprehensive, coordinated, patient- and family-centered, accessible, and accountable • Committed to quality and quality improvement using evidence-based medicine and clinical decision support tools (U.S. Department of Health and Human Resources, Agency for Health Care Research and Quality, n.d.)

BOX 3-1. RANGE OF SERVICES OFFERED AT A FEDERALLY QUALIFIED HEALTH CENTER: INTEGRATED CARE CENTER IN SAN FRANCISCO, CALIFORNIA

- Primary medical care
- Mental health counseling and medication management
- Dental care
- Substance use disorder treatment
- Pharmacy
- Housing referrals
- Employment counseling and training referrals
- Provided lunches
- Charter high school for adults
- Residential detox
- Computer literacy classes
- Chiropractic medicine and acupuncture

Adapted from Healthright 360. (2017, August 29). *California's first integrated health care center for low-income and homeless people opens in San Francisco* [Press release]. Retrieved from https://www.healthright360.org/news/californias-first-integrated-health-care-center-low-income-and-homeless-people-opens-san

Box 3-2. Food, Mood, and Move Group

The Food, Move, and Mood group was a 12-week program that was held two times per week in 2-hour sessions. The impetus for developing this program was twofold. First, service users of the community behavioral health services agency were asked to complete satisfaction and feedback surveys on a quarterly basis. These surveys repeatedly showed a strong interest in having groups on both exercise and nutrition. Furthermore, the surveys also showed a strong preference for activity-based, rather than verbal, groups. The second impetus came directly from the staff and administration, who expressed concern that most of the staff did not have the necessary expertise. The occupational therapist was then asked to develop a program to address these agency needs while providing reimbursable service—specifically, a group that addressed symptoms of mental illness through the use of exercise and diet/nutrition.

The group was purposely not limited to service users with specific diagnoses (such as mood disorders) because depression is a common symptom of many different disorders. Using a wellness perspective with diet and exercise, the goal was to minimize or prevent episodes of depression but also to prevent or manage chronic physical conditions, especially diabetes, heart disease, chronic pain syndromes, and arthritis. Therefore, this wellness- and prevention-oriented program addressed the interrelationship between physical and mental health.

The program used a variety of psycho-educational techniques to inform participants of the relationship between psychiatric symptoms management (especially mood stabilization), nutritional practices, and movement. In addition, practice-based skill development for improving diet and exercise (activities of daily living) were incorporated into every session as tolerated by the individual (based on baseline data and self-reported health history). A key feature of the design of this group was for participants to take responsibility for incorporating new learning into their daily routines. Guidelines were provided at the start of the program, and progress was discussed at every meeting.

Every group meeting began with simple stretching or other movement activity. There was also a check-in for each participant to share his or her related triumphs and struggles and to provide mutual support. Examples of the main activities included having game days in the park, using the Nintendo Wii, cooking healthy group lunches and snacks, playing self-designed games to explore calories and nutritional content of food items, grocery shopping, and creating an agency kitchen garden.

A self-designed set of scales were used to collect baseline data on awareness of mood, as well as both knowledge and practice of nutrition and exercise. Participants were informed that the scales would also be readministered at the end of this 12-week group to chart progress. At the end of the 12-week program, the scales were readministered. Significant progress was made in awareness of mood triggers and increase in movement activities. There was also an overall increase in nutrition awareness, but only minimal changes in actual dietary practices. At the participants' request, an ongoing support group was established at the adjacent wellness center.

includes behavioral health, and the occupational therapist has unique skills for understanding the impact of habits, roles, and routines that affect mental health. Consider the individual who is given a prescription for depression by his or her physician. Successfully taking this prescription requires that this individual change approximately seven health behaviors: he or she must fill the prescription, take it home, read the directions, and build it into his or her daily routine. The individual may or may not have to modify his or her diet. These steps all require significant health behavior change. The occupational therapist understands the importance of establishing new habits and routines and can work with the client on all aspects of achieving a positive outcome for effective medication management. Occupational therapy brings skills and expertise to contribute to the effectiveness of the primary care team in the care for clients with behavioral and mental health issues.

In the United States, the reported involvement of occupational therapists in primary care is so far minimal and primarily limited to university-based programs (Murphy, Griffith, Mroz, & Jirikowic, 2017). However, in Canada, the number of occupational therapists currently working in a primary care model appears to be growing (Donnelly, Leclair, Wener, Hand, & Letts, 2016). There are also reports of occupational therapy working in primary care elsewhere in the world (Fong, 2008), but actual statistics regarding prevalence could not be found. Regardless of the current status of occupational therapists in primary care, it is important to recognize that the practice of occupational therapy is historically and philosophically well aligned with the principles of the current primary care models, especially the focus on the provision of holistic and integrated services. Box 3-2 provides a description of group that was developed by the first author and co-led with a

Managing Chronic Pain

Are you struggling with pain and combined mental and physical conditions? Join us to learn the information and skills that you need to control your chronic pain (instead of the pain controlling you!). Each session is structured using a variety of methods (activities, discussion, lecture, and exercises). Emphasis is placed on applying what is learned to your daily life.

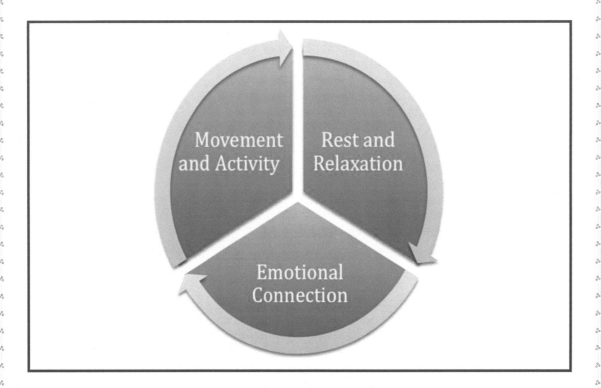

(Time and days)

(Location)

(Contact for further information)

Figure 3-2. Flyer template for pain management group.

BOX 3-3. THE ROLE OF OCCUPATIONAL THERAPY IN COMMUNITY MENTAL HEALTH

- Evaluating and adapting the environment at home, work, school, and other environments to promote an individual's optimal functioning
- Providing educational programs, experiential learning, and treatment groups or classes to address assertiveness, self-awareness, interpersonal and social skills, stress management, and role development (e.g., parenting)
- Working with clients to develop leisure or avocational interests and pursuits
- Facilitating the development of skills needed for independent living, such as using community resources, managing one's home, managing time, managing medication, and being safe at home and in the community
- Providing training in activities of daily living (e.g., hygiene and grooming)
- Consulting with employers regarding appropriate accommodations as required by the Americans with Disabilities Act
- Conducting functional evaluations and ongoing monitoring for successful job placement
- Providing guidance and consultation to persons in all employment settings, including supported employment
- Providing evaluation and treatment for sensory processing deficits

Reprinted with permission from Castaneda, R., Olson, L., & Cargill, R. (2013). *Fact sheet: Occupational therapy's role in community mental health.* Bethesda, MD: American Occupational Therapy Association.

Master of Social Work intern. Figure 3-2 is a template for a flyer advertising a group that was also developed by the first author and co-led with a marriage and family therapist. Both of these community interventions represent coordinated and collaborative services that address physical and mental health as well as overall functioning and recovery goals.

COMMUNITY BEHAVIORAL HEALTH CENTERS

The previous chapter explored the many reasons for the downsizing of psychiatric hospitals in the United States, but it is important to understand the historical context. The early 1960s was a time of optimism regarding social change, and there was support for the concept that people with mental illness are best served living in their communities. In 1963, President John F. Kennedy signed into law the Community Mental Health Centers Act. This legislation allocated funds for the construction of community mental health centers and provided the blueprint for comprehensive community mental health services (National Council for Behavioral Health, 2018). Although this legislation was well-intentioned, even visionary, the transition to community services did not live up to expectations. Chronic underfunding, poorly defined missions, lack of training/support for qualified providers, and fragmented service delivery have plagued community mental health services for decades. Funding for community-based behavioral health

care varies from region to region but is heavily dependent on government sources, which is primarily from the Medicaid Program in the United States but supplemented by any number of block grants from various governmental agencies. Still, these funds are often insufficient to deliver even mandated services, let alone comprehensive and state-of-the-art services. Therefore, funding and services may need to be supplemented with private nonprofit and for-profit organizations, as well as referrals or contractual arrangements with service providers in private practice. Despite many obstacles, services in the community remain a cost-effective option to hospitalization and, more importantly, are consistent with the goals of sustainable recovery. The American Occupational Therapy Association outlines a significant role for occupational therapists in community mental health care, which is highlighted in Box 3-3.

The term *behavioral health* has become the preferred term to designate service agencies because it describes the range of services provided. As shown in Figure 3-1, behavioral health care is an "umbrella term for care that addresses any behavioral problems bearing on health," including mental health and substance abuse conditions (Peek et al., 2013, p. 9). Specific interventions in a behavioral health service include medication and symptom management, case management, group and individual counseling, psychiatric rehabilitation, and addiction treatment. Although community agencies, especially in the United States, are now more commonly referred to as *behavioral health services*, the term *mental health service* is still appropriate and accurate when discussing services for specific populations.

CASE ILLUSTRATION 3-1: UYEN—PERFORMANCE IN THE COMMUNITY

Uyen is a 24-year-old woman with a 4-month-old baby. Her parents expressed concern about her ability to care for the child and took her to a psychiatrist. She was diagnosed as having obsessive compulsive disorder and was referred to a community behavioral health program. Several functional assessments were completed to document her skills and abilities. Treatment initially consisted of role playing various living skills for the purpose of providing practice in managing her anxiety. The occupational therapist felt that she was ready to try these skills in the community and accompanied her on a trip to the store. Uyen was able to negotiate the market effectively until she arrived at the checkout counter, where she dropped her intended purchases and ran from the building. She later told the therapist that the man at the counter scratched under his arm and she "knew" that the germs would be given to her and her baby and make them sick.

Discussion

Although Uyen was successful in carrying out simulated living skills in the safety of the clinical environment with a therapist she trusted, it is not possible to account for the behavior of all individuals or the levels of stimulation in the community at large. In order to master the necessary living skills needed for parenting, Uyen will need further intervention in the community, with the goal of developing coping skills for environments that she cannot change.

The Merger of Mental Health and Addiction Services

The combination of mental health services and what was formerly known as *alcohol and other drug* (AOD) services is beneficial to many service users (especially those with dual diagnoses) because, in theory, they would have a wider variety of care options. However, the rules and regulations guiding the delivery of services and the training and philosophy of service providers have historically been different between mental health and AOD providers. For example, AOD staff typically focus on abstinence from substances and often insist on a commitment to a clean and sober lifestyle before commencement of services (unless service is court mandated). On the other hand, mental health and rehabilitation specialists, as well as those in the social service sector, would be more likely to use a *harm reduction approach*. "Harm reduction is a public health philosophy and intervention that seeks to reduce the harms associated with drug use and ineffective drug policies" (Drug Policy Alliance, n.d.). Advocates of a harm reduction approach frame addiction as a public health threat; therefore, the aims of the approach are to reduce the spread of transmittable diseases and overdoses and reduce the mortality and morbidly rates of long-term substance use. Examples of harm reduction approaches include needle exchange programs and methadone clinics, as well as health education focused on health practices and safety consequences. Although the approach is controversial and at odds with the commonly accepted approaches used with substance use disorders, it provides a practical starting point when working with people who are not able or willing to commit to abstinence, and it is particularly useful when working with the homeless and those with dual diagnoses. Although research regarding the effectiveness of a harm reduction approach is not conclusive, there is evidence that certain specific intervention strategies have shown positive results. For example, participants in needle exchange programs are "actually more likely to attend long-term rehab than those who don't. European countries who have similar community programs, including Switzerland, Brazil and Norway, have seen a reduction in new cases of HIV contraction and the overall spread of AIDS" (Ackerman, 2015). Although there are many logistics yet to be sorted out regarding the merger of mental health and addiction services, all stakeholders ultimately agree that the primary goals are recovery oriented and focused on healthy, productive lives and community inclusion.

Limitations of Community Behavioral Health Centers

Other than the previously discussed limits in funding and poor coordination, a major pitfall of community behavioral health services is the faulty assumption that approaches and practices that worked in institutions can simply be transferred to the community. For example, with the establishment of community behavioral health centers, the expectation was that people in need of services would come to the providers and receive conventional services of individual meetings and groups, as well as medication management. Although this arrangement is a logistic and financial necessity, genuine community care must also include being in the community. Understanding how someone functions within his or her own community is essential for providing meaningful interventions, particularly from a psych rehab or occupational therapy perspective. Case Illustration 3-1 is an example of understanding function outside of the clinical environment of a center.

Because occupational therapy focuses on daily living skills and social inclusion, we are in an ideal position to provide intervention in any number of neighborhood settings, including homes, schools, jails, streets, parks, and businesses. Unfortunately, due to antiquated reimbursement schemas, there are sometimes limits placed on how and when professional services can be provided outside of the clinical setting. One solution is to procure funds, such as grants, specifically for the purpose of community integration and social inclusion. Another solution is for occupational therapists to seek employment opportunities outside of the medical model, with community organizations such as employment centers, criminal justice settings, social and human service providers, and schools (for specific behavioral health interventions not limited to academic performance). Yet another solution is to use the energy and creativity of occupational therapy interns to develop and facilitate specific interventions carried out in the neighborhood. One such intern-led endeavor was called *the community exploration project*, which included visiting parks, hiking trails, and stores, as well as attending special events in a small rural town.

HEALTHY COMMUNITIES

Where you live matters to your health. In fact, your ZIP code may be more important to your health than your genetic code. The communities where people live, learn, work, and play shape how well and how long they live. (Robert Wood Johnson Foundation [RWJF], n.d.)

Physical and mental health is dependent on many complex and interacting factors, including community dynamics, housing quality, social support, employment opportunities, economic stability, neighborhood, built environment, and work and school conditions (Office of Disease Prevention and Health Promotion, n.d.; WHO, 2014). WHO further identifies determinants specific to mental health: "Multiple social, psychological, and biological factors determine the level of mental health. ... Poor mental health is also associated with rapid social change, stressful work conditions, gender discrimination, social exclusion, unhealthy lifestyle, physical ill-health, and human rights violations" (2018).

One model to both foster the development of healthy communities and provide prevention/early intervention services is trauma-informed care. As discussed throughout this text, especially in Chapter 7, trauma-related symptoms can be triggered by any number of recent and past events, and traumatic experiences must always be considered in any treatment setting. However, it is in the community that prevention and early identification can best take place. SAMHSA launched a community trauma initiative in 2015 to address these issues.

Building resilient and trauma-informed communities is essential to improving public health and well-being. Communities can be places where traumatic events occur, and they can also help keep us safe. They can be a source of trauma, or they can buffer us against the negative effects of adversity. Communities can collectively experience trauma much like individuals do, and they can be a resource for healing (SAMHSA, 2017).

Despite the fact that many well-respected governmental and nonprofit organizations have advocated for healthy communities, health services have been slow to incorporate community-level responses. This is especially true in the United States, which has fragmented service delivery dominated by the medical model. Occupational therapists are in a unique position to be leaders in advocacy and in the development of healthy communities because our scope of practice and theory base encompasses all aspects of community functioning. Fossey and Krupa (2016) advocate for an occupational justice perspective, especially linked to community development. One model guided by an occupational justice perspective is the participatory occupational justice framework. This model not only focuses on occupational justice, it especially supports collaboration and partnerships in achieving sustainable community development (Whiteford & Townsend, 2011).

COMMUNITY PARTNERS

Community behavioral health services are typically seen as therapeutic interactions occurring within a designated center or clinic. These centers may be geographically in the community but not necessarily of the community. Therefore, it is important to identify realized or potential partnerships for the improvement of mental health in the community. As previously mentioned, occupational therapy is poised to play a major role in these partnerships because of our scope of practice, which emphasizes social inclusion and full participation. However, we need to take a more proactive role in developing community partners for positive change.

Interagency Collaboration

Collaboration is essential to not only meet the recovery goals of individual service users but also to promote healthy, inclusive communities. For example, Health and Human Services organizations are generally responsible for housing and food subsidies, child and adult protective services, foster care, back-to-work initiatives, and in-home help services. All of these tasks overlap with the goals of behavioral health intervention, but unfortunately it is all too common for services to be provided on parallel tracks without any coordination or even communication. Laws regarding confidentiality often interfere with such cooperation, but these rights can be waived by the service

Box 3-4. The Social Services Transportation Advisory Council

This council includes representation from all of the major social and health-related service organizations in the county, along with representatives from the board of supervisors and the transportation department. An occupational therapist was the spokesperson for the local behavioral health service because of her familiarity with the laws and regulations regarding access (e.g., Americans with Disabilities Act) and a knowledge of the process for determining "reasonable accommodations." The occupational therapist also shared her particular interest in advocating for people with so-called "hidden disabilities," which include mental illness and many other conditions that do not necessarily have outward signs of a disability, such as diabetes and cardiovascular disease, yet can be remarkably limiting in one's ability to access transportation and other services.

The advisory council collaboratively agreed upon several recommendations that were accepted and implemented by the transportation department with positive results. Among these recommendations were the following:

- Adjusting bus schedules to improve access to services
- Advertising schedule changes widely, including postings at social and health service agencies
- Publishing policy and procedures for receiving transit discounts
- Training bus drivers for sensitivity and management of behaviors on public transit
- Educating service users about public transit offered in cooperation with transit employees
- Providing peer travel companions for people with disabilities to negotiate the transit system

user provided that protocols are initiated by the behavioral health service provider. Another avenue for interagency collaboration involves the use of task forces or advisory councils to create community-wide agendas. Task forces are typically time limited, whereas advisory councils are usually convened intermittently (such as quarterly meetings). Task forces and advisory councils are both designed to clarify roles and responsibilities, establish or strengthen lines of communication, and make recommendations for action. They are generally organized around a substantial community issue, such as homelessness, safety, or drug use epidemics, in which all task force members have a stake. Box 3-4 is an example of an advisory council with behavioral health representation that focuses on community transportation issues.

Local Government

Besides the obvious role that local government may have in the disbursement of state and federal funds, the local government can also provide leadership in recognizing the contributions of behavioral health services and combating stigma. For example, "May Is Mental Health Month" started as a grassroots movement in 1949 (Mental Health America, 2018). There has been substantial growth in the number of local governing bodies officially sponsoring related events and issuing declarations of recognition and support. Behavioral health staff can enhance the governmental support by voluntarily serving on task forces or boards that are government sponsored. Conversely, it is highly desirable to have a government official, such as a city or county board member, serve on the local behavioral

health advisory board. Another effective way to demonstrate the strength of a government partnership is to work with individual service users and their families to take an active role in government. This may include attending public council meetings, serving on boards, and, perhaps most importantly, engaging in one's right to vote.

Faith-Based Community

In an upcoming chapter, the complex relationship between religion, spirituality, and behavioral health is explored in terms of personal and social identity. For the purposes of this chapter, the discussion is confined to the potential partnership between the faith-based community and behavioral health services.

Faith and community leaders are often the first point of contact when individuals and families face mental health problems or traumatic events. In fact, in times of crisis, many will turn to trusted leaders in their communities before they turn to mental health professionals. When leaders know how to respond, they become significant assets to the overall health system (U.S. Department of Health and Human Resources, n.d.).

It is also an unfortunate reality that some faith-based groups have discouraged members of their congregations from seeking help for mental illness or psychosocial distress, espousing that only spiritual intervention is needed. It is, of course, an individual's right to choose forms of intervention and support, but considering the authority of faith-based groups and the vulnerability of many people with mental illness, there is an inherent power inequality that can greatly hinder recovery goals.

TABLE 3-2. RECOMMENDATIONS FOR IMPROVING RELATIONSHIPS BETWEEN CONSUMERS, FAITH-BASED ORGANIZATIONS, AND COMMUNITY MENTAL HEALTH SERVICES

RECOMMENDATIONS TO SAMHSA/CMHS	RECOMMENDATIONS TO FAITH-BASED ORGANIZATIONS	RECOMMENDATIONS TO CONSUMERS AND CONSUMER ADVOCATES
• Provide education to faith-based and community organizations. • Enhance education for health care and social service providers. • Create ongoing dialogue and foster partnerships between mental health agencies and faith-based communities. • Encourage consumer involvement. • Promote best practices models. • Provide federal assistance, monitoring, evaluation, and feedback.	• Create a welcoming, supportive environment for mental health consumers. • Introduce instruction on mental health and mental illnesses as required topics in seminary education. • Use CMHS's *Participatory Dialogue* guide to organize dialogues in local communities. • Create partnerships between consumers and faith-based organizations for education. • Develop curricula to address and demythologize mental illness for adults and children suitable for use and adaptation by faith-based organizations. • Develop a fact sheet on faith and spirituality in mental health. • Increase awareness and skills related to cultural competence.	• Develop a compendium of best practices and lessons learned about engaging faith communities. • Develop guidelines for faith-based organizations on factors involved in creating a supportive, welcoming environment. • Educate consumers and consumer groups on techniques to engage with faith-based organizations and to create change. • Contribute to the development of curricula about the needs of persons with mental health issues. • Volunteer to share faith-based stories with congregations to put a face on recovery and the role that spirituality plays in recovery. • Present at consumer conferences on the role of spirituality in recovery and how to create positive change in faith-based organizations *(continued)*

To minimize obstacles and maximize the benefits of behavioral health and faith-based community partnerships, SAMHSA published recommendations for (1) SAMHSA/ Center for Mental Health Services, (2) faith-based organizations, and (3) consumers and consumer advocates (SAMHSA, 2004). A summary of these recommendations can be found in Table 3-2. A subsequent document entitled, *Mental Health: A Guide for Faith Leaders*, was published by the American Psychiatric Association Foundation (2014) and is available through their website.

Law Enforcement

Implied in the previously quoted SAMHSA community trauma initiative, community entities can be valuable partners, but it is also important to acknowledge that these same entities can be the root of significant barriers to recovery by engaging in negative practices that stigmatize and marginalize people with mental illness, sometimes even putting their lives in danger. The challenge for all people concerned about behavioral health issues is to recognize and confront barriers while engaging in activities that promote healthy, inclusive communities. One of the most prominent community entities responsible for both significant barriers and supports for people in psychosocial distress is law enforcement.

While police brutality against racial and ethnic groups is well documented and routinely seen in the news, incidents involving people with mental illness of all backgrounds is not as clear in the public discourse. For example, there appears to be bias in reporting that both people of color and people with mental illness involved in cases of police violence must have instigated the violent response in some way. This is a blatant and damaging stereotype, and although there is pushback from communities against such discrimination, there is not sustained resistance against labeling people with mental illness as violent (see Chapter 2 for a discussion on violence and behavioral health disorders). According to Fuller, Lamb, Biasotti, and Snook (2015), the

TABLE 3-2 (CONTINUED). RECOMMENDATIONS FOR IMPROVING RELATIONSHIPS BETWEEN CONSUMERS, FAITH-BASED ORGANIZATIONS, AND COMMUNITY MENTAL HEALTH SERVICES

RECOMMENDATIONS TO SAMHSA/CMHS	RECOMMENDATIONS TO FAITH-BASED ORGANIZATIONS	RECOMMENDATIONS TO CONSUMERS AND CONSUMER ADVOCATES
• Foster research.	• Address issues of discrimination and stigma. • Educate mental health providers about the role of chaplains in psychiatric hospitals as part of the treatment team. • Provide support for the grieving process related to having a disability, which includes mental illnesses. • Consider the social ramifications of mental illnesses and work to improve conditions such as housing and employment. • Include consumers on committees and governing boards of faith-based organizations. • Provide transportation resources to enable consumers to participate in the activities of faith communities.	• Organize dialogues between faith-based organizations and mental health consumers. • Volunteer in community efforts (e.g., in homeless shelters) to demonstrate the hope and reality of recovery and to give back to the community. • Generate publicity for the positive role that faith communities play in the recovery of persons with mental illnesses. • Create and disseminate templates for consumer letter-writing campaigns to clergy and lay leaders of faith-based organizations. • Encourage consumer participation at all levels of planning, research, education, program development, and policy. • Mobilize consumer groups to prepare reference manuals on mental health and other social support resources. • Promote consumer participation on governing boards and committees of faith communities.

Abbreviation: CMHS, community mental health services.

Adapted from Substance Abuse and Mental Health Services Administration. (2004). *Building bridges: Mental health consumers and members of faith-based and community organizations in dialogue* (DHHS Pub. No. 3868). Rockville, MD: Author.

four million adults in the United States with untreated severe mental illness account for:

- 1 in 4 of all fatal police encounters
- 1 in 5 of all jail and prison inmates
- 1 in 10 of all law enforcement responses

There are potentially many mental health consequences of police-inflicted violence, including an increase in symptoms such as anxiety and paranoia. A study conducted by DeVylder et al. (2017) concluded that there is a strong association between police victimization and suicide attempts and that "[p]reventing such victimization through trauma-informed trainings for police officers, and otherwise addressing the widespread trauma in many urban communities, may improve community mental health and potentially even reduce suicide attempts" (p. 635). Given the increased awareness in the behavioral health arena of

trauma-related symptoms, it is imperative that behavioral health providers not only continue to research the effects of police victimization, but also strongly advocate for the rights and safety of service users and participate in providing training for law enforcement.

Police violence and abuse of power does not only affect and potentially traumatize the people who are directly threatened, injured, or killed; the whole community may be traumatized. After a violent incident involving law enforcement, members of the community may experience rational and irrational fear of the police. Kendall (2015) documents numerous incidents of community members mistrusting the police and, therefore, refusing to cooperate with investigations. These scenarios are classic examples of how a community becomes unhealthy and will not recover without substantial changes in policy, consequences for actions, training programs, and interagency collaboration.

One reason there is a high degree of interaction between police and those with mental illness is that, because of the paucity of comprehensive behavioral health services in many locales, the police are often the first responders in mental health crises. Unfortunately, many police forces do not offer sufficient training to handle psychiatric emergencies. To address this situation, the National Alliance on Mental Illness supports the use of Crisis Intervention Team (CIT) programs:

> In over 2,700 communities nationwide, CIT programs create connections between law enforcement, mental health providers, hospital emergency services, and individuals with mental illness and their families. Through collaborative community partnerships and intensive training, CIT improves communication, identifies mental health resources for those in crisis, and ensures officer and community safety. (2018)

In addition to national initiatives, the local community can do much to foster positive relationships with law enforcement. Behavioral health services are uniquely qualified to develop mutually beneficial partnerships. For example, local police or sheriff offices may assign an officer or officers to liaison with local behavioral health services, serve on advisory boards, be a first responder to agency emergencies, or facilitate community meetings. In turn, the behavioral health agency can provide expert training on deescalation techniques and communicating with people experiencing severe symptoms.

THE FUTURE OF OCCUPATIONAL THERAPY IN COMMUNITY BEHAVIORAL HEALTH SERVICES

As this chapter illustrates, there is a natural fit between the mission of community behavioral health services and occupational therapy. However, we are significantly underrepresented in community behavioral health services. Because of many years of underrepresentation, many agencies throughout the country are not even aware of the potential contributions of occupational therapy. This is especially unfortunate in underserved areas where it is difficult to attract and retain qualified behavioral health specialists and where the needs of the community include multiple social and occupational injustices. In order to establish and protect the place of occupational therapy in community behavioral health, several actions need to be taken:

- Prepare educational material and engage in extensive outreach to behavioral health organizations to explain the role of occupational therapy and the benefit of including us on teams

- Expand occupational therapy roles beyond direct service to include consultation and program development (see Chapter 5 for further discussion of these roles)
- Create alternative models of service delivery, including the establishment of new nonprofit organizations and private practice (see Chapter 10 for discussion of a child behavioral health private practice)
- Develop new internship programs in areas that currently do not have an occupational therapy presence but have access to potential occupational therapy supervisors for a minimum of 8 hours per week

This last action is particularly effective in not only demonstrating the value of occupational therapy, but also in encouraging student occupational therapists to pursue positions in community behavioral health. Because many universities are faced with a shortage of fieldwork placement sites, it is imperative that new internship programs are developed for this vital area of practice.

Box 3-5 presents an abbreviated proposal for establishing a new occupational therapy internship program in a rural area. Not only was this program considered highly successful, it paved the way for an expansion of occupational therapy services in this community. The initial contract allowed for payment of 8 hours per week of occupational therapy supervision for two interns, but the number of hours in subsequent contracts was increased multiple times to include intern supervision and to provide direct services and consultation.

SUMMARY

Occupational therapy has an important place on both primary care teams and in community behavioral health services. Occupational therapists have skills in providing assessment and intervention for physical and behavioral health issues that directly impact function and quality of life. We are also highly trained in assessing the environment, which allows us to understand the inner workings and interrelatedness of a community. (See Chapters 6 and 7 for further discussion.) Our theory base includes occupational justice, which provides a framework for intervention with marginalized and underserved people. Furthermore, we can conduct outreach to individuals identified as at risk or vulnerable for medical compromise due to behavioral or mental health issues and can provide services in a variety of settings to ensure continuity of care for optimal outcomes.

In order to establish the value of occupational therapy in the community, we must become better skilled at interprofessional collaboration and articulating the expertise and unique contributions the occupational therapist brings to the team. The volatile and ever-changing health care reimbursement system presents uncertainty about the future, and how community models will be financially supported in the United States is unknown. Occupational therapy

Box 3-5. Internship Program Proposal

SITUATION STATEMENT

It is well-documented that there is a recurrent shortage of health care professionals in rural areas throughout the country. For occupational therapy in California mental health services, the disparity is extreme. No occupational therapists were identified as working in public community mental health in any of the California counties designated as rural. In some ways, this is not surprising. All of the occupational therapy schools in California are located in greater metropolitan areas, and occupational therapy internship sites are largely within commuting distance of these universities. Also, the majority of students attending occupational therapy school are from metropolitan areas. Therefore, occupational therapy students in California have little or no experience with rural culture or the health issues encountered in rural areas. Conversely, because of the lack of occupational therapy presence in rural counties, the benefits of having occupational therapy as part of a community mental health team are not well understood.

PROCEDURES AND PLANNING

Given the rural context, the first step in developing this program is to elicit the support of the community behavioral health services board as well as agency administrators and staff. Several presentations have already been given with an emphasis on educating board members, administrators, and staff about occupational therapy and explaining how occupational therapy could fit into the agency.

A second, equally important planning step is to ensure that the internship structure is practical and desirable. The challenge is to find occupational therapy interns who are willing to abandon their familiar environments, relocate to a place where they had no support system, and work in a program that is not yet developed and does not have an occupational therapist on staff. To partially address these concerns, it is preferable to take two interns at a time so they would have each other for support. This model has worked well in a variety of internship placements and is frequently used by occupational therapy programs throughout the country. However, the real linchpin for a practical and desirable rural internship is supplied housing. Several ideas for providing housing are being explored. In addition to housing, there is a request in the budget for a reasonable daily living stipend because financial incentives are critical in recruiting qualified applicants.

The selection of interns is set up to be a competitive process because a pilot program internship is bound to be somewhat unstructured. Qualifications include an interest in program development, an ability to be flexible, and a willingness to take initiative and be self-directed. Also, applicants should show a willingness to learn about rural culture and a desire to potentially practice in a rural environment.

BENEFITS TO THE AGENCY

The addition of two full-time occupational therapy interns along with a part-time consulting occupational therapy supervisor will enrich the agency by providing a strong rehabilitation perspective and by diversifying the philosophy, approaches, and strategies of the service. Additional benefits are as follows:

- Staff will benefit by receiving much-needed assistance, especially in planning and leading groups that are activity based.
- Clients will benefit by having specific practical skill development and through occupational therapy assessments that can identity both strengths and functional problems influencing recovery.
- The agency will benefit by being able to expand services and provide new offerings to settings beyond the center, including the continuation school, senior center, juvenile hall, county jail, and wellness center.

OBJECTIVES

The overall objective of this pilot program is to provide a quality educational and clinical experience for two occupational therapy interns. Related objectives include the following:

- Develop a supervision model that meets or exceeds all requirements yet is suitable for an agency that does not have occupational therapists on staff.
- Develop an occupational therapy program, including assessment and intervention protocols, as well as documentation formats.

(continued)

Box 3-5 (continued). Internship Program Proposal

OBJECTIVES (CONTINUED)

- Provide direct occupational therapy services to the clients of the agency as well as to several other organizations in the county through individual assessment and intervention, as well as group interventions.
- Provide indirect occupational therapy services through consultation and collaboration with staff and clients.
- Establish mechanisms for sustaining the introduced occupational therapy procedures and methods.

SUPERVISION MODEL

The traditional model of supervision dictates that the occupational therapy supervisor is a member of the professional staff and continuously on site. Because this model is not possible, a consultation contract is requested to cover the supervision hours. The minimum time requirement for supervision of occupational therapy interns is 8 hours per week, which is a line item in the budget. For the pilot of this program, it is expected that additional time will be needed to establish a program and policies and to educate the staff about occupational therapy. However, the occupational therapist agrees to volunteer extra time for the initial (pilot) offering of this internship program. If the program is sustained, the hours of supervision and other service can be renegotiated. Furthermore, mechanisms are needed to ensure the quality of the supervision for this nontraditional arrangement and to ensure that the lack of an occupational therapist continually on site is not a detriment to the learning experience. Staff of the community behavioral health services are requested to provide orientation to all components of the agency and to take responsibility for providing on-site support for the interns. The occupational therapy supervisor will be available on call for urgent concerns or emergencies.

---

must be ready to address these uncertainties and be prepared to take its place as a valued member in community service.

References

Ackerman, M. (2015). *The pros and cons of needle exchange programs.* Retrieved from https://www.recovery.org/the-pros-and-cons-of-needle-exchange-programs

American Psychiatric Association Foundation. (2014). *Mental health: A guide for faith leaders.* Arlington, VA: Author. Retrieved from https://apafdn.org/impact/community/faith-based-guide

American Psychological Association. (n.d.). *Growing mental and behavioral health concerns facing older Americans.* Retrieved from http://www.apa.org/advocacy/health/older-americans-mental-behavioral-health.aspx

Bahorik, A. L., Satre, D. D., Kline-Simon, A. H., Weisner, C. M., & Campbell, C. I. (2017). Serious mental illness and medical comorbidities: Findings from an integrated health care system. *Journal of Psychosomatic Research, 100,* 35-45. doi:10.1016/j.jpsychores.2017.07.004

Centers for Medicare & Medicaid Services. (2018a). *Federally qualified health center.* Retrieved from https://www.cms.gov/Outreach-and-Education/Medicare-Learning-Network-MLN/MLNProducts/downloads/fqhcfactsheet.pdf

Centers for Medicare & Medicaid Services. (2018b). *Next generation ACO model.* Retrieved from https://innovation.cms.gov/initiatives/Next-Generation-ACO-Model

Dahl-Popolizio, S., Manson, L., Muir, S., & Rogers, O. (2016). Enhancing the value of integrated primary care: The role of occupational therapy. *Families, Systems, & Health, 34*(3), 270-280.

DeVylder, J. E., Frey J. J., Cogburn, C. D., Wilcox, H. C., Sharpe, T. L., Oh, H. Y., … Link, B. G. (2017). Elevated prevalence of suicide attempts among victims of police violence in the USA. *Journal of Urban Health, 94,* 629-636. doi:10.1007/s11524-017-0160-3

Donnelly, C. A., Leclair, L. L., Wener, P. F., Hand, C. L., & Letts, L. J. (2016). Occupational therapy in primary care: Results from a national survey. *Canadian Journal of Occupational Therapy, 83*(3) 135-142. doi:10.1177/0008417416637186

Drug Policy Alliance. (n.d.). *Harm reduction.* Retrieved from http://www.drugpolicy.org/issues/harm-reduction

Fong, K. (2008). Occupational therapy in primary health care: A new era for involvement and contributions in the new health system in Hong Kong. *Hong Kong Journal of Occupational Therapy, 18,* i-ii.

Fossey, E., & Krupa, B. (2016). Developing occupational just communities. In T. Krupa, B. Kirsh, D. Pitts, & E. Fossey (Eds.), *Bruce & Borg's psychosocial frames of reference: Theories, models, and approaches for occupation-based practice* (4th ed., pp. 285-301). Thorofare, NJ: SLACK Incorporated.

Fuller, D. A., Lamb, H. R., Biasotti, M., & Snook, J. (2015). *Overlooked in the undercounted: The role of mental illness in fatal law enforcement encounters.* Retrieved from http://www.treatmentadvocacycenter.org/storage/documents/overlooked-in-the-undercounted.pdf

Halle, A. D., Mroz, T. M., Fogelberg, D. J., & Leland, N. E. (2018). Occupational therapy and primary care: Updates and trends. *American Journal of Occupational Therapy, 72*(3), 1-6.

Healthright 360. (2017, August 29). *California's first integrated health care center for low-income and homeless people opens in San Francisco* [Press release]. Retrieved from https://www.healthright360.org/news/californias-first-integrated-health-care-center-low-income-and-homeless-people-opens-san

Institute of Medicine. (1994). *Defining primary care: An interim report.* Washington, DC: National Academy Press.

Kathol, R. G., Patel, K., Sacks, L., Sargent, S., & Melek, S. P. (2015). The role of behavioral health services in accountable care organizations. *American Journal of Managed Care, 21*(2), e95-e98.

Kendall, M. (2015, April 10). The police can't police themselves. And now the public is too scared to cooperate with them. *The Washington Post.* Retrieved from https://www.washingtonpost.com/posteverything/wp/2015/04/10/the-police-cant-police-themselves-and-now-the-public-is-too-scared-to-cooperate-with-them/?noredirect=on&utm_term=.623481d149d9

Mental Health America. (2018). *Mental health month.* Retrieved from http://www.mentalhealthamerica.net/may

Murphy, A. D., Griffith, V. M., Mroz, T. M., & Jirikowic, T. L. (2017). Primary care for underserved populations: Navigating policy to incorporate occupational therapy into federally qualified health centers. *American Journal of Occupational Therapy, 71,* 1-5.

National Alliance on Mental Illness. (2018). *Crisis Intervention Team (CIT) programs.* Retrieved from https://www.nami.org/Get-Involved/Law-Enforcement-and-Mental-Health

National Council for Behavioral Health. (2018). *Community Mental Health Act.* https://www.thenationalcouncil.org/about/national-mental-health-association/overview/community-mental-health-act/

Office of Disease Prevention and Health Promotion. (n.d.). *Social determinants of health.* Retrieved from https://www.healthypeople.gov/2020/topics-objectives/topic/social-determinants-of-health

Patient-Centered Primary Care Collaborative. (2018). *CMS comprehensive primary care plus (CPC+).* Retrieved from https://www.pcpcc.org/initiative/cms-comprehensive-primary-care-plus

Patient Protection and Affordable Care Act, 42 U.S.C. 18001 (2010).

Peek, C. J., & the National Integration Academy Council. (2013). *Lexicon for behavioral health and primary care integration* (AHRQ Publication No.13-IP001-EF). Rockville, MD: Agency for Healthcare Research and Quality. Retrieved from http://integrationacademy.ahrq.gov/sites/default/files/Lexicon.pdf

Robert Wood Johnson Foundation. (n.d.). *RWJF Commission to Build a Healthier America.* Retrieved from https://www.rwjf.org/en/how-we-work/grants-explorer/featured-programs/rwjf-commission-to-build-a-healthier-america.html

Substance Abuse and Mental Health Services Administration. (2004). *Building bridges: Mental health consumers and members of faith-based and community organizations in dialogue* (DHHS Pub. No. 3868). Rockville, MD: Author.

Substance Abuse and Mental Health Services Administration. (2011). *Consumer-operated services: Building your program* (HHS Pub. No. SMA-11-4633). Rockville, MD: Author.

Substance Abuse and Mental Health Service Administration. (2017). *SAMHSA spotlight: A series on building resilient and trauma-informed communities* (HHS Pub. No. SMA-17-5014). Rockville, MD: Author.

Tello, M. (2017, August 30). *Patient-centered medical home: A new model for medical care* [Web log post]. Retrieved from https://www.health.harvard.edu/blog/patient-centered-medical-home-a-new-model-for-medical-care-2017083012260

U.S. Department of Health and Human Services. (n.d.). *For community and faith leaders: Creating community connections for mental health.* Retrieved from https://www.mentalhealth.gov/talk/faith-community-leaders

U.S. Department of Health and Human Services, Agency for Healthcare Research and Quality. (n.d.). *Defining the PCMH.* Retrieved from https://pcmh.ahrq.gov/page/defining-pcmh

Whiteford, G., & Townsend, E. (2011). Participatory occupational justice framework (POJF 2010): Enabling occupational participation and inclusion. In F. Kronenberg, N. Pollard, & D. Sakellariou (Eds.), *Occupational therapies without borders: Towards an ecology of occupation-based practices* (Vol. 2, pp. 65-84). Edinburgh, Scotland: Churchill Livingstone.

World Health Organization. (2008). *Integrating mental health into primary care: A global perspective.* Geneva, Switzerland: Author.

World Health Organization. (2014). *Social determinants of mental health.* Geneva, Switzerland: Author. Retrieved from http://apps.who.int/iris/bitstream/10665/112828/1/9789241506809_eng.pdf

World Health Organization. (2018). *Determinants of mental health.* Retrieved from http://www.who.int/news-room/fact-sheets/detail/mental-health-strengthening-our-response

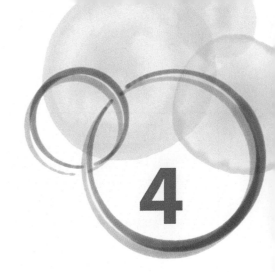

Direct Service Provision

Anne MacRae, PhD, OTR/L, BCMH, FAOTA

The primary role of occupational therapists has historically been the provision of direct services, including assessment, treatment, and discharge. The terminology and process has somewhat changed because of the new emphasis on collaboration and peer-driven services and the transition to a more social model of practice. The differences between the conventional (medically oriented) occupational therapy process and a socially oriented process are shown in Figure 4-1. For the purposes of this chapter, the emphasis is on social orientation, but as described in Chapter 1, occupational therapy is a rehabilitation profession that bridges the medical and social model. Therefore, the medically oriented process is also discussed as indicated.

There is some debate regarding how much of occupational therapy practice should be devoted to direct service. The source of this debate at least partially stems from the changing educational levels of occupational therapists around the world. Many countries are considering a master's degree–level entry to the profession, and some countries are moving toward a doctoral-level entry. The American Occupational Therapy Association (AOTA) has the official position that "the profession should take action to transition toward a doctoral-level single point of entry for occupational therapists, with a target date of 2025" (AOTA, 2014a). However, this is not a uniformly accepted position. Some have argued that such a move will decrease the number of therapists available for direct service provision and increase the cost of service. Advanced education

for the profession has allowed for the production of quality research and also opened up many opportunities for consultation, program development, and other positions of leadership. These roles are explored in the subsequent chapter. However, in order to maintain our identity and credibility, direct service must remain the backbone of the profession. Even limiting this discussion to direct services, the range of possible settings necessarily influences the scope of assessments, access to sources of information, and selection of interventions. Therefore, every effort is made in this chapter to highlight the service process in a variety of settings.

REFERRAL TO SERVICES

Within the medical model, a psychiatrist traditionally initiated referrals to psychosocial occupational therapy services. This is primarily because there is historical precedent for a hierarchical model of service with clearly defined roles and responsibilities. However, it is also tied to the common reimbursement criteria that requires a physician, or other licensed diagnostic clinician, to request, determine, and initiate the services to be provided. Even within medically oriented services, referrals are now often initiated as part of a team process in which all interdisciplinary team members, including occupational therapists, make recommendations for referrals.

MacRae, A. (Ed.). *Cara and MacRae's Psychosocial Occupational Therapy: An Evolving Practice, Fourth Edition* (pp 49-71). © 2019 Taylor & Francis Group.

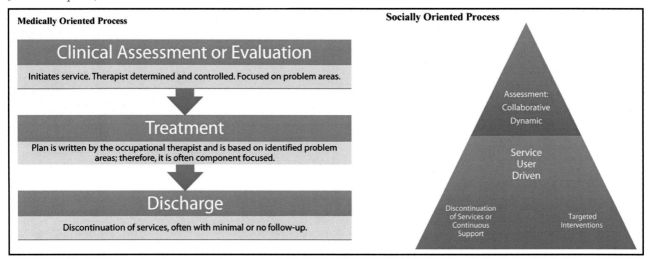

Figure 4-1. Medically oriented process and socially oriented process.

In settings that operate on a social model, or with a recovery perspective, the ideal situation is for service users to self-refer. However, practitioners often have the role of educating service users about available programs, groups, and one-on-one intervention, as well as their potential usefulness for the individual. Although professionals make recommendations and certainly encourage participation in a variety of services, the choice is ultimately with the service user and should not be mandated or coerced in any way, except under very specific circumstances. These circumstances include when a court order is in place or when sedation in a medical (psychiatric) emergency is necessary for safety.

CORE VALUES AND INTERPERSONAL STRATEGIES

Every aspect of occupational therapy service provision, beginning with the referral, requires adherence to our professional values and the purposeful use of interpersonal strategies. The AOTA (2015) identifies the seven core values of occupational therapy as altruism, equality, freedom, justice, dignity, truth, and prudence. Many occupational therapy professional organizations have also adopted statements of similar core values. Thomas and Menage (2016) suggest that compassion, although neglected in the literature, should also be acknowledged as a core value of occupational therapy because "it lies at the heart of professional relationships and person-centred practice" (p. 3). Having these core values is often the reason that people are attracted to the field of occupational therapy. Nevertheless, mentoring is needed for students and novice therapists to understand how these values are manifested in practice.

Interpersonal strategies are specific techniques for applying core values into practice and are defined in

Table 4-1. These strategies may be cognitively understood and emotionally embraced but still can be quite difficult to apply in practice. Again, students and novice therapists can best master these skills through mentoring by experienced practitioners that goes beyond the teaching of specific content, but rather role models the therapeutic relationship.

THERAPEUTIC RELATIONSHIP

In developing an occupational profile, the therapeutic use of self is as important as the information obtained. Therapeutic use of self involves a therapist's "planned use of his or her personality, insights, perceptions, and judgments as part of the therapeutic process" (Punwar & Peloquin, 2000, p. 285). Rapport-building and therapeutic alliance start from the first contact with the service user. It is important to nurture trust from the outset. Trust can be gained through practicing nonjudgment. Throughout the provision of services, a lot of personal and intimate information will be requested. How the practitioner responds will determine whether the service user will continue to open up or shy away from sharing due to a fear of rejection or shame. Carl Rogers (1951), a noted humanistic psychologist, argued that client progress can only be made in a therapeutic relationship that embodies unconditional positive regard, defined as basic acceptance and support of a person regardless of what the person says or does. The need for unconditional positive regard is especially true in the context of client-centered therapy. Questions need to be asked in a nonjudgmental way that avoid using "why" questions, which might make someone defensive or hesitant. It is also important to be mindful of facial expressions and nonverbal body language in response to the information received. Case Illustration 4-1 presents the therapeutic relationship from the perspective of a service user.

TABLE 4-1. INTERPERSONAL STRATEGIES

VALIDATION	The conveyance of respect for an individual's experience or perspective and that the individual is a valued human being. Validation could be a simple action, such as greeting a person and saying you are glad to see him or her or acknowledging his or her distress about talking to himself or herself around others. It could be nonverbal, such as sitting with and listening to a person, although he or she may seem to make little sense.
SETTING LIMITS	The identification of behavior that cannot be tolerated or is inappropriate for the setting. Limit setting also necessitates the provision of clear expectations and feedback about how to change the behavior. It is therapeutic in that it addresses behavior that is a barrier to satisfying occupational performance, roles, habits, or successful relationships.
ENCOURAGEMENT	Providing emotional support and assurance for clients' actions, behaviors, or choices. In a mental health setting, encouragement is often needed for clients to engage in activities, try out new occupations or new situations, or move to the next level of treatment. Although it seems a simple and commonsense technique, it also has to be timed and specific to individual situations and service users so as not to seem that the occupational therapy practitioner is merely a cheerleader. A practitioner's desire to instill hope, whether conscious or unconscious, must be balanced with the needs of the individual client and his or her worldview.
ADVICE	Recommending a course of action or choice, and may not necessarily be consistent with client-centered, collaborative practice unless used cautiously and within a clear clinical reasoning framework. Occupational therapy practitioners may advise clients when establishing realistic goals, based on information gained through the occupational profile. Advice is also given regularly during intervention when service users seek help to achieve their goals. Although it is tempting to offer advice to discourage action that does not appear to be in the service user's best interest, it is important to present this in a neutral way so that the individual is able to accept or reject it while still maintaining a working therapeutic relationship. Care must be taken to ensure that advice is given in a manner that conveys respect for service users and also the choices that they make.
COACHING	Demonstrating, guiding, or prompting when necessary for service users to accomplish tasks. It also fosters collaboration between the practitioner and the service user and can be viewed as more supportive than an "expert" model. Therefore, it is consistent with occupational therapy's core values. Coaching can also be a motivating factor because it redirects individuals to performance aspects that may be satisfying or validating of their skills or habits.
CONFRONTATION	To oppose or bring together for examination or comparison or to present for acknowledgment or contradiction. Occupational therapy practitioners may have face-to-face conversations with clients that are frank discussions of clients' behaviors, actions, skills, or performances that may be harmful or destructive. Confrontation is carried out with honesty and directness, often with an appraisal of clients' actions or behaviors. Confronting also conveys caring, that the practitioner cares enough about the client to notice and attempt to intervene when the client may be harming him- or herself.

(continued)

Table 4-1 (continued). Interpersonal Strategies

REFRAMING	Providing alternative interpretations of behaviors, actions, performance patterns, or skills. Very often in mental health settings, clients are unsure of their strengths and very knowledgeable about their weaknesses. This useful cognitive therapy technique highlights other aspects of individual's behaviors, actions, skills, or patterns when he or she can only see usually negative aspects.
METAPHORS	The use of metaphors allows the service user to quickly grasping a concept without having it explained with lengthy words. It is particularly effective with people experiencing mental illness because metaphors are usually concrete examples that can readily be identified in everyday life. Using metaphors in conversations may not be a natural way of talking but can be learned and practiced.
REALITY TESTING	Offering an explanation of a situation that occurs in real life to counter obvious distortions or denials that service users may use. The understanding of what is actually happening is offered in such a way that the therapist encourages the individual to think about and reflectively examine a situation.

CASE ILLUSTRATION 4-1: CEDRIC'S STORY IN HIS OWN WORDS—RECEIVING OCCUPATIONAL THERAPY SERVICES

When I got referred to occupational therapy, I was hesitant to go in and didn't know what to expect. When we first met, very quickly my occupational therapist was able to disarm me and show me that there was nothing to worry about. She showed me that anything we were going to do in therapy would help me greatly and organize my life.

I feel like a lot of therapists might go, "Here's what you need to do," and my occupational therapist didn't do that at all. If you are just telling someone what to do, I feel like it would be a temporary solution to a longer-term problem. To be honest (no offense), my occupational therapist didn't do much, if you look at it that way. It's kind of like her job is to show the clients they can do this on their own, they don't need you. You have to do this in an intelligent way, you don't just tell them, "You don't need me," but, "Let me show you how you don't need me" and teach them the tools to succeed on their own.

My occupational therapist made me feel like I could be myself and didn't judge me. Oftentimes I would admit my faults and I wouldn't be afraid to say I took two steps back this week. I wasn't afraid because I knew my occupational therapist would say, "Okay, well, let's see how we can get back on track." Also, humor is everything. If my therapists didn't use humor, I feel like they would have been robots. I think my occupational therapist picked up on the cues. I was silly first, and then she was like, "Oh okay, that's okay to do with this guy." I don't think it's for everyone. I think it benefitted me greatly because my occupational therapist picked up on it early on and went with it.

Anytime I brought up something that made me happy, she would fully 100% encourage it and push me toward it. That's what I needed—what everyone needs. Go after what you love. If they're not getting 100% encouragement from the occupational therapist, then they might not go after it.

Discussion

Starting occupational therapy can be confusing and anxiety producing. It was important to Cedric that the therapist was approachable and clearly communicated the benefit of the service for the client. He valued that the occupational therapist did not give advice but encouraged his own creative problem solving, seeing him as the expert. Cedric has a strong value for humor, so this was a useful tool for the occupational therapist to use in strengthening the relationship. To establish a strong rapport and therapeutic alliance, the therapist was open and nonjudgmental, using unconditional positive regard. This also involved "holding the hope" for Cedric and seeing his potential, even when he was unable to see it himself.

Goal Development, Refinement, and Attainment

In the conventional (medical) service delivery approach, the establishment of goals is considered the final product of assessment. However, in the socially oriented approach, goals are viewed as a process on a continuum that overarches all aspects of service delivery (Figure 4-2). Goal development needs to begin with at least a rudimentary level of self-awareness. It is quite common for an individual to go through an exploratory process before being able to identify any goals. As self-awareness increases, goals can be developed, refined, or changed, and new goals can be added. Typically, the service user may start with a "grand vision." Although this can be exciting and motivating, it is usually vague and therefore not measurable. The recovery goals are more manageable and specific but still may not include the steps necessary to achieve these goals. Objectives provide the mechanism to reach goals through a step-by-step process with the just-right challenge that is geared toward success. It is then that the individual has the opportunity to create even more challenging goals that may or may not require professional assistance. This approach is consistent with the conclusions drawn from research conducted by Yarborough, Yarborough, Janoff, & Green (2016):

> Mental health recovery is complex and dynamic; individuals' recovery goals can be expected to change over time. Person-centered care must accommodate changing consumer priorities, services must be flexible and responsive, and outcomes need to match consumers' objectives. Clinicians can assist in (a) identifying recovery goals, (b) monitoring progress toward and recognizing movement away from goals, (c) tailoring support to different phases/ stages, and (d) supporting transitions between phases/stages. (p. 97)

While it is accurate that several formal assessment tools do result in the establishment of goals, the practitioner has the responsibility to assist the service user in refining and revising goals and documenting the outcome or attainment of goals. There are several variations of the Goal Attainment Scale, which is the most commonly used method in mental health service for measuring and quantifying progress. It has also shown to be a motivating and valued tool in occupational therapy practice (Cairns, Kavanagh, Dark, & McPhail, 2015).

Assessment

There is some confusion in the literature about the proper terminology for this step of information gathering. The AOTA (2014b) refers to this as *evaluation*. However, the term *assessment* is preferred by many other psychosocial

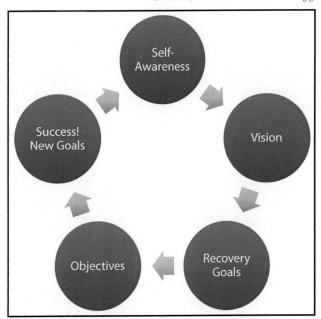

Figure 4-2. The process of goal development, refinement, and attainment.

professions and occupational therapy associations in other parts of the world. The term *assessment* is also used in non-health care–related fields. For example, the education literature uniformly defines *evaluation* as summative, final, and judgmental, whereas *assessment* is formative, interactive, and continuous. Viewing the process as collaborative and ongoing is a better fit for recovery-oriented services; therefore, the term *assessment* is used in this chapter. Despite the confusion with terminology, the *Occupational Therapy Practice Framework* (*Framework*) also supports the defining principles of the term *assessment* with the following statement: "Information related to the occupational profile is gathered throughout the occupational therapy process" (AOTA, 2014b, p. S13). However, readers, particularly in the United States, should be aware that the terms *evaluation* and *assessment* are perhaps used incorrectly and are sometimes used interchangeably.

The essence of assessment is information gathering, but this process is often viewed by service users as intrusive, judgmental, and possibly even secretive. Within the recovery perspective, every effort is made to conduct assessment in collaboration with the service user with transparency and agreed-upon focus. This approach does not diminish the importance of the unique expertise of the occupational therapist. Rather, it increases the responsibility of the practitioner to clearly explain the results of any formal evaluation tools and to share observations and interpretations.

Initial Assessment

Intake summaries or other data collected upon initiation of services, along with reports by others on the team with prior contact, are often the first source of information.

Although this information can sometimes be helpful in understanding some details of the service user's history and the events that triggered the need for services, as well as recommended precautions (such as suicidal ideation), it is rarely complete and too often contains factual errors. Furthermore, the information will most likely lack the details of the individual's daily living issues necessary to develop an occupational profile. In other words, the professional responsibility of the occupational therapist is to engage in an assessment process that is client centered and occupational based (World Federation of Occupational Therapists, 2010).

The initial assessment often has to be cursory for a number of reasons, including time limits imposed by the agency or reimbursement sources, but the most compelling reason is to meet the service user's needs. Many people with mental illness or in psychosocial distress are not able or willing to engage in lengthy verbal exchanges and benefit the most when a trusting relationship can evolve. Furthermore, there is often limited tolerance for this aspect of care and an expressed desire to get started in addressing the causes of current occupational problems. Therefore, as soon as some jointly identified problems and preliminary goals are identified, intervention services can commence with the understanding that assessment will be ongoing through dynamic and continuous assessment.

Dynamic and Continuous Assessment

Dynamic assessment refers to an interactive process that is used in many educational and health professions (Haywood & Lidz, 2007). Occupational therapists need to assess what the individuals can achieve on their own, but they are also interested in the extent to which performance can be improved. Dynamic assessment is useful for this purpose because it focuses on individual variations in function under different circumstances rather than comparing the person to normative data or a criterion reference.

Due to the nature of occupational therapy practice, which focuses on *doing*, dynamic assessment blurs the boundaries between *assessment* and *intervention*. In some settings, this may be problematic, especially for coding or billing of services. However, in many psychosocial settings, dynamic assessment is an ideal way to develop a therapeutic relationship, work on goals in a timely manner, and get a more accurate picture of an individual functional abilities. Case Illustration 4-2 shows an example of a dynamic assessment.

Dynamic assessment is closely related to another concept called *continuous assessment*, which simply means that assessment is an ongoing process. In psychosocial practice, there are many reasons why important information may not be forthcoming in a specific time frame. Service users may exhibit many symptoms, such as paranoia, psychosis, or cognitive deficits. They also may have a traumatic past that leaves them wary of disclosure and limits their ability to trust others. As the therapeutic relationship develops, further information may come to light through observation or verbal disclosure that leads the therapist to a better understanding of the presenting problem or to the identification of additional problems.

The recommended approach for assessment in recovery-oriented service is top-down, meaning beginning with the big picture. In occupational therapy, this means the focus is on occupations, client factors, performance skills, and performance patterns as well as context and environment (AOTA, 2014b). As part of the dynamic and continuous process, information may be uncovered that requires further investigation. This often entails using tools associated with a more medical or bottom-up approach—in other words, component-based assessments such as those focusing on cognition or sensory processing. Assessments that are commonly used in behavioral health settings include the Executive Function Performance Test (Baum, Morrison, Hahn, & Edwards, 2007) and the Adolescent/Adult Sensory Profile (Brown & Dunn, 2002). The occupational therapy and interdisciplinary assessments used in behavioral health settings are too numerous to comprehensively discuss in this chapter. Although a few additional assessments are highlighted in this chapter as they relate to particular topics, many other assessments are discussed in subsequent chapters as they relate to specific settings or populations.

Group Assessment

In the medical model, assessment is viewed as a closed and private relationship between a clinician and a service user, with the clinician leading the process. However, in a social model, assessment is collaborative and can include family members, peers, or other support. Therefore, it is possible for assessments to be conducted in a group setting that overlaps with interventions. In occupational therapy, the latter model is valued because many of our assessment tools are interactive and occupation focused. Furthermore, it is a very efficient use of time and fosters a sense of personal responsibility and group leadership roles because peer participants help each other. One legitimate rationale for the former (private) approach is protecting client confidentiality. When occupational therapists use assessments as a group intervention, it is critical that options are available to protect privacy. For example, in a group session using the Canadian Occupational Performance Measure (Law et al., 2015), some participants may be reluctant to share their specific occupational problems. The occupational therapist should avoid a round-robin approach to group sharing that would expose the reluctant individual. However, once some volunteers share their results, others are often inspired to further complete and possibly even share their own forms. In addition to fear of disclosure, there may be other reasons that an individual may not want to participate in the process or share his or her responses. Most often, it is because the group member does not understand the instructions

CASE ILLUSTRATION 4-2: DOUBLE OT ASSESSMENT—EXAMPLE OF DYNAMIC PROCESS

Clare, an 18-year-old woman with difficulties in managing her anger, was referred to occupational therapy by her probation officer. During the initial meeting with Elena, the occupational therapist, Clare expresses an interest in work. Elena suggests that they engage in the the Double OT Work Skills Assessment (Haworth & Cyrs, 2017). Clare is initially hesitant, inquiring, "Are you going to be asking me a bunch of questions?" Elena explains that it's not a typical assessment and actually plays out like a secret agent game, where Clare will solve a mystery and demonstrate a different job skill with each step of the "investigation." Elena also mentions that her previous clients have liked being able to identify their skills and then use this information in job interviews.

After Clare agrees to try it out, Elena playfully initiates the dynamic assessment by reading the mission aloud and explaining the basic instructions. Clare's skeptical demeanor begins to soften as she giggles in response to the absurd plot. Clare then reads the prompt for the planning task and quickly starts drawing a line through the corresponding paper maze, slowing her pace gradually as she progresses along. In task, Elena observes Clare persevere in completing the maze despite intermittently running into dead ends.

In processing after completion, Clare is encouraged to identify the work skill she used in task. She calls the skill "strategy." After Elena agrees that she used strategy and clarifies that strategy is a type of planning, Clare is prompted to generalize how the skill of planning is used across occupations. This prompt opens the discussion, fostering reflection and awareness as Clare verbalizes that she is good at planning but "I often fall through." Elena responds by offering strategies to meet Clare's stated area for growth. Clare shares which ones she believes could work for her, and Elena takes notes in order to include them in a written summary, later shared with her work supervisor. Elena shares observed strengths based on Clare's performance in the task, explaining that Clare demonstrated the ability to problem solve, persevere in task, and recover from mistakes without exhibiting frustration, despite being "quick to anger."

The interaction between Clare and Elena follows this pattern for each subsequent task in the assessment, providing space after task completion to name the skill, apply it to work, and appraise personal performance. Upon completion of the assessment, Clare announces, unprompted, "I would definitely recommend that all of my friends do that. It was fun and helpful."

Discussion

The playful and collaborative nature of this dynamic assessment facilitates the development of a therapeutic relationship, allowing Clare to perform each task to the best of her ability, thereby rendering the results of the assessment more accurate. This is particularly vital when working with adolescents, who are notorious for their disengagement in similar situations. Additionally, Clare is asked to perform various tasks under differing fictional circumstances throughout the assessment, and although this is not a change of physical environments, the structure allows for Elena to witness the range of Clare's functioning. This enables Elena to identify how her performance can best be enhanced or supported at her job. Furthermore, both by increasing Clare's awareness of her skills and by seeking her input on useful strategies to support her continued development, Elena blends the principles of assessment and intervention. Beyond serving as a way in which to establish rapport, this assists in challenging the hierarchical nature of assessment and honors the value of the client's self-knowledge. The reported results of this assessment are provided in Figure 4-3.

or is confused by the process. It is obviously the occupational therapist's responsibility to provide clear step-by-step instructions at a pace that is suitable for the group member's ability. It is also extremely helpful to have a coach available to assist participants in a one-on-one situation within the group. The coach may be a designated peer group member, a peer specialist, an invited case manager, an occupational therapy assistant, or an intern. Sometimes, symptoms such as delusions or paranoia may also interfere with an individual's ability to complete this activity. The coaching process may assist this individual, or it may be that the individual is not capable of completing the assessment in a group setting. However, there is still value in listening to the instructions and hearing other group members share their results. In all cases, the occupational therapist should offer participants the opportunity to follow up individually to clarify problems and goals and create a plan based on them.

CASE ILLUSTRATION 4-3: RICKY'S EXPERIENCE IN THE KAWA MODEL GROUP

Instructions for completing the Kawa exercise were provided, both verbally and in writing, to the group of 10 people. One of the participants, Ricky, initially moved his chair away from the table and appeared to be uninterested in the activity. However, after seeing all the other members begin the activity, he moved his chair closer and began to look at the instructions. He then posed several questions but did not initiate drawing. Instead, he watched others in the group engage in the activity for approximately 10 minutes. He then began drawing but continued to ask clarifying questions and seek reassurance that he was doing it right.

Participants were asked if they wished to share their drawings. Ricky shared several aspects of his drawing, including large "boulders" representing unemployment, extensive debt, recent breakup with his girlfriend, and chronic pain. Ricky was initially unable to identify any assets (driftwood), but with coaxing from other participants, he added "sense of humor" and "good listener." He also added an original element of a school of fish pushing up a boulder, which he identified as his friends at the center helping him.

Discussion

Although conducting this exercise in a group did have a certain element of exposure, the group also provided encouragement and role modeling. This helped Ricky to not only complete the exercise, but to practice his social skills and enhance friendships as well.

One of the most commonly used assessment tools used in psychosocial occupational therapy groups is an exercise using the Kawa Model (Iwama, 2006). It is especially effective as group intervention because it has a nonverbal, visual component that can be very creative, it allows the individual to self-assess their strengths as well as obstacles to recovery, and it is personalized so there is no right or wrong answer. Therefore, many group participants are comfortable sharing their Kawa drawings and encouraging other group members to expound on their own drawings. As with the Canadian Occupational Performance Measure, it is preferable to have available assistants or coaches to help individuals within the group. It is the occupational therapist's responsibility to train all assistants with informational and practice sessions prior to service user groups. Case Illustration 4-3 describes the experience of a participant in a group Kawa Model exercise. Box 4-1 shows instructions that are used to begin training helpers in Kawa Model groups.

Observation

Observation is a traditional cornerstone of all occupational therapy assessment but is especially valuable in the psychosocial arena. As previously discussed, people in psychological distress or with mental illness often have limited tolerance for verbal exchange and may also have limited ability to accurately report their symptoms or experiences. Observational assessment focuses on multifaceted and complex actions; therefore, it is helpful to have a framework to organize observations. The previously mentioned Executive Function Performance Test is observational in nature and provides a specific framework. However, there are limitations with formal tools, including the following:

- The occupational therapist may not have sufficient time to conduct assessment with observational tools.
- A continuous assessment protocol necessitates using one's observational skills during a wide variety of interventions.
- Many formal tools, although concerned with occupational functioning, do so by focusing on very specific aspects or components of function.

Unlike component-based tools, most observations for assessment look at the big picture. As MacKenzie and Westwood (2013) state: "Observation patterns used by occupational therapists are presumably related to top-down influences that are not necessarily related to domain-specific knowledge" (p. 4). Often, both the individual's strengths and occupational problems are readily identified through observation. However, it is not uncommon for observation to trigger more specific component-based assessments because the reason for the identified occupational problems may be subtle and elusive.

Considering the value of observation in daily occupational therapy practice, every effort should be made in occupational therapy educational programs to provide observational practice opportunities and to encourage students to increase their observational skills in their everyday lives. This may seem obvious, but there is an unfortunate societal trend to spend an inordinate amount of time focused on a tech device screen (such as a smart phone) rather than attending to the environment all around. This issue is discussed in several chapters of this book but perhaps has special significance for this chapter because one cannot help but wonder if overattachment to screen time will diminish the observational skills of future generations.

Box 4-1. Instructions for Kawa Model Exercise

THE KAWA MODEL EXERCISE

An evidence-based tool for understanding the relationship between the person and the social and physical environment.

- Provides a visual representation of a personal narrative within a context, identifying both strengths and areas of concern as perceived by the individual
- Applicable cross culturally, as well as with people of various learning styles and functional/developmental levels, through the use of universal, metaphorical, and naturalistic concepts
- Adaptable for individuals, groups, communities, and organizations

Instructions

1. Provide worksheet with description of Kawa elements and sample picture, as well as colored pencils, crayons, or markers to complete drawing.

   OR

   Create/provide a white magnet board with pre-cut magnetized pieces for Kawa elements, as well as dry erase markers for labeling. For example:

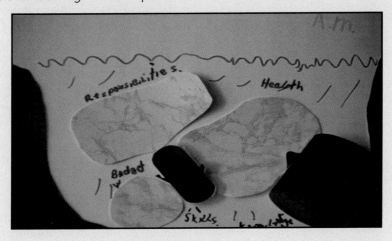

2. Explain/review the Kawa metaphor to understand the purpose and meaning of the exercise:
   - It symbolizes the journey through life; the river upstream represents the past, whereas the lower stream represents the future.
   - A free-flowing river represents good health.
   - A river impeded by rocks and driftwood, or a shallow bank, represents a problem and ill health.
3. Review the elements of the Kawa Model throughout the exercise:
   - Water: Life energy and health; shaped by surrounding environment; changeable
   - (River) bank/base: The physical, economic, political, social, and cultural environment
   - Rocks: Life difficulties, circumstances, symptoms, and issues; each has a unique size and is difficult to remove
   - Driftwood (assets or liabilities): Personal attributes, resources, values, and character; can either block the water or move rocks away
   - Spaces: Life energy (water) flows through spaces
4. Encourage yourself and others to be thorough and creative.
5. Assure yourself and others that there are no right or wrong models. Perceptions and interpretations are varied and personal.

Adapted from Iwama, M. (2006). *Kawa Model: Culturally relevant occupational therapy.* London, England: Churchill Livingstone.

Box 4-2. Motivational Interviewing: Different Types of Change Talk

MNEMONIC: DARN CAT

Preparatory Change Talk

Desire (I want to change)

Ability (I can change)

Reason (It's important to change)

Need (I should change)

Implementing Change Talk

Commitment (I will make changes)

Activation (I am ready, prepared, willing to change)

Taking Steps (I am taking specific actions to change)

Interview

The first step in a mental health interview, no matter how informal, is to seek permission of the service user. In order for such permission to constitute informed consent, the purpose of the questions and the length of expected time must be clearly conveyed. It is also the appropriate time to discuss how or with whom information may be shared. Although the laws involving health care confidentiality are quite stringent, they are not absolute, and the service user needs to know who may be covered by umbrella confidentiality, such as members of the treatment team within the same organization. They also need to be informed of circumstances that would require a legal breach of confidentiality, which are generally limited to situations when there is a threat of violence. It is not uncommon for some negotiation to ensue regarding the parameters of interviews.

Motivational Interview

A common myth regarding people with mental health challenges is that they are unmotivated. It is true that some people with schizophrenia experience negative symptoms of avolition-apathy and diminished expressiveness (Velligan & Alphs, 2014). However, this is not the majority of people with mental illness or those in psychosocial distress. Some individuals just might not be motivated to do what a professional or service wants them to do at that moment.

Motivational interviewing is an evidence-based treatment featuring change talk, which is defined as statements by the client revealing consideration of, motivation for, or commitment to change. Research indicates a clear correlation between client statements about change and outcomes. The more someone talks about change, the more likely he or she is to change. It is highly recommended that

occupational therapists wanting to use motivational interviewing attend a formal training session. (See Suggested Resources.) However, there is a brief mnemonic device, DARN CAT, summarizing the key components of change talk (Box 4-2).

Motivational interviewing can be a strategy to help activate the motivation a person already has and help him or her move toward positive behavior change. The spirit of motivational interviewing is collaborative, evocative, and honoring of individual autonomy. In order to make sure that the therapist is not leading the service user too strongly, the therapist must *resist the righting reflex*, which is our drive to fix things and give advice. Although there is a place for giving information and providing education, this is usually with an invitation where the service user can accept of refuse. The preferred approach is to allow the service user to solve his or her own problems, generate solutions, and experiment with different approaches. Using a strengths-based approach, the occupational therapist explores what the service user is motivated to do. To ensure accuracy, active listening strategies in motivational interviewing involve asking open-ended and evocative questions to inspire change while using affirmations, reflection, and summarizing. Motivational interviewing can be used in the initial interview, while setting goals, and throughout intervention when the prospect of behavior change is relevant to the individual. Table 4-2 is an example of a motivational interview dialogue.

Assessment Results

Occupational therapists use a wide variety of assessment tools and strategies, including formal and self-designed instruments, observation, and interview methods. In fact, it is rare for occupational therapists to depend on a single assessment tool, technique, or strategy. For example, one study examining whether self-report or observation is preferred for assessing task performance concluded that using both together provided more accurate and detailed results (Nielsen & Waehrens, 2015). The totality of our professional skills and unique expertise is required to choose, administer, and interpret assessments and then report the results.

Because it is common for occupational therapists to use multiple tools and methods to conduct a thorough assessment, techniques must be chosen to synthesize and summarize the assessment data. The most common approach is to document with an assessment summary note. This document may be limited to occupational therapy or part of a document that represents an interdisciplinary team.

In addition to, or instead of, a narrative note, occupational therapists may use a template of an occupational profile, such as the one provided by AOTA (2017a). A sample of a completed occupational profile is provided in Table 4-3.

An occupational profile is "a summary of a client's occupational history and experiences, patterns of daily living, interests, values, and needs" (AOTA, 2014b, p. S13).

TABLE 4-2. MOTIVATIONAL INTERVIEW WITH TREVOR: A SAMPLE SCRIPT

SPEAKER	RESPONSE	COMMENT
Occupational therapist	It's great to see you again, Trevor. Last time we spoke, you were discussing how you would like to be more successful in work and have better work/life balance. Is this something you would like to discuss again today, or is something else on your mind?	Asking for permission; giving multiple options
Trevor	Yeah, that's still on my mind. Work is just too much. I find it hard to unwind, but I need to figure out something.	Change talk: need
Occupational therapist	Can you tell me more about what it means for you to unwind?	Open-ended question; exploratory
Trevor	Putting my feet up, watching the game, having a few beers, nothing crazy. I don't know why my wife is on my case about it. I don't see the problem with drinking weeknights. Are you going to tell me to stop drinking?	
Occupational therapist	It's about what you think is right for you. So you are a hard worker, and in order to relax at home, you watch sports and drink beers, and you don't have any concerns about this.	Resisting the righting reflex; strengths-based; affirmation; simple reflection; amplified statement
Trevor	Well, sometimes I am a bit hung over the next day, and this affects my work.	
Occupational therapist	You mentioned last time we met that your work was a strong value of yours.	Linking client behavior to values
Trevor	Yeah, but I need to relax too!	
Occupational therapist	So on the one hand, being successful at work is really important to you, and on the other hand, being able to unwind after a long day is also important.	Using a double-sided reflection to highlight two behaviors and discrepancy between them
Trevor	Both are, but I don't want to feel so crummy all the time.	
Occupational therapist	You enjoy relaxing with a few beers but hate the feeling the next day. What are other ways you have tried to relax in the past that have worked?	Simple reflection; evocative question; calling on past success
Trevor	Working out, music, stuff I dropped a long time ago. There's just no time!	
Occupational therapist	Okay, to summarize, you work long, hard hours at your job and you drink to relax at home, but this has impacted your work performance. You have tried other strategies in the past with success but are concerned about how you will find time to do these. Would you like to explore ways to unwind that fit into your schedule?	Providing summary; open-ended question
Trevor	Sure, I guess I'm open to exploring it.	Contemplation stage of change

TABLE 4-3. CEDRIC'S OCCUPATIONAL PROFILE

CLIENT REPORT

Reason the Client Is Seeking Service and Concerns Related to Engagement in Occupations	Cedric (age 21) referred by disability services counselor for time management and organization skills to improve his performance in education occupations
Occupations in Which the Client Is Successful	Cedric thrives on performance art (break dancing, improvisation, acting); he is a pre-med major experiencing a lot of stress with limited time for social/creative occupations
Personal Interests and Values	Cedric values creativity, humor, and family
Occupational History (i.e., life experiences)	From suburb of Los Angeles, third year of college, improvisation acting on the side
Performance Patterns (i.e., routines, roles, habits, and rituals)	Struggles with time management: arriving to class/appointments on time, organizing calendar, procrastinating with assignments; difficulty with sleep routine due to internet use/schoolwork in the evening

ENVIRONMENT	SUPPORTS TO OCCUPATIONAL ENGAGEMENT	BARRIERS TO OCCUPATIONAL ENGAGEMENT
Physical (e.g., buildings, furniture, pets)	Supportive home environment, quiet and conducive to studying	Living alone reduces engagement with peers/roommates
Social (e.g., spouse, friends, caregivers)	Interest in performance arts, dance/acting groups	Anxiety with trying new activities, decreased time due to major requirements

CONTEXT	SUPPORTS TO OCCUPATIONAL ENGAGEMENT	BARRIERS TO OCCUPATIONAL ENGAGEMENT
Cultural (e.g., customs, beliefs)	Culturally Jewish, nonpracticing	Decreased engagement with family cultural activities due to school requirements
Personal (e.g., age, gender, socioeconomic status, education)	Gender identity: male Age 21 Pursuing bachelor's degree	Perceived high expectations from parents about medical career
Temporal (e.g., stage of life, time of year)	Young adult, junior in college, mid-semester	College requirements increase stress; increased autonomy in time use
Virtual (e.g., chat, email, remote monitoring)	Strong digital skills and experience	Would like to decrease virtual occupations that lead to procrastination

CLIENT GOALS

Client's Priorities and Desired Targeted Outcomes	Improve participation in creative occupations such as dance and acting Improve social occupations and create new friendships Improve time management and organization related to academic performance

Adapted from American Occupational Therapy Association. (2017a). *AOTA occupational profile template.* Bethesda, MD: Author.

The occupational profile is gathered through conversation, interview, and observation. Although the service user's perspective is the most highly valued, information can also be gathered from family and service provider perspectives. These key informants are especially important when a service user has impairments in memory and difficulties in communication.

For service users who find it difficult to express their goals and share about their occupations, the occupational therapist can gather information through creative means such as a picture collage or photography project. This visual representation of the client's occupations and goals can complement the AOTA occupational profile.

Some formal assessments also include a template for reporting results, some more detailed than others. The Double OT Assessment, introduced in Case Illustration 4-2, has a particularly thorough reporting form; a sample of a completed form, based on the case of Clare, is shown in Figure 4-3.

In the interest of time, some occupational therapists create their own reporting form that allows for the concise recording of information obtained through multiple methods. Figure 4-4 presents one such form: an occupational therapy summary checklist. It is based on Case Illustration 4-3 on the Kawa Model group, but it is important to recognize that such a form is not based on a single assessment tool but is rather a compilation from the Kawa Model, observation and interview, and other selected instruments. The form does not cover every aspect of the *Framework*; it focuses on the problem areas most likely to be found in people with mental illness or distress. Using a dynamic and continuous assessment process, a reporting form such as this may be continually revised as new assessment tools are completed and new information comes to light. Depending on the employer's documentation requirements, it is often necessary to post a preliminary checklist, with revisions then added at set intervals.

INTERVENTIONS

Occupational therapists around the world pride themselves on conducting occupation-based practice, where the intervention involves doing an occupation. However, not all interventions are occupation based; some are occupation focused, where the focus of intervention and/or purpose of assessment is on occupation (Fisher, 2013). Psychoeducational groups or individual teaching about occupations, targeted interventions addressing components, and a plethora of activities are all under the umbrella of occupational interventions. The potential interventions provided by occupational therapists are too numerous to list here, and a wide variety are presented in various chapters of this book. For the purposes of this chapter, which highlights the dynamic association between assessment and intervention, a sampling of potential interventions is provided.

Narrative Interventions

One method of narrative used by occupational therapists is a life history approach, where various methods are used to reconstruct and interpret the individual's life, which can be chronological or developmental (Frank, 1996). Life stories can include case histories, life charts, and life stories. Life charts are used to display a linear account of key life events. Life stories are first-person narratives, involving the collaboration of the researcher or therapist to create an assisted autobiography.

Other narrative approaches are occupational storytelling and storymaking (Mattingly, 1991; Clark, 1993). In *occupational storytelling*, the narrative itself is part of the intervention. Intervention involves facilitating the creation of a life history and chronological narrative for service users to make sense of their lives (Frank, 1996, p. 251). Occupational therapists help to imagine new possibilities and to connect with the meanings of past occupations. These sessions are therapeutic because they give the opportunity for reflection. *Occupational storymaking* involves the therapist and service user creating stories that are "enacted in the future, rather than telling them" (Clark, 1993, p. 1074). Case Illustration 4-4 demonstrates occupational storytelling and storymaking within the occupational therapy process.

Groups

Groups are by far the most common structure for psychosocial occupational therapy interventions, and the majority of them use activities as modalities. The *Framework* defines *activities* as "actions designed and selected to support the development of performance skills and performance patterns to enhance occupational engagement" (AOTA, 2014b, p. S41). There are many groups focused on specific activities of daily living skills, such as cooking and shopping or hygiene and grooming, as well as movement and other areas of healthy living. Other activity groups are focused on social inclusion and may involve planning and carrying out events either in the agency setting or in the community. Still other groups are part of a larger "packaged" and time-limited programs, some of which are highlighted in Chapter 5.

The Group Protocol

Writing a group protocol is a way of organizing one's thinking about a group. In a narrow sense, it is an aid for the occupational therapist; in a broader sense, it is an aid for colleagues or others involved in the delivery of services or making referrals. In these different ways, the group protocol contributes to the functioning of the organization by describing its services to prospective clients. The group protocol can serve to demystify psychological treatment by linking the content of the group to practical issues of daily life. Providing this information can relieve the fears and satisfy the curiosity of new group members. Often it

Double OT Assessment Summary

Name: ___Clare Johnson___   Date of Birth: ___5/13/00___   Administrator: ___Elena Marcus, OTR/L___

Date of Double OT Assessment: ___1/12/18___

Skills & Corresponding Notes	Area for Growth	Functional	Independent
Self-care – (see 1)		X	
Community mobility – (see 2)			X
Financial management – Wants to work on developing this skill. Able to use fiscal resources to meet short-term goals (see 3)			X
Generalization – Able to create general ideas, qualities, or characteristics out of, and distinct from, concrete realities or actual instances (see 4)		X	
Organization – Wants to work on developing this skill (see 5)			X
Planning – Able to develop a method of proceeding or acting. She often begins quickly, then slows her pace (see 6)			X
Time management – Clare values getting things done fast (see 6,7)		X	
Cognitive flexibility – Able to change strategies to solve problems			X
Insight			X
Judgement – Able to discriminate between and evaluate different options to form an opinion			X
Problem solving – Able to identify, analyze, and integrate information into a solution			X
Attention		X	

Skills & Corresponding Notes	Area for Growth	Functional	Independent
Emotional regulation – (see 8)		X	
Confidence – (see 9)		X	
Impulse control – Able to regulate and resist sudden intense urges to do something		X	
Motor skills – (see 10)		X	
Direction following – Wants to work on developing this skill (see 11)		X	
Clarification – Able to seek needed verbal or written information by asking questions or reading directions			X
Initiation – Able to start the next action or step without hesitation			X
Sequencing – Able to perform steps in an effective or logical order. Wants to work on developing this skill (see 6,12)			X
Social interaction skills – Offers professional eye contact			X
Conflict management – Able to maintain and manage interactions with other people			X
Coping skills – (see 8,9)		X	

Recommendations:

1. Positively reinforce professional attire and self-care choices. Offer curriculum that explores how image and personal presentation informs others' impressions and responses.

2. Provide hands-on, timed scenarios that promote planning to arrive at new places, reinforcing and further developing this skill. Assist her in planning out how to navigate to new places, offering strategies and support. Help her to break down the steps of how to visit and experience new places. Process which strategies worked best and why.

3. Because Clare expressed a goal of wanting to save money, help her to set financial goals and create a budget in order to visualize how to reach them. Support growth in terms of financial literacy by providing activities that encourage money management, such as breaking down financial resources into daily increments. Assist her in monitoring progress toward financial goals through regular check-ins and by providing a tracking method that can be used independently.

Double OT

Figure 4-3. Double OT Assessment reporting form. *(continued)*

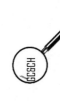

4. Provide opportunities to use professional language; encourage and support use. Encourage Clare to think of how a particular skill set could be used across professions. When teaching specific job skills, provide her with opportunities to identify how each skill can be applied to jobs she has had in the past, has now, or hopes to acquire in the future. Provide space and time for reflection. Offer activities that promote imagination.

5. Clare does well organizing when she is able to label or make lists. Provide her with structure by which to organize items or ideas and ample time to complete tasks. Encourage her to begin making modifications to the organizational structure as she sees appropriate, reinforcing this strength.

6. Encourage Clare to notice her pace if she hurriedly starts an activity without a plan. Prompt her with phrases such as, "It seems like you are in a rush; what is going on?" Follow by helping her create a step-by-step plan. Provide her with sufficient time to engage in planning. Collaborate to identify helpful ways to ensure she remembers important information and deadlines (she finds sticky notes helpful). Work on goal setting. Collaboratively prioritize what is important.

7. Clare is able to leave the house 15 minutes earlier than she needs, showing personal recognition of this area for growth while enacting compensatory strategies to build skills. Promote time management skill development through writing in a planner, keeping a schedule online, setting alarms, or wearing a watch she has chosen. Offer time-sensitive activities that require her to monitor her own time. Verbally reinforce successful time-sensitive task completion. Encourage her to review her work. Provide checklists to mark off tasks as completed. Reflect on the benefits of completing work quickly versus deliberately and where utilization of each approach is appropriate.

8. Provide environmental support for emotional regulation through consistency, provision of a safe space, and empathic listening. If Clare becomes overwhelmed, help break down tasks into manageable steps for achievement. Help her to identify triggers to dysregulation and collaborate to develop coping strategies to help regulate her emotions. Positively recognize and reinforce implementation. Positively reinforce openness to experience and self-expression. Support her in working to remove dysregulating influences in their life. Point out progress. Facilitate new, positive activities and experiences. Process how the media, including news, social media, movies, and TV, and regular notifications, such as on a cell phone, influence behavior and mood. Brainstorm healthy strategies to address this influence. Assist Clare in identifying who she can reach out to when feeling upset.

9. Reflect on strengths. Provide consistency and stability. Increase Clare's ability to articulate value to employers through self-exploration activities and strengths-based curriculum. Review with her what is working well, reinforcing learned skills. Affirm independent decisions she makes and recognize progress. Explicitly praise her for the skills and strengths she is developing.

10. Offer activities that strengthen fine motor skill development, such as origami, baking, knitting, or playing an instrument. Work on puzzles, play cards or Jenga, or do arts and crafts to further develop fine motor coordination.

11. Repeat verbal directions, encourage attention to steps, and check for understanding. Rephrase as needed and provide visual cues. Provide space and support for her to process and ask questions. Positively reinforce or incentivize complete work.

12. Provide tasks that require creating order, allowing Clare to plan arrangements where one element leads to another. Positively reinforce optimal sequencing. Reflect on cause and effect. Provide support to assist her in identifying patterns. Encourage Clare to outline plans in advance, facilitating a daily to-do list or writing out of personal and professional goals. Collaborate to identify helpful ways to ensure she remembers important information and deadlines.

Summary:

Through assessment, Clare reported that she would like to work on financial management, specifically budgeting, saving, and opening and managing a bank account. She also reported wanting to work on organization (also a strength of hers), direction following, sequencing/prioritization, and time management. In areas where Clare exhibits independent strengths, promote her as a model for her peers, supporting increased confidence and leadership skills. Provide written directions as reference. She prefers thorough instructions given up front and structure provided to carry out work tasks. Allow her to read aloud.

Clare presents in the preparation stage of change. Identify and help lower barriers to change. Help her to identify social support and verify that she has the underlying skills for change. Clarify her goals and strategies for change and offer expertise and advice. Provide options and negotiate a plan. Encourage small initial steps and manage expectations. Review past successes and have her publicly announce any plans for change.

Administrator's Signature _____*Elena Marcus, OTR/L*_____   Date ____*1/28/18*____

Double OT

Figure 4-3 (continued). Double OT Assessment reporting form.

Occupational Therapy Summary Checklist

Client Name: _____Ricky S. _____**Date:** _____May 2, 2018_____

| **AREAS OF OCCUPATION**
(Check problem areas, comment) | **PERFORMANCE SKILLS**
(Check problem areas, comment) |

AREAS OF OCCUPATION				PERFORMANCE SKILLS	
Activities of Daily Living (ADL)				**Motor and Process Skills**	
☒Bathing, showering States he showers daily but has pronounced body odor				☐Positioning	
☐Dressing				☐Coordination	
☒Personal hygiene and grooming Hair is uncombed and greasy, clothes unwashed				☐Balance	
☒Sexual activity Recently broke up with girlfriend. States he has "no one."				☐Sequencing	
☐Other (specify)				☐Pace	
Instrumental ADL				☐Manipulation of objects	
☐Care of others (pets/people)				☒Attending to task Short attention span	
☐Community mobility				☐Lifts	
☐Home establishment and maintenance				☐Heeding	
☒Financial management Significant personal debt on credit cards. Monthly expenses consistently exceed SSI payments.				☒Endurance Complaints of fatigue in all groups	
☒Health management and maintenance Chronic pain and Hx of opioid abuse; currently using prescribed.				☐Initiation	
☐Meal preparation and shopping				**Social Interaction Skills**	
☐Safety procedures and emergency responses				☒Approaches/starts Hesitant to begin activities	
☐Religious or spiritual activities				☐Concludes/disengages	
☐Other (specify)				☐Produces speech fluently	
Rest and Sleep				☐Culturally appropriate touch	
☒Rest Often appears agitated				☐Expresses emotion	
☒Sleep preparation Does not use routine or strategies				☐Transitions	
☒Sleep participation Complains of not being able to sleep because of pain				☐Empathy	
	Education	**Work**	**Leisure**	☐Gestures & eye contact	
☐ Exploration				**Performance Patterns**	
☒Participation		States he cannot work because of prior injury	Watches TV; no active hobbies or leisure pursuits	☒Routines Does not have regular routines or schedules. States he has "a lot of time on his hands."	
☒Performance	Poor reading skills			☐Rituals	
Social Participation				☒Roles Due to lack of work and recent separation from girlfriend, he has minimal roles. States that he tries to "be a friend."	
☒Community Isolated				**Signature and date:**	
☒Family Estranged				*Darlene Johnson, MS. OTR/L*	
☒Peer, friend States he has some friends at Wellness Center					

Figure 4-4. Occupational therapy summary checklist.

CASE ILLUSTRATION 4-4: JORDAN—OCCUPATIONAL STORYTELLING AND STORYMAKING

Karen is an occupational therapist working in a nonprofit private practice occupational therapy clinic. She shares that the most memorable client referral she ever received stated the reason for referral as "leaving a cult." The phone number provided connected her with the client's girlfriend, who informed Karen that her partner, Jordan, was planning to leave the church and that she would like to find a coach to support him in this transition.

Karen's initial evaluation revolved around Jordan telling stories of childhood occupations: being involved in the church and in theater and going to movies. He never graduated from high school and obtained a job in the film industry due to his church connections. Jordan's narrative detailed a disruption in his life course: meeting his girlfriend, who was not in the church and whom his family disapproved of. This relationship was a pivotal change in his narrative; he began to have doubts about his involvement in the church and wanted to leave, but he feared retaliation by the church, loss of work, and rejection from family. When Jordan decided to leave the church and move in with his girlfriend, these fears came to fruition.

This chapter in his life was difficult for Jordan; he had lost his meaningful occupation of work and church service, as well as his family support. He struggled with his spiritual identity. Was he still religious? Occupational therapy was a place to explore previous occupations and create new ones. Jordan had a passion for film and began to write film review blogs. He wanted to maintain his faith but needed new occupations and rituals to express his spirituality. Together, Karen and Jordan explored prayer, meditation, and yoga. They explored how to obtain his General Equivalency Diploma and eventually apply for a degree in film at a major university.

Discussion

It was important for the occupational therapist working with Jordan to understand his life history. Karen used occupational storytelling, starting with his past occupations and leading to his present occupations while highlighting his values and meaning. The next stage involved active engagement in occupations, with reflection following each engagement. Karen questioned: Did I enjoy this activity or find it meaningful? Would I incorporate this activity into my daily life and routines? Jordan was in the process of recomposition and redefining his future self and identity. Together, Karen and Jordan engaged in storytelling and storymaking, using occupation in the process.

favorably disposes the new member to the group and aids in the rapid cohesion and integration. Group members may share protocols with their families, often giving relief to worried or curious family members and providing a basis of discussion regarding the client's difficulties and experiences.

There are many potential variables in a group protocol, which are identified and discussed in Table 4-4. Depending on the purpose and audience, the therapist may desire a very brief description and limit the variables of a protocol. However, for students, interns, or novice therapists, a detailed description containing many variables provides for a thorough understanding of the process (Cole, 2012).

Craft Groups

One of the most traditional forms of an occupational therapy group is an open-ended craft group. These groups fell out of favor when occupational therapy became aligned with the medical model and the profession sought to distance itself from our rich historical activity base on an effort to enhance our acceptance and status. This is unfortunate because craft groups, when properly designed, have great potential for continuous assessment and skill building. Table 4-5 provides tips for facilitating craft groups to fit the needs of service users and maximize therapeutic benefits.

Nevertheless, there is a legitimate concern about the use of occupational therapy craft groups. All too often, the therapeutic purpose and intended benefits are not made clear to either service users or reimbursement sources. It is the responsibility of the occupational therapist to not only design craft groups to facilitate occupational engagement, but to also communicate the professional service being offered. For example, during the referral process or as part of an orientation to the group, the occupational therapist should explain to potential participants that, although the group is relaxing and fun, it has a therapeutic purpose. Figure 4-5 shows a handout given to participants in a craft-based workshop group as part of their orientation. Handouts such as the one presented have the dual role of providing a type of protocol as previously discussed, in a format that it is visually inviting and, therefore, is a communication and marketing tool for the group.

TABLE 4-4. POTENTIAL ELEMENTS OF A GROUP PROTOCOL

ELEMENT	COMMENTS
Group leader	Name and credentials as appropriate
Title of group	Should be both inviting and descriptive
Setting	Type of organization (e.g., hospital, wellness center); designated space (e.g., community room, workshop, outdoor space)
Frequency	Length of each session; times per week; number of weeks (if time-limited group)
Population	Can be identified by age groups, symptoms, functional issues; also note number of participants
Contraindications*	Serious concerns regarding participant safety should be noted. It is common in group protocol to suggest who is not appropriate for a particular group or would not benefit from it.
Purpose of group	Therapeutic reason for providing group (may not be necessary if obvious in title)
Goals	Long- and/or short-term depending on group; also may be written as expected outcomes
Structure and logistics	Rules, guidelines, expectations, roles of all participants and leaders
Content and methods	Include the role of the group leader and skills to be used; depending on purpose of protocol, content may be quite specific with a timed schedule or open ended.
Supplies	Needed for preparation, especially if someone else will be leading actual group; may include a budget for supply expenses
Frame of reference, model, or approach*	May be implied in title or content but could also be elaborated to provide the rationale for group
References*	Especially important if group is theory based or if content and process is credited to an outside source

*These elements are rarely included in professional protocols but are important for students, interns, and novice therapists to learn the process of writing group protocols.

Creative and Expressive Arts Groups

Although craft activities may enhance creative expression, it is not necessarily the central focus or therapeutic purpose of the groups. Occupations that are specifically expressive have been used extensively in occupational therapy since the profession's inception, but they fell somewhat out of favor as occupational therapy attempted to align with the medical model. There is some recent evidence suggesting that the use of arts and expressive modalities is again on the rise in occupational therapy (Eschenfelder, Gavalas, Pendergast, & Gorman, 2018). During the decades that they were out of favor in occupational therapy, several new therapies, such as music, art, and drama, were developed to fill the void. In the current health care climate, there is some understandable tension between these various therapists as they attempt to carve out or protect their professional domains. However, occupational therapists have a significantly different focus than the various expressive art therapies and can work well in collaboration because the disciplines complement each other's skills. For example, expressive art therapists tend to have mastery of their specific area of practice (e.g., drama, music), whereas occupational therapists may be learning skills with clients. Occupational therapists use expressive modalities for generalized skill development as well as specific leisure, social, and other occupational skills. "Expressive art can strengthen the occupational profile and information-gathering process [and] can facilitate the development of client-centered goals and individualized intervention planning, creating an overall positive service delivery process" (Eschenfelder et al., 2018).

TABLE 4-5. TIPS FOR FACILITATING CRAFT GROUPS

PLANNING	PREPARATION
• Balance the information in terms of why one would want to do this (fun, satisfaction, meaningful) and why someone would need to do this (therapeutic outcome, expectations of setting). • Explore interests and motivations prior to developing groups. • Determine a set time and place for the activity and stick to the planned schedule as much as possible. • Use flyers or a bulletin board as well as verbal reminders for reinforcement of groups. • Familiarize yourself with the equipment, and create a sample of the completed activity for demonstration.	• Set rules for the group (attendance, participation, minimize outside interference). • Observe safety protocols (many activities have inherent risks [e.g., sharp edges, fumes]). • Arrange the environment for maximum participation and client comfort. • Make sure equipment is accessible to all participants. • Have written/visual instructions and/or provide demonstration. • Encourage group members to be involved in setup. • Assign jobs/tasks to participants as appropriate.
FACILITATION	**CLOSURE**
• Decide the role of the leader (e.g., participant, role model, observer, etc.). • Encourage participants to take on leadership roles (e.g., role model, assistant). • Be adaptable! Change the directions or grade the task depending on the participants' needs; be sensitive to the individual's learning styles, frustration tolerance, and cognitive/motor abilities. • Allow for different timelines (availability to complete the task later).	• Perform a check-in (assess the group members' wants and needs). • Remind participants of purpose of activity, and provide your observations of how the goals were met. • Clean up with the participants. • Observe time limitations and allow for follow-up and completion. (Does the individual need to be allowed an opportunity in the future to complete the activity?) • Provide supplies for participants to take home if desired. • Plan for future activities.

Music Groups

Music may be used in groups in a passive way to enhance the environment and provide sensory stimulation or relaxation. However, actual music groups are focused on the active process of music making. Cohn, Kowalski, and Swarbrick (2017) describe three primary benefits of using music as an occupational therapy modality: "(a) music as a means of increasing group cohesion toward common goals, (b) music as a means of increasing socialization, and (c) music as a meaningful occupation can empower individuals to enhance and embrace wellness and recovery" (p. 168).

TamboRhythms, a company founded by occupational therapist Jorge Ochoa in San Antonio, Texas, offers several music-making programs. The programs are for all ages and are specifically aligned with the principles of occupational therapy. For example, "group drumming can be used to promote/support the occupations of play, social participation, instrumental activities of daily living (health management and maintenance), and rest & sleep" (TamboRhythms, n.d.). An important point posted on the TamboRhythms website is that no previous musical experience is required to take part in the programs, which is consistent with the previously provided description of occupational therapy's incorporation of expressive modalities.

Performance Arts Groups

Occupational therapists have used performance art in their practice since the turn of the 20th century. Puppetry and drama were used in the 1920s and 1930s in the mental health setting to work on social skills and keeping patients active (Phillips, 1996). Occupational therapists still use drama, role playing, mime, and theatrical games in psychosocial practice today. The key is to harness the strengths and interests of service users so that the dramatic art is

Welcome to the Occupational Therapy Workshop!

What is a workshop?

A workshop atmosphere provides a safe and relaxing environment to explore a wide range of activities and hobbies. By working with the manual arts (arts and crafts), you can feel better about yourself and help others while having fun! All group participants are involved in planning and choosing group and individual projects. You will also be given supplies to continue projects at home, if you desire.

How does a workshop help people with mental illness?

Job and Life Skills	Emotional Benefits
<ul><li>Find a new hobby</li><li>Replace destructive habits</li><li>Improve time management</li><li>Increase budgeting skills</li><li>Take responsibility</li><li>Develop leadership roles</li><li>Prepare for work roles</li><li>Manage the environment</li></ul>	<ul><li>Increase motivation and self-esteem</li><li>Engage in physical and mental relaxation</li><li>Develop stress management techniques</li><li>Discover coping strategies</li><li>Build confidence</li><li>Take pride in accomplishments</li></ul>
Cognitive Benefits	Social Skills
<ul><li>Practice following directions</li><li>Engage in problem solving</li><li>Increase planning and organization skills</li><li>Improve frustration tolerance</li><li>Take care of supplies and equipment</li><li>Learn new skills</li></ul>	<ul><li>Work well with others</li><li>Communicate effectively</li><li>Cooperate with tasks</li><li>Teach and role model for others</li><li>Share learning process and outcomes</li></ul>

How does a workshop work?

The expectation of the workshop is for everyone to participate in every session. However, there are several ways that you can do this, so your choices are honored.
- Work with the group to learn a new activity.
- Work on an individual project. (Group leader or member can help you get started)
- Work on an ongoing group project. (Back-up plan – to be determined by the group)
- Teach others a new activity.
- Help others by doing a part of a larger project. (For example, sanding wood pieces)
- Help the group by doing assigned work tasks. (For example, organizing, labeling, cleaning, or cutting fabric, wood, and paper for future projects)

Figure 4-5. Orientation to a workshop (craft) group.

not just working on underlying skills, but is a meaningful occupation itself.

Participating in theater is an occupation that provides purpose, structure, and new roles, routines, and habits. Wasmuth and Pritchard (2016) studied the use of an interdisciplinary occupation-based theater project for veterans in substance use recovery. They found improvements in social and occupational participation after a 6-week intervention, and 86% of the participants in the production were drug free for 6 weeks following the performance. Being part of a theater production involves an aspect of self-accountability, requiring punctuality, dependability, and preparation. Other examples of theater in mental health recovery include a drama project in Wexford, Ireland, titled *A Face in the Crowd*. This production is led by an occupational therapist and mental health nurse and tells the true story of what it is like to live with a mental illness. In Berkshire County, Massachusetts, Shakespeare & Company artists engage adolescent offenders to provide an alternative to traditional punitive measures. Juvenile offenders work with artists and engage in classes, rehearsals, and performances of Shakespeare's plays. (See Suggested Resources for websites.)

INTERVENTION DOCUMENTATION AND OUTCOMES

Because occupations or activities are often viewed as commonplace, it is sometimes difficult for a person reading documentation to see the therapeutic value. Although it is perfectly acceptable to name the chosen activities in a progress note (e.g., specific game or craft), it is important that the professional service being offered is made clear. Box 4-3 provides tips for documenting activity groups.

One of the most important ways to demonstrate the worth of occupational therapy is by defining clear outcomes and measuring those outcomes to provide clear evidence of the effectiveness of the intervention. In many countries, the drivers for outcome measurement are increasing. Funders of services and managers expect evidence of occupational therapy outcomes to be collected and available. As Unsworth (2000) states, "current pressures to document outcomes and demonstrate the efficacy of occupational therapy intervention arise from fiscal restraints as much as from the humanitarian desire to provide the best quality health care to consumers" (p. 147). The AOTA (2017b) further states that "[o]utcomes for people with mental health needs in occupational therapy may include a focus on improvement of individual skills and abilities that enable increased competence and participation in valued roles" (p. 13).

DISCONTINUATION OF SERVICES OR CONTINUOUS SUPPORT

Ideally, the discontinuation of services (or discharge) occurs when the service user and the occupational therapist collaboratively agree to end services, preferably because all identified goals have been achieved. Unfortunately, discontinuation of services often happens because of policy and insurance limits or because time limits for the meeting of goals have been exceeded. Sometimes, especially in the acute hospital setting, a person may be discharged from service without the occupational therapist even being informed. Other times, the service user leaves services without notice or closure for any number of reasons, including dissatisfaction with progress, exacerbation of symptoms, or life circumstances unrelated to service.

In the social model service delivery, there is not an automatic expectation that service will end. Some critics assert that without an enforced ending date, people are less likely

BOX 4-3. TIPS FOR DOCUMENTING OCCUPATION-BASED OR ACTIVITY GROUPS

WORD SAMPLES FOR PREPARATION

- Cueing (specify frequency and type: verbal, visual, kinesthetic)
- Modifying (such as making the task simpler or deleting steps); specify the level of assistance required
- Adapting (changing the activity to facilitate participation; e.g., changing to large print for someone with a visual impairment)
- Grading (providing various levels of increasing complexity to provide a balance of success and challenge); in groups, this often means that participants may have different roles such as helper

WORD SAMPLES FOR ASSESSMENT (OBSERVATION)

- Ability to follow directions
- Sequencing
- Frustration tolerance
- Endurance
- Energy level
- Ability to request assistance
- Ability to be redirected
- Ability to cooperate and interact with others
- Ability to take initiative and responsibility

WORD SAMPLES FOR INTERVENTION (GOALS AND ACTUAL OUTCOME)

- Increased:
  - Self-esteem
  - Confidence
  - Socialization
  - Use of productive time
- Assumed (or developing) leadership role
- Improved:
  - Coordination
  - Balance
  - Endurance
  - Communication
- Changes in affect (e.g., bright, calm, engaged)

to work on goals. This assertion minimizes the genuine desire of many people with mental illness to manage or overcome their problems. Nevertheless, it is true that some people get comfortable in their situation or role as a service user, but forced discharge is not the most effective (or humane) technique to motivate individuals toward recovery. Rather, it is up to the providers to grade the services to best meet the changing needs of service users, provide services that are motivating and engaging, and arrange support as needed.

Some service users express concern about discharge because they reasonably fear that without the structure of a program, they will decompensate and be isolated from support. It may not be financially realistic to have unlimited professional services, but a social orientation emphasizes peer service provision and support.

Ideally, professionals such as occupational therapists can stay involved in service provision throughout a continuum of levels of care and community entities. However, in order to do so, occupational therapists must at times minimize the direct service role and instead focus on referral and linkage agents as well as consultation.

SUMMARY

This chapter outlines the provision of occupational therapy direct services from a recovery perspective. The occupational therapy process includes referral, goal development, assessment, intervention, and discontinuation of services or continuous support. However, unlike the conventional medically oriented process, which is linear and controlled by the therapist, this chapter focuses on a social orientation, which acknowledges that the process is cyclical and driven by the service user.

The presented interventions are not meant to be all-encompassing. Rather, it is hoped that they inspire creative thought for developing and adapting a wide range of offerings suitable for the specific needs of service users in a multitude of settings.

ACKNOWLEDGEMENTS

Elizabeth Cara, PhD, OTR/L, MFT, contributed Table 4-1 and to the discussion of group protocols. Karen McCarthy, OTD, OTR/L, contributed to several sections, cases, and tables. Genevieve Cyrs, MS, OTR/L, and Christine Haworth, MA, OTR/L, contributed Case Illustration 4-2 and Figure 4-3.

REFERENCES

American Occupational Therapy Association. (2014a). *Board of Directors position statement on entry-level degree for the occupational therapist*. Bethesda, MD: Author.

American Occupational Therapy Association. (2014b). Occupational therapy practice framework: Domain and process (3rd ed.). *American Journal of Occupational Therapy, 68*(Suppl.1), S1-S48. doi:10.5014/ajot.2014.682006

American Occupational Therapy Association. (2015). Occupational therapy code of ethics. *American Journal of Occupational Therapy, 69*(Suppl. 3), 6913410030. doi:10.5014/ajot.2015.696S03

American Occupational Therapy Association. (2017a). *AOTA occupational profile template*. Bethesda, MD: Author.

American Occupational Therapy Association. (2017b). Mental health promotion, prevention, and intervention in occupational therapy practice. *American Journal of Occupational Therapy, 71*(Suppl. 2), 7112410035. doi:10.5014/ajot.2017.716S03

Baum, C., Morrison, T., Hahn, M., & Edwards, D. (2007). *Executive Function Performance Test: Test protocol booklet. Program in occupational therapy*. St. Louis, MO: Washington University School of Medicine.

Brown, C., & Dunn, W. (2002). *Adolescent/Adult Sensory Profile*. London, England: Pearson Education.

Cairns, A., Kavanagh, D., Dark, F., & McPhail, S. (2015). Setting measurable goals with young people: Qualitative feedback from the Goal Attainment Scale in youth mental health. *British Journal of Occupational Therapy, 78*(4), 253-259.

Clark, F. (1993). Occupation embedded in real life: interweaving occupational science and occupational therapy. *American Journal of Occupational Therapy, 47*(12), 1067-1078.

Cohn, J., Kowalski, K. Z., & Swarbrick, M. (2017). Music as a therapeutic medium for occupational engagement: Implications for occupational therapy. *Occupational Therapy in Mental Health, 33*(2), 168-178.

Cole, M. B. (2012). *Group dynamics on occupational therapy: The theoretical basis and practice application of group intervention*. Thorofare, NJ: SLACK Incorporated.

Eschenfelder, V. G., Gavalas, C. M., Pendergast, T. M., & Gorman, C. A. (2018). Expressive art to facilitate the development of the occupational profile: A scoping review. *The Open Journal of Occupational Therapy, 6*(1), Article 8. Retrieved from https://doi.org/10.15453/2168-6408.1360

Fisher, A. G. (2013). Occupation-centred, occupation-based, occupation-focused: Same, same or different? *Scandinavian Journal of Occupational Therapy, 21*(Suppl. 1), 96-107.

Frank, G. (1996). Life histories in occupational therapy clinical practice. *American Journal of Occupational Therapy, 50,* 251-264. doi:10.5014/ajot.50.4.251

Haworth, C., & Cyrs, G. (August 21, 2017). Supporting transitions to the workforce for at-risk youth: Developing and using an occupation-based work skills assessment. *OT Practice,* 21-24.

Haywood, H. C., & Lidz, C. S. (2007). *Dynamic assessment in practice: Clinical and educational applications*. New York, NY: Cambridge University Press.

Iwama, M. (2006). *Kawa Model: Culturally relevant occupational therapy*. London, England: Churchill Livingstone.

Law, M., Baptiste, S., Carswell, A., McColl, M. A., Polatajko, H., & Pollock, N. (2015). *Canadian Occupational Performance Measure (COPM)* (5th edition). Toronto, Canada: Canadian Association of Occupational Therapists.

MacKenzie, D. E., & Westwood, D. A. (2013). Occupational therapists and observation: What are you looking at? *OTJR: Occupation, Participation and Health, 33*(1), 4-11.

Mattingly, C. (1991). The narrative nature of clinical reasoning. *American Journal of Occupational Therapy, 45,* 998-1005.

Nielsen, K. T., & Waehrens, E. E. (2015). Occupational therapy evaluation: use of self-report and/or observation? *Scandinavian Journal of Occupational Therapy, 22*(1), 13-23. doi:10.3109/11038128.2014.961547

Phillips, M. E. (1996). The use of drama and puppetry in occupational therapy during the 1920s and 1930s. *American Journal of Occupational Therapy, 50*(3), 229-233.

Punwar, J., & Peloquin, M. (2000). *Occupational therapy: Principles and practice*. Philadelphia, PA: Lippincott.

Rogers, C. R. (1951). *Client-centered therapy: Its current practice, implications and theory*. Boston, MA: Houghton Mifflin.

TamboRhythms. (n.d.). *Music and occupational therapy*. Retrieved from http://tamborhythms.synthasite.com/music-and-occupational-therapy.php

Thomas, Y., & Menage, D. (2016). Reclaiming compassion as a core value in occupational therapy. *British Journal of Occupational Therapy, 79*(1), 3-4.

Unsworth, C. (2000). Measuring the outcome of occupational therapy: Tools and resources. *Australian Occupational Therapy Journal, 47*(4), 147-158.

Velligan, D. I., & Alphs, L. D. (2014). Negative symptoms in schizophrenia: An update on identification and treatment. *Psychiatric Times, 31*(11).

Wasmuth, S., & Pritchard, K. (2016). Theater-based community engagement project for veterans recovering from substance use disorders. *American Journal of Occupational Therapy, 70*, 7004250020. doi:10.5014/ajot.2016.018333

World Federation of Occupational Therapists. (2010). *Position statement on client-centredness in occupational therapy*. Forrestfield, Western Australia, Australia: Author. Retrieved from http://www.wfot.org/ResourceCentre.aspx

Yarborough, B. J. H., Yarborough, M. T., Janoff, S. L., & Green, C. A. (2016). Getting by, getting back, and getting on: Matching mental health services to consumers' recovery goals. *Psychiatric Rehabilitation Journal, 39*(2), 97-104. doi:10.1037/prj0000160

SUGGESTED RESOURCES

Canadian Occupational Performance Measure: http://www.thecopm.ca
First Fortnight: The Art of Mental Health: https://www.firstfortnight.ie
Kawa Model: http://www.kawamodel.com
Motivational Interviewers Network of Trainers (MINT): http://www.motivationalinterviewing.org
Shakespeare & Company: http://www.shakespeare.org/education/shakespeare-in-the-courts
Tamborhythms: http://tamborhythms.com

Consultation and Program Development

Anne MacRae, PhD, OTR/L, BCMH, FAOTA

In the previous chapter, the position was taken that occupational therapists must not only maintain but also expand their roles in direct service delivery in order to retain credibility. However, the changing landscape of health care and social services has also afforded occupational therapists the opportunity to develop new leadership roles in administration, management, research, consultation, and program development. In keeping with the practice-based focus of this text, the latter two roles, consultation and program development, are presented in this chapter.

CONSULTATION

The advantages of hiring a consultant include having someone who has expertise that may not otherwise be available or affordable to the hiring agency and having someone who can offer an objective perspective on a particular problem. Although it is expected that a consultant provides advice, suggestions, or recommendations, the most important skill of a consultant is the ability to listen, and hence gain the trust of the recipients of the consultation and understand their perspective.

Within the British National Health Service, there is an official post of Consultant Occupational Therapist (College of Occupational Therapists, 2010). The core function of this role is expert clinical practice, with supporting functions that include practice and service development and professional leadership. Because of the privatized and fragmented health care services in the United States, there are no uniform standards for qualifications or formal recognition of an occupational therapy consultant on a governmental level. On a professional level, there are also no specific standards or qualifications established. Nevertheless, it stands to reason that, at the very least, a consultant should have substantial practical experience in the area of consultation.

Although it is difficult for an occupational therapist to support oneself solely on the income of a consultant, it can be a very rewarding role for someone in retirement; for an individual who has the means and/or desire to work part-time; or for occupational therapists who have flexibility in their jobs, significant expertise, and the support of their employers. I have had the honor of engaging in many forms of occupational therapy consultation and share my personal story in Box 5-1.

Consultation is particularly important for occupational therapists in the behavioral health arena to reclaim and advance our roles in the field in the face of our minimal presence and limited recognition of the profession within behavioral health services. Beins (2009) further states that a "consultant model of practice offers a means of survival for mental health therapists who have long been limited by the constraints of medically based service delivery models" (p. 1).

MacRae, A. (Ed.). *Cara and MacRae's Psychosocial Occupational Therapy: An Evolving Practice, Fourth Edition* (pp 73-91).
© 2019 Taylor & Francis Group.

Box 5-1. Personal Journey of an Occupational Therapy Consultant

Like many professionals, my initial consulting experiences were on a very informal basis: former students asking for advice, colleagues asking for second opinions, and follow-up from presentations, for example. I enjoyed it (still do) and took advantage of every opportunity that came my way.

My first formal consultation role was in 1997, when I had the honor of receiving a Fulbright Fellowship. The consultation consisted of providing assistance in upgrading a diploma-level occupational therapy program operated by the Institute of Health Care to a Bachelor of Science degree that would be accepted by the University of Malta. I was also asked to consult with the then-fledgling mental health day treatment program and received two additional short-term Fulbright awards over the next several years to continue this work. I have had the pleasure of witnessing the establishment of a thriving baccalaureate degree program at the University of Malta, and the Maltese community mental health service expand from one small center to a total of five centers. I would like to think that my consultations also played some role in the advancement of innovative teaching strategies and content, as well as new models of practice in mental health. I continue to visit Malta on a regular basis to provide further consultations and to see dear friends and colleagues whom I have come to know so well.

Through the years, my name became known for consultation services, and the opportunities expanded. Some of my most rewarding consultations were conducted directly with service users and peer specialists, as well as professional staff working in recovery-oriented community programs. Other opportunities arose when I was hired as a contract consultant by the California Institute of Behavioral Health Solutions to deliver webinars and full-day trainings/workshops on topics related to recovery for counties throughout California.

In full disclosure, consultation was never my primary employment, and I am not a good role model for consulting as a business. My skills and expertise are a better fit for struggling community entities rather than health care businesses, so I often accepted honoraria on a sliding scale and asked for nothing else other than expenses (e.g., travel and daily per diem). I am able to do this because I maintained other primary employment that not only paid me a salary, but also provided benefits, such as health insurance. Although I am now officially retired from the university, I maintain an active guest lecture and consulting schedule.

My advice to occupational therapists wishing to do consulting work is to focus on establishing your expertise and continue to refine the personal skills of leadership. Also be patient: a career trajectory can be developed as a student or novice therapist but may take years to come to fruition. On the other hand, always stay open to possibilities. Unexpected opportunities are around every corner. Most important, find your passion and follow your heart.

Leadership

Although the topic of consultancy is minimally addressed in the occupational therapy literature, components of consultation are more thoroughly addressed. The most prominent of these components is leadership.

The Governance Institute (2009) states, "In most organizations, there are two groups of leaders: the governing body, and the chief executive officer and other senior managers" (p. 2). This is a rather typical definition that often assumes leaders are essentially synonymous with *managers* or *administrators*, which is not the focus of this chapter. However, there is also a whole body of literature that defines leadership as a configuration of qualities, values, and behaviors that inform and guide performance in a wide variety of roles. In other words, leadership is a rather nebulous concept that is not tied to a specific role. Kouzes and Posner (2017) propose that being able to recognize the contributions of others is a key factor in successful leadership.

These qualities include expecting high standards of others, being clear about goals, personalizing and individualizing the recognition given (which implies taking the time in getting to know the recipients of consultation), and being appreciative of everyone's contributions. Galuska (2014) identifies several additional qualities, including a tolerance for ambiguity and the ability to learn from adversity as well as success. West et al. (2015) adds the following to the list of leadership qualities as personality traits: high energy, self-confidence, emotional maturity, and personal integrity.

The occupational therapy literature tends to fall in line with the broad-based definitions of leadership, focusing on the qualities of effective leaders. The American Occupational Therapy Association (AOTA) sponsors an Emerging Leaders Development Program, which hosts leadership institutes. Yamkovenko (2014) identified tips from participants attending one such institute, including being better at listening, being self-aware, dealing with conflict, managing time, and learning how to delegate and mentor. These are consistent with leadership qualities defined in the interdisciplinary literature. However, Yamkovenko also includes some that are unique to occupational therapy, including expanding one's professional network and promoting the benefits of AOTA membership.

Servant and Transformational Leadership

According to Savel and Munro (2017):

> One of the key differences between standard autocratic leadership and servant leadership is that the latter is a bottom-up approach, whereas the former is more top-down. Of course, the classic style of leadership is that someone high up in a business structure makes the decisions and the people below simply follow them. In a servant leadership structure, this approach is inverted, with the primary job of the leaders being to foster, nurture, and nourish the associates in an organization so they can be the best they can be. Not only are the voices of the associates heard, but their ideas are communicated, disseminated, and implemented much more easily to those in positions of leadership. (pp. 97-98)

Trastek, Hamilton, and Niles (2014) suggest that servant leadership is the best model for use in health care settings because of its focus on trust and empowerment, which increases the ability of service users to make decisions in their best interest. Thomas, duToit, and van Heerden (2014) agree and specifically define its importance in occupational therapy practice as a means to ensure that individuals reach their full potential.

Related to servant leadership is the concept of *transformational leadership*, which specifically applies to leaders engaged in organizational change. "Transformational leaders work to inspire their followers to look past their own self-interest and to perform above expectations to promote team and organizational interests" (Trastek et al., 2014, p. 379). Whitmer and Mellinger (2016) suggest that organizational resilience is the hallmark of servant and transformational leadership, defining such resilience as "the ability to respond productively to significant disruptive change and transform challenges into opportunities" (p. 255). The dire need for health care reform and the emphasis on collaboration and client centeredness found in psychosocial practice fits with servant and transformational leadership as the most philosophically consistent leadership models for occupational therapy.

Mentorship

Another related concept or role associated with both consultation and leadership is *mentorship*, which is defined by Milner and Bossers (2005) as "a relationship in which the mentor, who is usually a more experienced individual, works closely with a mentee for the purposes of teaching,

guiding, supporting, and facilitating professional growth and development" (p. 205). However, Milner and Bossers, as well as several other occupational therapy authors, confine their discussion of mentorship within the profession, either with occupational therapy practitioners or students (Ellison, Hanson, & Schmidt, 2013; Lapointe, Baptiste, von Zweck, & Craik, 2013; Yamkovenko, 2014). Nevertheless, the concepts put forth in these publications can and should be applied to mentorship relationships that cross professional boundaries. As discussed in Chapter 1 and highlighted in Case Illustration 5-1, a role for occupational therapy in the social model of practice is to provide mentorship for peer specialists as they embark on leadership roles in peer-driven services. In Case Illustration 5-1, the mentorship was provided to a group of already-hired peer specialists to enhance their professional growth. However, sometimes mentorship is deeply intertwined with an occupational therapist's practice as preparation for service users embarking on new roles. Case Illustration 5-2 is a hypothetical story based on several occupational therapy service recipients that exemplifies the overlap between direct service and mentorship.

MODELS OF CONSULTATION FOR OCCUPATIONAL THERAPISTS

Internal Consultation

Occupational therapists who are internal consultants are employed by an organization that has multiple services and then consults for other units or components within the same parent organization. Beins (2009) describes her experiences with this form of consultation and credits, among other factors, her unique expertise in sensory processing and credentials in sensory integration as the vehicle that helped her develop her consultant role. This is consistent with the British definition of a consultant occupational therapist as a person with expert clinical practice. Examples of internal consultation include the following:

- Consultation on multiple psychiatric units of the same hospital, sharing specific expertise on assessments or techniques
- Consultation conducted by an occupational therapy mental health specialist on a medical surgical unit or primary care service sharing perspectives on grief, emotional trauma, and/or recognition of warning signs of psychological decompensation
- Consultation across sectors of a health care organization such as outpatient and inpatient units, as well as home health services. This is especially helpful in establishing protocols for the continuity of care, referrals, and cross communication.

CASE ILLUSTRATION 5-1: GROUP MENTORSHIP FOR PEER SPECIALISTS

As part of a larger grant project, meetings were scheduled once per week, with the occupational therapist as mentor and a group of peer specialists as mentees. Although the group was initially dependent on the occupational therapist to provide information, training, and suggestions, there was an agreement from the outset that all decisions would be made in collaboration and all points of view would be explored before coming to any decisions regarding new roles and responsibilities of the peer specialists.

Topics of ongoing mentoring included documentation, communication skills, boundaries and limits, understanding symptoms, environmental and social obstacles to recovery, specific activities and interventions (such as worksheets), and interviewing technique. Role play was often used to understand particularly difficult situations with service users and provide feedback to each other regarding methods to address problems. The peer specialists provided feedback about their sense of growing competence but were also sufficiently comfortable to share their perceived limitations and fears.

Discussion

It is quite common for mentees to initially over-rely on the expertise of the mentor, so it is essential for the mentor to immediately lay the groundwork for developing a collaborative partnership with shared responsibility. In this case, there is no doubt that the mentoring occupational therapist has significant content expertise on specific topics. However, the peer specialists have the lived experiences in common with service users and greater access to service users. The mentor does not need to minimize his or her content expertise but does need to show respect for the unique expertise of the mentees and to facilitate the further acquisition of knowledge and skills through practice with various educational strategies.

External Consultation

The term *external consultation* is sometimes used to denote any form of consultation that is conducted by a specialist brought in from outside the hiring agency. However, there is benefit in further refining the definition to limit external consultation to people who, although not on staff of the hiring agency, are members of the same profession as those receiving the consultation, such as occupational therapists. External consultation within one discipline offers the added benefits of professional role modeling and motivation for undertaking a successful change process.

This form of consultation is typically conducted by recognized leaders in the field, including authors and researchers. However, it is rare that it is a primary or full-time employment, even among the most prestigious occupational therapy consultants. As with all forms of consultation, significant and specific expertise is essential. External consultants are often hired to introduce new models of practice, such as adopting a trauma-informed care approach. They may also be tasked with helping develop reliable outcome measures and data collection strategies that are specific to a discipline such as occupational therapy. Providing assistance for the development or enhancement of occupational therapy academic programs is also within the realm of an external consultant, and for the occupational therapist with a significant background in direct practice and academic teaching, it is a service that is in high demand around the world.

It should also be noted that many roles undertaken as part of the professional responsibilities of an occupational therapist are in essence external consultation, even if the role or service is not formally recognized as such. For example, many experienced occupational therapists routinely offer workshops and conference presentations for their colleagues.

Interdisciplinary Consultation

In the United States, it is not common for psychosocial occupational therapists to be involved in interdisciplinary consultation. This is partly because of the previously stated lack of uniformed standards for qualifications or formal recognition. Nevertheless, there are many areas in which an occupational therapy expert can offer invaluable assistance in enhancing existing services and developing new services. Box 5-2 describes the role of an occupational therapist in interdisciplinary consultation for the development and implementation of a new grant-funded project.

In the course of a consultation, it is not uncommon for additional needs to arise that may spawn new grants, contracts, or projects. For example, during the Milestones Outreach Support Team (MOST) project presented in Box 5-2, the need for a recovery-oriented work evaluation specifically for peer specialists was identified. A subsequent project to develop such an instrument was launched, initially designed for the MOST project, but then used in a variety of settings and new projects. The new evaluation was specifically designed to help peer specialists develop skills in self-evaluation, handling negative feedback, communication, and self-advocacy. Although many occupational therapists are familiar with the supported employment

CASE ILLUSTRATION 5-2: KELLY AND THE PEER SPECIALIST JOB

Kelly is a current service user of the behavioral health agency who was encouraged by several clinical staff to apply for a newly created peer specialist position. She initially declined the offer. However, her clinical coordinator asked her to reconsider and recommended that she meet with the occupational therapist for work skills development. A referral to occupational therapy was made with Kelly's permission.

At the initial meeting with the occupational therapist, Kelly questioned if she was ready for employment, even though she had apparently told several staff that it was her dream job. She presented as quite agitated and anxious and made several self-deprecating comments regarding her own "worthlessness" and how she was "disappointing everybody," especially the staff. In addition to informal observation and interview, initial assessments included the Canadian Occupational Performance Measure (COPM; Law, 2015), the KAWA Model drawing exercise (see Table 4-1), and the Transition-to-Work Inventory (Liptak, 2012).

Kelly had no difficulty identifying multiple obstacles with her Kawa drawing but struggled to identify assets/liabilities (driftwood), eventually listing "kindness" and "empathy." On the COPM, getting a job was listed as her highest priority. Other goals included managing symptoms, improving communication skills, and learning to set boundaries.

The results of the Transition-to-Work Inventory were particularly illuminating. Almost all of Kelly's responses represented helping professions such as nursing and social work. However, she did not feel able to return to school for appropriate training and was unclear about related options.

Initial recommendations for intervention included continuation of one-on-one occupational therapy to address coping skills and refinement of goals, as well as referrals to a work readiness group, symptom management group, and communication skills groups, all of which were led or co-led by the occupational therapist. Each group was offered in 12-week cycles. At the end of that time, a reevaluation took place that showed significant improvement in symptom management and some improvement in self-esteem, especially in relation to her level of confidence in her abilities. She continued to show difficulties in setting limits, which presents challenges in relationships and roles involved in helping others. Despite her difficulties with boundaries, she did show some improvement in her ability to be more assertive in communication. At the reevaluation, Kelly decided that she would negotiate with the director about the peer specialist job. She requested and was granted accommodations that included limited hours.

Discussion

Given the anxiety that Kelly demonstrated, it was important to explore whether she was feeling pressured to take this particular job simply to please others or whether issues of trust and self-esteem were clouding her ability to make a decision regarding employment. Developing a trusting relationship and providing sufficient time, support, and opportunities for skill development were essential for Kelly to be able to come to her own decision. It is also important to recognize that getting a job was not the end of the process. Kelly needed ongoing mentoring and support in order to be successful with her new employment.

model, the term *supportive* was purposely chosen because it minimizes the stigma that has become associated with the term *supported employment*. Implicit in the term *supported* is the need for an individual to have greater than average guidance and supervision, usually ongoing, and provided by a behavioral health staff member. Alternatively, the term *supportive* denotes a positive working relationship that ideally should be found in any employment situation. This evaluation tool has subsequently been used in a variety of settings precisely because it is not based on a medical model that assumes the presence of a diagnosis or disability.

The Supportive Employment Evaluation is completed in a collaborative manner and is backed up with specific examples from both the employee and the supervisor. Within the process, employees are able to provide input on what they see as needed support, and then goals and plans are collaboratively determined. The instructions for completing this evaluation are presented in Box 5-3, and the template for the Supportive Employment Evaluation is provided in Table 5-1.

Interdisciplinary consultation is also an opportunity to instruct an outside group on the benefits of including occupational therapy in a mental health service team. For example, consultation aimed at developing a psych rehab service would position occupational therapists as psych rehab specialists and provide descriptions of the possible range of unique contributions of the discipline. (See Chapter 1 for further discussion of psych rehab.)

Box 5-2. The Milestones Outreach Support Team Project

The state of California funds various Innovation Projects through the Mental Health Service Act. In order to be funded, Innovation Projects must demonstrate that the proposal represents a new practice or approach or an adaptation for a new setting or community. In addition, the program must include new learning as it applies to quality of services, better outcomes, and access to services (Mental Health Services Oversight & Accountability Commission, n.d.).

A rural California County Behavioral Health Agency applied for Innovation Program funding in order to introduce a recovery-oriented respite bed program for people recovering from a mental health crisis. Besides addressing a critical service need, there was a goal to learn whether a reciprocal relationship between the respite bed program and peer specialist staff of the county wellness center produced better quality of service and improved recovery-oriented outcomes. The stated goals of the project were to help respite residents on their road to recovery, reconnect them to their community, and provide a mechanism for peer specialists to pursue their own personal growth, recovery, and/or wellness, as well as expand their employment skills.

An occupational therapist consultant was included in the initial grant for 8 hours per week to develop a protocol for implementation of the program. Qualifications for this position listed on the proposal included a practitioner who had extensive experience in both behavioral health and teaching/mentoring, as well as a strong belief in the value of employment and a knowledge base in developing employment skills.

The initial tasks of the occupational therapy consultant consisted of developing policies and procedures to generate referrals and communicate with both the clinical staff and the staff of the residential care facility operating the respite bed. It was jointly decided to create a toolbox of activities, interview scripts, and assessments to be used. The peer specialists showed a strong preference for worksheet activities such as interest checklists, an activity clock, and the Kawa Model. There was also an awareness that helping individuals develop goals was important, and after reviewing several tools, the group decided to use the COPM. Although the peer specialists administered the COPM for MOST project participants, all results were reviewed and continued assistance with rating and writing narrative summaries was provided by the occupational therapist.

The agency was also interested in having the MOST staff use formal, interdisciplinary, recovery-oriented outcome measures. After considerable review of the literature and formal and informal meetings with staff, The Client's Assessment of Strengths, Interests and Goals was chosen (Lecomte, Wallace, Caron, Perreault, & Lecomte, 2004). In addition, a recovery-oriented outcome tool for all staff (including clinicians and peer specialists) called the *Milestones of Recovery Scale* (n.d.) was chosen, and training was provided. Although all staff in the agency received the mandatory training, the occupational therapist also facilitated follow-up practice sessions with the peer specialists so they would be comfortable using this instrument with their MOST project service users.

Due to a small number of participants typical in a rural county, quantitative data solely from the MOST project was limited. Therefore, assessment results from MOST clients, who were also service users of the behavioral health agency, were recorded with the agency and is part of ongoing cumulative data collection. However, there was substantial anecdotal and qualitative evidence from peer specialists, referring clinicians, and recipients of MOST services that was overwhelmingly positive.

Because the program was considered a success, an additional grant was received, and the occupational therapist was once again asked to consult to expand this program and have peer specialists continue to follow people as they left the respite bed and became members of the wellness center. The MOST program was also opened up to all members of the wellness centers who requested additional support in their recovery. Because of this expansion, the peer specialists were not able to juggle all of their responsibilities, and the regular group offerings at the county wellness center were in jeopardy. In order to alleviate the work load of the peer specialists while enriching the program offerings of the wellness centers, new procedures were developed for formalizing volunteer roles. These procedures were approved by the leadership committee and were put into place. Along with the new volunteer program, the agency funded an additional peer specialist position.

Box 5-3. Directions for Completion of the Supportive Employment Evaluation

The purpose of this employment evaluation is to identify areas that may need improvement in your work performance and acknowledge areas of strength. Working with a recovery perspective, the goal is to provide you with both opportunities and support for personal growth. It is not meant as a judgment on you as a person; rather, it is a helpful tool to be used collaboratively with your employer. Depending on your job description, some of the rated items may not apply to you. It is OK to leave them blank.

DIRECTIONS

1. Circle the description next to each item that best fits how you see your own performance. Try to give specific examples in the box below the rated items. Also try to give specific ideas of the kinds of help you think you may need to improve. (NOTE: If you do not want to do this step alone, you can do it together with your employer.)
2. Meet with your supervisor with the completed form and discuss your observations and comments. Clarify any differences between your perceptions. (Specific examples help the most.)
3. Develop goals and a plan together with your supervisor.

Table 5-1. Supportive Employment Evaluation

Employee name (please print) _____

WORK SKILLS, HABITS, AND TOLERANCE

Interest, motivation, or enthusiasm	Hesitant, slow to interest	Generally good but inconsistent	Eager, absorbed in all aspects of job
Ability to initiate activities, energy output	Slow to get started, needs multiple cues and prompts	Applies self to tasks with minimum prompts	Energetic, initiates tasks, shows leadership
Ability to follow through, concentration, attention span	Needs frequent reminders	Generally adequate attention, some lapses	Good attention and follow-through
Ability to take directions, response to authority	Avoids, openly defies authority, debates suggestions	Accepting, tolerant, responds to suggestions	Responds well to feedback, able to initiate change
Quality of workmanship, neatness, accuracy,	Below average, multiple errors	Acceptable, improving skills	Exact, few mistakes, careful attention to detail
Quantity of work, production	Below standard, less than required	Average or acceptable	Above average, considerable work
Attendance, punctuality, regularity	Unpredictable, often late, inconsistent	Usually prompt, fairly consistent	Regular, punctual, stays overtime when needed

Specific examples of items:

Employee:

Supervisor:

(continued)

TABLE 5-1 (CONTINUED). SUPPORTIVE EMPLOYMENT EVALUATION

Support needed (employee perspective):

Goals/plan:

SOCIALIZATION, ATTITUDE TOWARD OTHERS

Social participation	Little involvement with others at worksite	Tries to control social situations or is marginally involved	Enjoys interaction and enthusiastically participates
Verbalization, quantity and content	Often tangential or off track, avoids conversation	Responds to conversation but either dominates or does not initiate conversation	Enjoys conversation and displays balance between listening to others and contributing to conversation
Aggressiveness, hostility	May negatively affect work environment	Occasionally demonstrated, may cause minor difficulties but generally able to resolve	None noticed, pleasant and cooperative
Thoughtfulness, peer adjustment	Doesn't share, indifferent, unsupportive	Notices others and recognizes their needs	Actively interested in others; praises and motivates others
Ability to work with others, cooperativeness	Stubborn, distant, aloof, critical, irritable	Friendly; may at times be overly passive or overly involved	Stimulates others, active and friendly, group participant

Specific examples of items:

Employee:

Supervisor:

Support needed (employee perspective):

Goals/plan:

(continued)

TABLE 5-1 (CONTINUED). SUPPORTIVE EMPLOYMENT EVALUATION

PERSONAL CHARACTERISTICS

Anxiety	Overly sensitive or otherwise shows anxiety that interferes with work	Moderately anxious, sometimes affects work	Able to control outward displays of anxiety, affect is conducive to a calm and supportive environment
Judgment, dependability, responsibility	Needs reminding, often inaccurate, not dependable	Average, accepts responsibility, usually reliable	Sound in judgment, eager to advance
Frustration tolerance, self-control, emotional control	Occasional poor control, moody, easily frustrated	Mood seldom affects work, shows control	Very stable, well controlled

Specific examples of items:

Employee:

Supervisor:

Support needed (employee perspective):

Goals/plan:

GENERAL OBSERVATIONS

Work appearance	Poor hygiene, clothes not appropriate	Occasionally careless with attire/grooming	Appropriate presentation, well groomed
Learning capacity	Slow to catch on, poor retention	Able to learn with instruction	Learns rapidly, remembers well
Knowledge of safety and agency policies	Partial knowledge, some mistakes, needs ongoing supervision	Learns correct procedures, a safe worker	Prevents safety problems, protects others
Use of time	Wastes time, poor organization, slow at decisions	Usually able to handle workload and manages situations	Efficient, busy, accurate

(continued)

TABLE 5-1 (CONTINUED). SUPPORTIVE EMPLOYMENT EVALUATION
Specific examples of items: Employee: Supervisor:
Support needed (employee perspective):
Goals/plan:
Additional comments (employee):
Additional comments (supervisor):
Employee signature/date _____ Supervisor signature/date _____

PROGRAM DEVELOPMENT

Program development is the process of formulating, improving, and expanding educational, managerial, or service-oriented work plans. The process is similar to the development of a group protocol (as described in Chapter 4) but is more extensive and usually implies planning that goes beyond the offering of a single topic group.

The multiple steps involved in the process of program development can vary depending on the nature of the program but are typically presented in a written proposal for the purpose of planning, organization, approval, and funding. The specific elements that may be found in a program proposal are presented in Table 5-2. The crux of a program proposal is the plan, which is often presented in graphic form as an attachment to the program proposal. One such program plan format that is widely recognized is the logic model developed by the W. K. Kellogg Foundation (2006) and shown in Figure 5-1. Models such as these are somewhat redundant in content to the overall program proposal, but graphic representations are especially appreciated by outside reviewers or those who are not familiar with the topic.

Programs may be intra-agency, which usually means coordinating several different services with a unifying theme, or inter-agency, which results in programs offered to multiple organizations or populations. The latter are often "packaged" programs with a set curriculum that may be offered directly by an occupational therapist or may involve training and mentoring others to conduct the program. The benefits of packaged programs are listed in Box 5-4. The following sections present examples of both an intra-agency and an inter-agency program developed by an occupational therapist.

TABLE 5-2. ELEMENTS OF A PROGRAM PROPOSAL

ELEMENT	COMMENTS
Needs assessment	This process may be quite informal or based on specific tools such as surveys and focus groups. It also may include a review of the literature that documents need on a societal level. The needs assessment sets the stage for why a supporting agency or funding source would want to proceed with this program. Depending on the format and audience for the proposal, this section may be combined with the statement of purpose.
Statement of purpose	Also called a *situation statement*, this element expands on the findings of the needs assessment to present a clear picture of the scope of the program. Why is this program important? The statement may need to provide background to explain the current situation to be addressed. Use terminology known to the audience (avoid jargon) and provide definitions as needed.
Provider qualifications	Includes credentials, background, and experience. Some proposal formats require that a resume or curriculum vitae be attached. Brief narrative should include specific interests or qualities that may not be captured in a curriculum vitae. Emphasize unique skills that can provide efficient and effective service. Because occupational therapy may not be well known to the target audience, a focused description of the field relative to the program being proposed may need to be included.
Goals	Include short- and/or long-term goals depending on the nature of the program. Goals should be measurable and presented with clear terminology known to the target audience.
Funding	Some programs include specific reimbursable therapeutic services (e.g., through public or private insurance). However, more commonly, funding is obtained through grants or other designated operational funds by sponsoring agencies (or agency). Very often, multiple funding streams are used. For example, the program provider may be paid as a consultant or project manager, but supplies and equipment may be in-kind donations (by sponsoring agency) or community donations or purchased through a grant. It is common for program proposals, especially those that are for grants, to require an attached detailed budget.
Stakeholders	Even for programs that are intended to be in house (intra-agency), it is important to identify all stakeholders that will potentially be affected by the program. This may include referral sources (to and from the program), possible shared funding sources, family members, and other staff in the agency. Every effort should be made to collaborate with all stakeholders to maximize benefits and minimize disruptions caused by the introduction of a new program.
Populations	Who is the target audience for participation in the actual program? Identify age limits and how participants will be recruited. Although some programs identify populations by diagnostic category by necessity, such as a specific program for those with depression, it is preferable when possible to gear programs toward particular functional outcomes or skills (e.g., people who need or desire assistance with work, leisure, social inclusion, activities of daily living [ADL]).
Marketing and outreach	How will the program be advertised (e.g., newspaper or newsletter, website postings, flyers, word of mouth, other announcements)? Even with in-house programs, methods for inviting participants and explaining the benefits of the program should be provided.
Plan	Advance plans that are well organized and detailed with specific understandable steps and a realistic timeline are not only more likely to be approved and funded, they also facilitate successful program offerings. Nevertheless, the provider needs to be prepared for unexpected events and maintain flexibility with the plan.

(continued)

TABLE 5-2 (CONTINUED). ELEMENTS OF A PROGRAM PROPOSAL

ELEMENT	COMMENTS
Logistics	Identify an appropriate location for the program, including any environmental requirements or modifications that may need to be made. Address participant transportation (e.g., provided by agency or plans for public transportation, parking facilities). Provide a specific schedule, including frequency of program sessions (e.g., three times per week), length of session time (e.g., 90 minutes), and program duration (e.g., 12 weeks). Some programs may be ongoing and not tied to specific sessions, but information still needs to be provided to explain how participants can access program offerings (e.g., drop-in basis, rotating schedule to be announced).
Outcome measurement	Data for individual outcomes can be collected through a variety of assessments; however, program evaluations are strongly suggested and may be mandated. Surveys are common, but a wide variety of instruments, often self-designed, are also used.
Sustainability	Every effort should be made to ensure the continuity of the established goals, methods, and outcomes of created programs if they are still needed. This may require a change of roles for the occupational therapist from direct service provider to consultant or mentor.

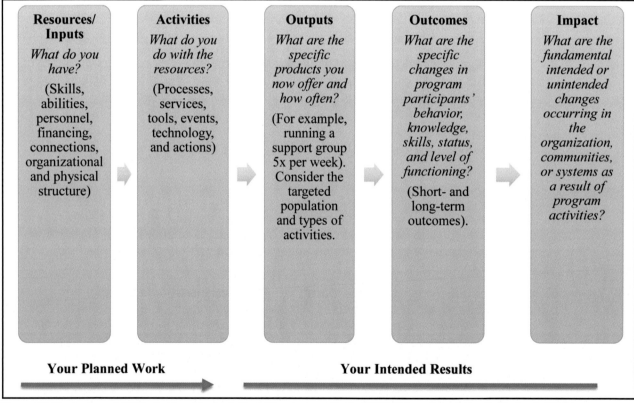

Figure 5-1. The logic model. (Adapted from The Logic Model Development Guide. [2004]. Kellogg Foundation. Battle Creek, Michigan.)

Intra-Agency Program Development: Value-Added Programming

One of the pitfalls of protocols focused on individual groups is that they are not necessarily effective in producing significant or enduring outcomes. For example, a single event group focused on self-care may impart some knowledge, provide encouragement, and facilitate motivation, but it is not likely to result in significant changes in skill level or be consistently incorporated in daily life routines. Value-added programming addresses this issue by creating mechanisms to reinforce new learning, practice skills, enhance

Box 5-4. The Case for "Packaged" Programs

- Single-session interventions rarely have measurable (related) outcomes.
- Ongoing (indefinite length) programs also present difficulties with outcome measurements and may be inefficient.
- Packaged programs can be replicated and/or carried out by others trained and mentored by the occupational therapist.
- The predetermined length of time can deliver services efficiently but also provides sufficient time for meaningful outcome measures.
- Programs can be flexible to meet the needs of various groups/populations.
- A set schedule provides participants with a sense of accomplishment.

opportunities for social inclusion, and meet recovery goals. The concept of value-added programming is that activities should address more than one recovery goal and that, whenever possible, activities, groups, or other program offerings, as well as the environment, should all be linked or coordinated to reinforce the development and attainment of healthy recovery goals. Therefore, the program is both efficient and effective—in other words, more bang for your buck. However, such coordinated, linked programming crosses the boundaries of all agency disciplines and stakeholders, requiring excellent communication skills and respect for interprofessional cooperation and collaboration.

Using the format previously described, a program proposal was developed to coordinate several different groups and activities for a wellness center for the purposes of enriching or adding value. Table 5-3 highlights the gratitude banquet, a value-added program that was organized within the *Eight Dimensions of Wellness* framework (Substance Abuse and Mental Health Service Administration, 2017). (See Chapter 1 for a description.)

The theme of the banquet rotated to celebrate holidays, seasonal changes, or other special events. In addition to all of the preparation for the banquet that occurred in groups, the program was enriched by various roles and responsibilities that can be assumed by the peer service providers and by service user volunteers, including setting up the environment, developing advertising flyers for the center, cooking, and cleaning up. Even service users with significant functional deficits were able to participate by performing simple tasks such as placing flowers on the table or arranging chairs. Individual therapeutic goals could also be met through engaging a participant in a specific task. For example, a service user who could benefit from social skills practice could be asked to be the greeter, waiting at the door to welcome people arriving to the banquet.

Inter-Agency Program Development: Work Readiness Program

Due to recognized expertise, the occupational therapist was asked to create a new county-wide work readiness project. This included being part of the team that wrote the initial grant and supplementary grants, then taking the lead on program development and implementation once funds were secured. As mentioned in Table 5-2, it is common to use multiple funding streams. This program was initially funded through a Mental Health Services Act grant, but additional funds, primarily for supplies and participant transportation, were sought through a community grant. Local funders typically request an abbreviated program proposal. In this case, the directions for the proposal requested a cover sheet, a one-page narrative, and a budget. Box 5-5 shows the narrative for the community grant.

Stakeholder Collaboration

Because of the scope of the grants, enrollment in the program needed to be open to the community beyond members of the behavioral health agency. Therefore, the first task undertaken by the occupational therapist was to identify potential stakeholders and partners. Meetings were organized with each of the identified agencies that were mentioned in the grant narrative to discuss the following agenda:

1. Provide an orientation of occupational therapy (not widely known or understood in this county).
2. Elicit their perspective on work-related problems with their constituents.
3. Build a trusting, reciprocal relationship and clear lines of communication.
4. Develop mechanisms for referral to the new work readiness group.

The description of occupational therapy provided was specific to work readiness and based on the domain descriptions found in the *Occupational Therapy Practice Framework* (AOTA, 2014). It was helpful to have a written description available for the audience for reinforcement. Therefore, a chart describing the unique occupational therapy skills relative to work readiness was created and disseminated when appropriate (Table 5-4).

Encouraging potential stakeholders to actively support a proposed project is a task that requires all of the consultant skills discussed in this chapter, including patience,

TABLE 5-3. EXAMPLE OF A VALUE-ADDED PROGRAM: THE GRATITUDE BANQUET

DIMENSION OF WELLNESS	DESCRIPTION
Financial	Practice with budget and shopping skills; determine available resources. **Related support groups:** Living skills, community group
Social	A sit-down meal with a specific structure encourages social interaction. Locate sufficient tables and chairs for group to sit together. Address stigma reduction and expand social inclusion. **Related support groups:** Social skills, community group, communication skills
Spiritual	Open meal with varied rituals (not necessarily of a religious nature). Spirituality is defined by Substance Abuse and Mental Health Service Administration (2017) as "expanding our sense of purpose and meaning in life." **Related support groups:** Rituals and traditions, self-affirmation/esteem group, recovery group
Occupational	Productive (work) roles are assigned for all participants in the actual banquet (setting table, serving, washing, cleaning up) and/or in the preparatory activities (menu planning, shopping, cooking). **Related support groups:** Living skills, job skills, cognitive skills
Physical	The banquet not only provides nutritious meals for overall health, it can also be used to share recipes to enhance healthy living and physical needs. Movement activities can be added before or after the meal. **Related support groups:** Living skills, cooking group (early prep of involved or time-consuming items such as breads), movement group (dance, exercise)
Intellectual	Preparatory activities require planning, budgeting, and researching (such as looking up recipes for menu planning) as well as creativity for pleasant presentation of the banquet (e.g., themed or seasonal decorating, centerpieces, personalized dinnerware). **Related support groups:** Living skills, cognitive skills, arts and crafts
Environmental	A well-arranged environment encourages cooperation and communication as well as a sense of comfort and belonging. The environment can also be enhanced to fit with the theme of the day (e.g., Mexican music in the background for the taco salad bar). **Related support groups:** Living skills, rituals and traditions, social skills, self-affirmation/esteem group, arts and crafts
Emotional	Many people with mental illness have difficulty with social settings and need practice with coping skills in a safe, nurturing environment. **Related support groups:** Communication group, social skills, symptom management

listening, clear communication, and understanding the roles and responsibilities of everyone involved in the consultation. Arranging meetings with stakeholders can often be difficult because of busy schedules and potential misunderstandings about the value of the meeting. There is often some resistance to a new player being put in the mix, and perhaps even some concern about protecting turf. However, with persistence and the support of at least one respected member of the community, such as the director of the behavioral health agency, the occupational therapist can get a foot in the door.

Once the stakeholders understand the unique focus of an occupational therapist and that collaborative relationship is valued, it is possible to identify common ground and quickly develop a referral network and other means of support for an effective partnership.

Box 5-5. Community Grant Program Proposal for Work Readiness Program

It is well-documented that having a personal identity as a worker, whether paid or volunteer, improves self-esteem and overall health, as well as increases a person's overall productivity and contributions to the community. However, many people are unprepared to develop a worker identity due to limited opportunities, a lack of role models, and poor skill development, especially the soft skills of behavioral expectations and norms, commonly referred to as *work culture*. This Work Readiness Program will focus on understanding work culture and practicing soft skills to prepare participants to enter or reenter the work force. Participants will assess their own readiness and create a plan with a timeline and tasks to fit one's own unique needs.

STATEMENT OF NEED

Although there are signs that the overall economy is slowly improving, rural areas have significant barriers to overcome. Rural communities in this state have a long history of underemployment, greater-than-average poverty rates, and health care disparities with above-average incidence of mental and physical illness, as well as alcohol and drug abuse. There are several programs in the county addressing employment, education, poverty, and health. However, what is lacking is a program specifically designed to prepare people to make best use of existing programs and to increase their employability by acknowledging existing barriers and focusing on soft skill development.

PREPARATION AND EXISTING RESOURCES

The developer and facilitator of this proposed program is a licensed occupational therapist with 35 years of experience in clinical interventions, academic teaching, research, and program development. Needed resources have been identified (see budget), and various community contacts have been made, including Health and Human Services, the Department of Rehabilitation, Probation Department, Department of Education (continuation school), and the local nonprofit job placement service. Representatives of all of these agencies, in addition to the mental health, wellness programs, and the Alcohol and Other Drug Program of County Behavioral Health Service, have acknowledged the need for this approach and have shown enthusiastic support for the Work Readiness Program. Indeed, a key to the long-term success of this proposed program will be ongoing communication and cross-referrals among the sister agencies/programs.

PROGRAM OVERVIEW

This no-cost program will be offered twice in this fiscal year (12 weeks each session in the fall and the spring). The goal is to offer the program at least once per year in the future. Enrollment is open to all county residents who are at least 18 years of age. Flyers and applications are being widely distributed throughout the county, and an announcement about the program will be published in the local newspaper. Attendance at the orientation is required to participate in the program, and a certificate of completion will be given to those who demonstrate consistent participation and attendance. Scheduling of the sessions was planned to minimize interference with other programs and maximize the accessibility of public transportation routes (see budget request for financial need bus vouchers). Sessions will be a mixture of lecture and small- or large-group discussions and activities. Participants will also be developing soft skills by the active engagement in group tasks. Participants will be provided with a workbook and binder for handouts to take home as a permanent resource and to carry out home assignments (see budget). Topics of the group sessions include the following:

- Understanding oneself: reflection and taking stock of skills, attributes, and challenges
- Understanding work culture (expectations and accountability)
- Self-esteem and confidence building, communication and social skills, conflict resolution
- Time management, planning, problem solving, budgeting
- Deportment and presentation (e.g., ADL skills, dressing, hygiene)
- Specific employment-related skills, including use of technology, resume development, and interview skills

TABLE 5-4. THE UNIQUE OCCUPATIONAL THERAPY SKILL SET FOR WORK READINESS

OCCUPATIONS	CLIENT FACTORS	PERFORMANCE SKILLS	PERFORMANCE PATTERNS	CONTEXTS AND ENVIRONMENTS
• ADL • Rest and sleep • Education • Work • Leisure • Social participation	• Values • Beliefs • Spirituality • Body functions and structures	• Motor and process skills • Social interaction skills	• Habits • Routines • Rituals • Roles	• Cultural • Personal • Physical • Social • Temporal • Virtual

Adapted from American Occupational Therapy Association. (2014). Occupational therapy practice framework: Domain and process (3rd ed.). *American Journal of Occupational Therapy, 68*(Suppl. 1), S1-S48. doi:10.5014/ajot.2014.682006

Outreach to Participants

The work readiness program was specifically designed for people who were falling through the cracks of traditional services. People with mental illness who were already being served through the county mental health agency were invited. However, the program was also marketed to nondiagnosed community residents who had significant issues with occupational engagement, specifically developing a sustainable work role. Targeted populations included the following:

- Released prisoners on parole/probation with little or no preparation or support for gainful employment
- People with a history of other legal complications, including loss of driver's license due to DUI charges and history of substance abuse
- People with limited skills due to poor education and dysfunctional support networks
- Women struggling to recover from abusive relationships and/or substance abuse, especially those who were attempting to regain their parental rights by demonstrating financial independence and productive, responsible roles

Because potential participants were from all over the county, a flyer was created to supplement the word-of-mouth and newspaper advertising. They were distributed in groups and posted in several community locations as well as in the behavioral health agency and wellness center. They were also provided to all collaborating agencies for distribution. The purpose of the flyer was to provide concise and inviting information in a visually pleasing format. The template for this flyer is presented in Figure 5-2.

Content

Although this packaged program consisted of 12 sessions, it was important to develop a far more extensive repertoire of activities and topics to accommodate the specific needs of the group participants and maintain flexibility as the population changes. There was some lecture involved, particularly in the initial session, but the majority of the sessions were highly interactive and occupation based. Methods included role play, mock interviews, discussions, board games, worksheets, other self-designed games and activities, and internet searches. A sampling of topics addressed in this program is provided in Box 5-6.

Outcomes

Results were measured using a pre- and post-work readiness scale, as well as a feedback/review form titled *Pulling It All Together*. This allowed the participants to not only provide feedback to the group leader, but also to personally reflect on the value of each topic/activity presented in the program and rate their impact on a scale of 1 to 10. Although the quantitative data from multiple group offerings all showed positive outcomes, the number of participants was too small to consider significant. Nevertheless, the qualitative responses were most illuminating and showed the overall success of the program. A sampling of narrative responses is listed in Box 5-7.

SUMMARY

"In the changing world of health care, a range of possibilities are open to occupational therapy" (Reed, 2016, p.11). This chapter focuses on the possibilities of engaging in consultation and program development to the betterment of not only the profession, but also the people we serve. As we move toward a social model of practice, occupational therapists need to apply the principles of servant and transformational leadership to be prepared to work in a collaborative and interprofessional manner. In the past, there was a sense of protectionism in occupational therapy that prevented occupational therapists from sharing any of their expertise with those outside the profession. However, at least in the mental health arena, sharing does not threaten our position. On the contrary, mentoring and training others may very well be our path to re-establishing our presence in mental health service.

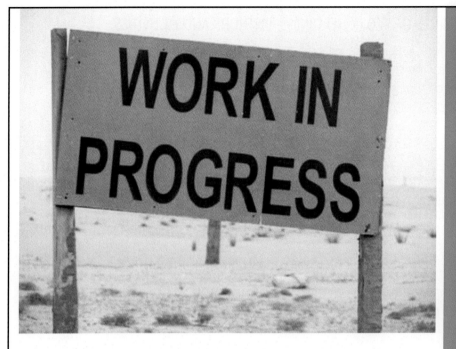

DO YOU WANT TO ENTER OR REENTER THE WORKFORCE?
Would you like to understand work culture better (what to expect of yourself and others; how to get and keep a job)?
Then explore your options! Apply for:

The Work Readiness Program

(Day and time)
(Inclusive dates of program)
(Location)

THIS IS A NO-COST PROGRAM OPEN TO ALL COUNTY RESIDENTS WHO ARE AT LEAST 18 YEARS OLD.

APPLICATIONS
* Applications are available at the county behavioral health service reception desk, as well as at various agencies and locations around the county.
* A completed application must be submitted by **(date)** to the behavioral health agency.
* Attendance at the first meeting (Orientation – date) is mandatory for continued enrollment in the program.
*A *Certificate of Completion* will be given to those who demonstrate consistent participation and attendance.
* This program is sponsored by …… and funded through ……..

Want more information?
Contact Person: (Name and credentials

Call (Phone number)
or e-mail

Figure 5-2. Work readiness program flyer.

Box 5-6. Examples of Work Readiness Methods and Activities

- ADL (e.g., choice of wardrobe for work)
- Role play (e.g., paired activity for interview practice)
- Board games (e.g., *Overcoming Employment Barriers*, available at http://jist.emcp.com)
- Self-created games (e.g., group activity "top 10 ways to get fired")
- Self-improvement (e.g., goal setting, education, self-esteem)
- Structured topic discussions (e.g., overcoming obstacles, handling rejection)
- Resource exploration (e.g., internet for application sources; support organizations)
- Guest speakers (e.g., legal advice for expunging criminal record)
- Worksheets (e.g., time management, communication/social skills)

Box 5-7. Feedback From Participants in the Work Readiness Program

WHAT, IF ANY, INTERNAL FACTORS HAVE YOU ALREADY CHANGED OR BEGUN ADDRESSING TO IMPROVE YOUR EMPLOYMENT OUTLOOK OR FUTURE?

Responses

Flexibility, confidence, improved attitude, improved time management, handling family and work, more upbeat, more self-esteem, can handle rejection better, motivation (wanting to do school work), being more positive

WHAT, IF ANY, EXTERNAL FACTORS HAVE YOU ALREADY CHANGED OR BEGUN ADDRESSING TO IMPROVE YOUR EMPLOYMENT OUTLOOK OR FUTURE?

Responses

Updated resume, established an email account, applied for jobs, developed resume, stayed clean and sober, had a successful interview, got a job

WHAT COULD BE DONE TO IMPROVE THE PROGRAM? ANY FEEDBACK IS WELCOMED!

Responses

More time, more games, more hands-on activities

Fun, enjoyable, supportive

"This class was amazing! Very informative. Offered new insights that can really help me immensely in my job seeking."

References

American Occupational Therapy Association. (2014). Occupational therapy practice framework: Domain and process (3rd ed.). *American Journal of Occupational Therapy, 68*(Suppl.1), S1-S48. doi:10.5014/ajot.2014.682006

Beins, K. M. (2009, December). From clinician to consultant: Use of a sensory processing framework in mental health. *Mental Health Special Interest Section Quarterly, 32*(4), 1-4.

College of Occupational Therapists. (2010). *Consultant Occupational Therapist.* London, England: College of Occupational Therapists. http://337492-web3.cot.co.uk/sites/default/files/general/public/Briefings_List.pdf

Ellison, J., Hanson, P., & Schmidt, J. (2013). Journey of leadership: Steps for a meaningful career. AOTA Learn Continuing Education Article. *OT Practice, 18*(19), CE1-18.

Galuska, L. (2014). Enabling leadership: Unleashing creativity, adaptation, and learning in an organization. *Nurse Leader, 12*(2), 34-38.

Governance Institute. (2009). *Leadership in healthcare organizations: A guide to joint commission leadership standards.* Retrieved from https://www.jointcommission.org/assets/1/18/WP_Leadership_Standards.pdf

Kouzes, J., & Posner, B. (2017). *The leadership challenge: How to make extraordinary things happen in organizations* (6th ed.). Hoboken, NJ: John Wiley & Sons.

Lapointe, J., Baptiste, S., von Zweck, C. M., & Craik, J. M. (2013). Developing the occupational therapy profession through leadership and mentorship: energizing opportunities. *WFOT Bulletin, 68*(1), 38-43.

Law, M., Baptiste, S., Carswell, A., McColl, M. A., Polatajko, H. J., & Pollock, N. (2015). *Canadian Occupational Performance Measure (COPM)* (5th ed.). Toronto, Canada: Canadian Association of Occupational Therapists.

Lecomte, T., Wallace, C. J., Caron, J., Perreault, M., & Lecomte, J.(2004). Further validation of the Client Assessment of Strengths Interests and Goals. *Schizophrenia Research, 66*(1), 59-70.

Liptak, J. (2012). *Transition-to-work inventory* (3rd ed.). St. Paul, MN: JIST Publishing.

Mental Health Services Oversight & Accountability Commission. (n.d.). *MHSA components.* Retrieved from http://www.mhsoac.ca.gov/components

Milestones of Recovery Scale. (n.d.). Retrieved from http://www.milestonesofrecoveryscale.com

Milner, T., & Bossers, A. (2005). Evaluation of an occupational therapy mentorship program. *Canadian Journal of Occupational Therapy, 72*(4), 205-211.

Reed, K. (2016). Frances Rutherford Lecture 2015: Possibilities for the future: Doing well together as agents of change. *New Zealand Journal of Occupational Therapy, 63*(1), 4-13.

Savel, R. H., & Munro, C. L. (2017). Servant leadership: The primacy of service. *American Journal of Critical Care, 26*(2), 97-99.

Substance Abuse and Mental Health Service Administration. (2017). *The Eight Dimensions of Wellness.* Retrieved from https://www.samhsa.gov/wellness-initiative/eight-dimensions-wellness

Thomas, C., du Toit, S. H. J., & van Heerden, S. M. (2014). Leadership: The key to person-centred care. *South African Journal of Occupational Therapy, 44*(3), 34-40.

Trastek, V. F., Hamilton, N. W., & Niles, E. E. (2014). Leadership models in health care—A case for servant leadership. *Mayo Clinic Proceedings, 89*(3), 374-381.

West, M., Armit, K., Loewenthal, L., Eckert, R., West, T., & Lee, A. (2015). *Leadership and leadership development in healthcare: The evidence base.* London, England: Faculty of Medical Leadership and Management.

Whitmer, H., & Mellinger, M. S. (2016). Organizational resilience: Nonprofit organizations' response to change. *Work, 54,* 255-265.

W. K. Kellogg Foundation. (2006). *Logic model development guide.* Battle Creek, MI: Author. Retrieved from https://www.wkkf.org/resource-directory/resource/2006/02/wk-kellogg-foundation-logic-model-development-guide

Yamkovenko, S. (2014). *Eight ways to be a better leader: Lessons learned from AOTA's Emerging Leaders Program.* Retrieved from http://www.aota.org/Publications-News/AOTANews/2014/Tips-from-Emerging-Leaders.aspx#sthash.02A8hFTq.dpuf

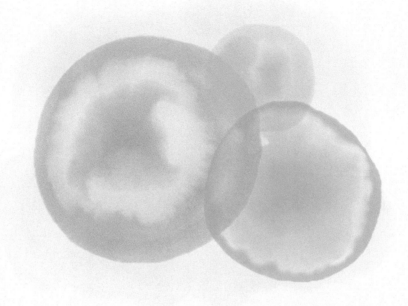

SECTION II

Understanding the Person in Context

Built, Virtual, and Natural Environments

Anne MacRae, PhD, OTR/L, BCMH, FAOTA

The role of environment in health is of critical importance in all of the health care disciplines and is discussed in both practice-based and theoretical terms throughout the scholarly literature. The *International Classification of Functioning, Disability and Health* (World Health Organization, 2018), as well as other World Health Organization documents, explicitly state that environmental factors are major determinants of mental health. Fritz and Cutchin (2017) state, "One environment that occupational scientists have not yet well investigated, but that should be of concern to researchers, is the neighborhood" (p. 140). The concept of *neighborhood* has various definitions, but the literature generally agrees that a neighborhood includes both the built and natural environments and, most importantly, the social connections created within the localized community. This concept is mirrored in the occupational therapy conceptual frameworks described in the following section. However, for the purposes of this chapter, the emphasis is on the built and natural environments, as well as the relatively new concept of a *virtual environment*. The subsequent chapter on personal and social identity expands on the interaction between individuals and groups within contexts and environments.

OCCUPATIONAL THERAPY CONCEPTUAL MODELS

"A unique concept within client-centered occupational therapy is the acknowledgment that clients are not divorced from the environments and community in which they live, work, and play" (Law & Mills, 1998, p. 15). This linkage between the person and the environment has been expanded and reinforced in revised definitions of client-centered practice (Sumsion, 2006).

In addition to the literature addressing client-centered practice, there are several conceptual and practice models that specifically address the role of the environment in occupational performance. Harrison, Angarola, Forsyth, and Irvine (2016) state, "the Model of Human Occupation provides clinical assessments and outcome measures that measure how the environment facilitates occupational participation" (p. 57). The Person-Environment-Occupation model was originally conceptualized by Mary Law and her colleagues in 1996 and has since been applied in occupational therapy extensively. Rigby and Kirsh (2016) emphasize that the Person-Environment-Occupation model is well-suited for mental health and provide an extensive review of the literature that supports this position. The Canadian Model of Occupational Performance and Engagement (Polatajko, Townsend, & Craik, 2007) is an expansion of the original 1997 Canadian Model of

MacRae, A. (Ed.). *Cara and MacRae's Psychosocial Occupational Therapy: An Evolving Practice, Fourth Edition* (pp 95-107).

Occupational Performance. This model explains that the physical, cultural, institutional, and social components of environment can influence occupational performance in a multitude of different ways. The Kawa Model (Iwama, 2006) also provides an excellent metaphoric and culturally sensitive framework for understanding the relationship between an individual and the social and physical environment. As discussed in Chapter 4, the Kawa Model can be used not only as a conceptual model, but also as an assessment and starting point of intervention in collaboration with service users.

An overarching conceptualization of the environment that can be used with other models is the occupational justice perspective. At the very heart of this perspective is an understanding of the relationship between a person and society and the interrelatedness of all aspects of humanity, both individual and community. Furthermore, an occupational justice perspective is not limited to observing and understanding the environment, but rather focuses on the actions required to empower individuals and communities to create or facilitate positive change in their environments (Standnyk, Townsend, & Wilcock, 2010).

Environmental Sustainability

Occupational therapy has traditionally focused primarily on individual occupational needs and has only recently considered broadening that focus to include families, significant others, communities, and other stakeholders. However, there is a growing awareness that occupational therapists also need to be involved in a political global effort to protect the environment in which we all engage in occupations. The World Federation of Occupational Therapists produced a position paper (2012a) declaring a core role for occupational therapists in working towards environmental sustainability. Simó Algado and Townsend (2015) proposed an ecosocial occupational therapy that connects the concepts of occupational justice to ecological issues. They called for occupational therapists to engage not only in dialogue, but also in action directed at helping communities achieve economic and environmental sustainability. Rushford and Thomas (2016) also called for occupational therapists to be actively involved with environmental sustainability, specifically focusing on "rising disaster risk and the consequences of human occupations on the environment" (p. 295).

THE BUILT ENVIRONMENT

The *built environment* includes all structures created by human beings. Obviously, there are tremendous variations depending on the purpose and age of the structures, as well as the population density of the town, city, or neighborhood. However, there are some commonalities across different societies and within the spectrum from rural to urban. One of the most essential built environments is housing, but other important buildings include schools, libraries, health care agencies, governmental and private business offices, public service facilities (e.g., police and fire stations), courts and jails, recreation facilities, places of worship, utility services, and commercial businesses and services (e.g., grocery and other stores, restaurants, senior or wellness centers). The built environment also includes the infrastructure needed to connect the buildings, including roads, bridges, tunnels, sewer, and water transport, as well as digital or electrical grids for heating and cooling, light, and a wide range of electronic and communication devices.

As previously mentioned, housing is one of the most important features of the built environment, and it is addressed throughout this book as it relates to behavioral health. However, a particular environmental issue that is garnering significant attention is the perceived increase in homelessness. It is difficult to estimate the number of homeless people with any precision because there are a multitude of different definitions of homelessness. For example, Tipple and Speak (2005) suggest that homelessness is not limited to "rooflessness" or "houselessness" but also includes various short-term (nonpermanent) housing arrangements and people residing in substandard housing. Other confounding issues in determining accurate data on the number of homeless people is the relative mobility of the population, the common desire to stay hidden from authorities, and the inability to access services, particularly in rural areas. Although homeless encampments are often hidden from the public eye, visibility is increasing. In some situations, the increased visibility is because of the overwhelming number of homeless people in areas of extreme poverty or affected by war, genocide, or other societal disruptions. (See Chapter 7 for further discussion.) However, there is also increased visibility of homelessness in high-income nations. For example, in the United States, even in very affluent communities, visible homelessness has increased dramatically partially because of poorly designed safety nets that limit services and minimize social support, but also because the high cost of living in such areas has prevented many people from procuring affordable housing. Figure 6-1 shows an example of a visible homeless encampment, known as a *tent city*, in an affluent American urban area.

Universal Design

Occupational therapists are particularly focused on the ability to perform occupations within the built environment. However, planning for functional buildings is not the sole domain of occupational therapists, or even health care providers. Many non–health-related professionals, such as architects, city planners, and public policy authors, are at least initially involved. The American Occupational Therapy Association (AOTA, 2015) has affirmed the unique

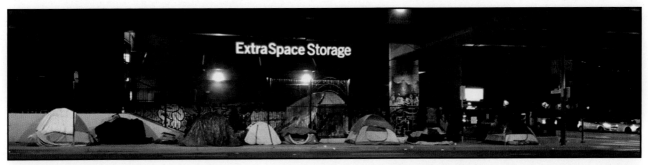

Figure 6-1. Tent city.

PRINCIPLE	TITLE	DESCRIPTION
1	Equitable Use	Useful for people with diverse disabilities; avoids stigmatizing or segregating users
2	Flexibility in Use	Accommodates a wide range of preferences; provides choice and adaptability
3	Simple and Intuitive Use	Easy to understand; accommodates range of literacy and language preferences; provides prompting
4	Perceptible Information	Communicates information using different modes (e.g., pictures, tactile, verbal)
5	Tolerance for Error	Minimizes hazards and provides warnings; also has fail-safe features
6	Low Physical Effort	Comfortable and efficient; minimizes fatigue and repetitive actions
7	Size and Space for Approach and Use	Allows for use regardless of body size and mobility

TABLE 6-1. THE SEVEN PRINCIPLES OF UNIVERSAL DESIGN

Adapted from National Disability Authority. (n.d.). *The 7 principles of universal design.* Retrieved from http://universaldesign.ie/what-is-universal-design/the-7-principles/the-7-principles.html

qualifications of occupational therapy practitioners to engage in complex environmental modifications and to be part of interdisciplinary teams addressing such issues. Although occupational therapists have always been and will continue to be involved in adapting existing environments, there is now a trend toward *universal design*, which is "the design and composition of an environment so that it can be accessed, understood and used to the greatest extent possible by all people regardless of their age, size, ability or disability" (National Disability Authority, n.d.).

The benefits of universal design are in its ultimate cost-effectiveness and reduction of stigma often associated with adapted environments for people with disabilities. Occupational therapists are urged to increase their awareness and use of universal design because it "contributes to health and well-being by enabling engagement in self-care, productivity, and leisure" (Canadian Association of

Occupational Therapists, 2009, p. 1). The World Federation of Occupational Therapists (2012b) concurs with this position and clarifies the significance of the position to occupational therapy by acknowledging that it is a human rights and occupational justice concern and that occupational therapists are experts in the interaction between the person and the environment and have the skills to maximize inclusion and participation. "Occupational therapy practitioners are particularly qualified and well suited to consult with architects, planners, and community agencies, as well as local, state, and federal policymakers with regard to universal design for livable communities" (Young, 2013, p. 3).

The seven principles of universal design are outlined in Table 6-1. These well-developed universal design concepts, particularly the principles of simple and intuitive use, perceptible information, and tolerance for error, are not limited to the physical needs of individuals; they also take

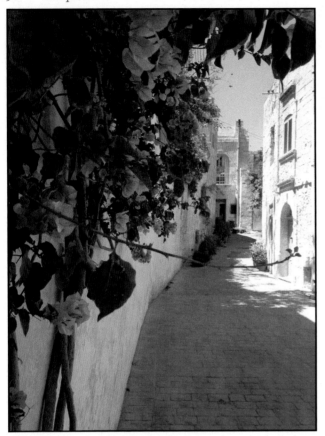

Figure 6-2. Accessibility challenges: European city.

independence in the community is necessary for accessibility. In other words, everyone, regardless of disability, deserves to be included in all aspects of home and community. In some cultures, depending on each other rather than the external environment is the norm and is not a cause of shame or stigma.

In addition to the issues of large-scale infrastructure, there are also cultural variants in one's own choices in the home that may run counter to universal design. Religious icons or altars as well as cultural symbols in artwork and crafts may seem to some people like clutter or a possible safety risk. Even one's choice of cooking utensils may seem impractical. However, such items may hold significant cultural meaning.

A broader cultural and environmental nexus can be represented by an overarching philosophical approach. For example, feng shui is a Chinese art form that is concerned with how energies of the environment interact with individuals and their dwellings. People use the principles of feng shui to strive to attain an emotional and spiritual balance in fast-paced and stressful environments. Although it is a specific cultural practice, feng shui and universal design both propose simplifying the environment. This is in direct contrast to the often cluttered and chaotic physical environments in which people with mental illness may live. Social, particularly economic, realities may limit the ability to create an optimal environment, but even small changes may assist people with mental illness in feeling more calm, safe, and organized.

Personal Choices in the Built Environment

Although universal design can improve quality of life and reduce stigma, the occupational therapist must balance these considerations with individual preferences when making recommendations. The personal meaning of objects or the emotional attachment to part of the environment may take precedence in any decision to change the environment. In many situations, the clutter found in service users' homes is potentially unsafe, and in some cases, the attachment to objects is considered pathological hoarding. However, whether or not the hoarding behavior is a symptom of a known mental illness, a sensitive approach to an individual's beliefs and needs is required in all home modification. According to McIntyre (2018), enforced clearing (of clutter) is not effective and can be a trauma that increases hoarding behavior. Case Illustration 6-1 shows an occupational therapy session in the home focused on creating a safe environment.

THE VIRTUAL ENVIRONMENT

According to the *Occupational Therapy Practice Framework (Framework)*:

into account the personal, social, emotional, and cognitive contexts of the inhabitants (Joines, 2009). For example, appliances with unfamiliar or complicated components may add to confusion or agitation, which ultimately will affect an individual's ability to function in the environment. People with poor judgment, impulsivity, or memory deficits may also experience falls, burns, electrical shock, or other trauma through interaction with poorly designed elements in the built environment.

Cultural Variants and Universal Design

The concepts of universal design are especially suited to new construction or major reconstruction that is undertaken in an effort to modernize. In fact, some countries require adherence to universal design for new building permits. However, there are also many places in the world that have historic architecture and ancient infrastructure that would literally need to be torn down to the ground to create structures in accordance with universal design. For example, many villages and cities in Europe, especially those built in the 1500s and 1600s, have extensive history and are representative of the culture and character of the locations (Figure 6-2). Although some physical adaptions are possible in historic structures, efforts also need to be made to preserve the historical and cultural value of the site. Accessibility then often depends on the human element, where the trait of interdependence rather than

CASE ILLUSTRATION 6-1: DECLUTTERING JESSICA'S HOME

Jessica is a 57-year-old woman with a history of depression. Although there are no documented issues suggesting hoarding behavior, she feels overwhelmed by all of her "stuff." She recently moved to a small assisted living apartment and rented a storage unit as a temporary placement for her many possessions. However, she feels that she cannot afford the monthly fee for the storage container and misses some of her more "precious" items that are in storage. While visiting Jessica's home, the case manager became concerned about the clutter and safety of the apartment and requested that the occupational therapist, Connie, conduct a home visit.

During the home visit, Connie asked Jessica to share stories about her favorite possessions, and they also discussed the placement of various objects. For example, one of Jessica's most treasured possessions is a braided rug that was handmade by her mother. However, the rug has become uneven and somewhat frayed over the years. Jessica and Connie discussed the potential for tripping over the rug and sustaining an injury. They then problem solved solutions together and decided to use the rug as a wall hanging. They planned a future occupational therapy session to build a frame for the rug and install it on the wall with nondamaging hardware.

Connie and Jessica also planned an additional session to visit the storage container and go through the stored items. Jessica repeated that she couldn't afford the storage fees and there was no room in her small apartment. She appeared distraught and overwhelmed, stating, "I feel like I have to throw my life into the trash." The occupational therapist suggested that there are alternatives to disposal of items, including organizing items in her apartment in a more efficient way. She also suggested that when they go to the storage unit, Jessica might find some possessions that could be gifted to others. Jessica hesitantly said, "Maybe my niece would like some of the family stuff." She then brightened considerably and added, "The senior center could really use some of my extra chairs!"

Discussion

People experiencing depressive symptoms can become easily overwhelmed, particularly in times of change. The occupational therapist needs to be aware of the trauma involved in upheaval of one's living situation and not rush the process. It is also common for people with depression to have low self-esteem and, therefore, sometimes judge self-worth based on material possessions. The personal meaning of objects should be respectfully explored, and finding ways for Jessica to feel safe and comfortable in her new home should be the overriding concern of intervention. Connie's approach allowed Jessica to set the pace of the intervention and determine for herself the value of her possessions. The intervention also addressed safety and set up the potential of social and productive roles in determining the fate of her possessions.

[V]irtual context refers to interactions that occur in simulated, real-time, or near-time situations absent of physical contact. The virtual context is becoming increasingly important for clients as well as occupational therapy practitioners and other health care providers. Clients may require access to and the ability to use technology such as cell or smartphones, computers or tablets, and videogame consoles to carry out their daily routines and occupations. (AOTA, 2014, p. S9)

Technology has dramatically facilitated the ability of people with mental illness to be informed and involved in their choice of treatments. The internet is not only a source of information about conditions; it also provides access to support and advocacy groups, legal advice, and networking sites. Many sources acknowledge that a substantial and growing number of service users specifically use the internet for health information. Wellness centers and other community-based services for people with mental illness often have internet-capable computers for service users and routinely offer computer classes. An occupational therapist can evaluate for universal accessibility, such as ergonomically correct workstations and keyboards, as well as speech and vision adaptations.

Technology also provides access to direct services through telehealth. It is well documented that there is great shortage of psychiatric services, especially in rural areas (Weiner, 2018). Telepsychiatry, a subset of telehealth, is one innovative technology developed to reduce this disparity. It is used to provide an array of services, including diagnosis and assessment and individual and group therapy. However, it is most widely used for medication management. Although primarily found in rural areas, it has also been introduced in areas with other underserved populations. A systematic review conducted by García-Lizana and Muñoz-Mayorga (2010) suggests that there is "a strong hypothesis that videoconference-based treatment obtains the same results as face-to-face therapy" (p. 1).

Box 6-1. Arrangements for Telepsychiatry Appointments

The interval between telepsychiatry appointments varies depending on the concerns of the service user, new symptoms, side effects of medication, or any changes in medications, but the average length of time between appointments ranges between 2 and 12 weeks. Children are usually seen at more frequent intervals. The length of each session is also dictated by the individual needs of the service user, but routine appointments are generally between 15 and 30 minutes. The initial telepsychiatry appointment, or an appointment after a major change in status such as discharge from the hospital, is typically at least 90 minutes. This allows for a thorough review of all medications, including those prescribed by primary care physicians, as well as the ordering of new prescriptions and necessary lab work. This investment of time is also crucial for relationship building between the psychiatrist and client.

The service user is encouraged to prepare a list of questions prior to the session and a brief report on his or her health. This may be done informally or with the use of a specifically designed tool. It is also a potential topic for an occupational therapy living skills or communication group or individual session.

The technology includes a video screen with camera and audio capability for both the service user and the psychiatrist. The environment is arranged for adequate light, minimal noise interference, and privacy. Although the service user has the right to a private session with the psychiatrist, it is strongly recommended that another care provider, such as the psychiatric nurse or case manager, be present to later clarify communication from the psychiatrist and provide additional information to the psychiatrist as needed. Some sessions may also include family members or other support persons for the service user.

In general, there is a high level of client satisfaction with telepsychiatry after an initial period of adjustment to the technology. The older population, who have less experience with technology, as well as people who may be quite symptomatic tend to require greater time to adjust to telepsychiatry, but they do eventually appear to gain equal benefit. Box 6-1 describes a typical arrangement for a telepsychiatry appointment.

Although there is a growing body of evidence of the effectiveness of telehealth/telepsychiatry for addressing mental health needs, there is a paucity of literature specifically involving occupational therapy. Considering the tactile, experiential, and observational nature of occupational therapy, especially for mental health, it might well be that telehealth is not the best fit for occupational therapy, but further research needs to be conducted. Also, there are many differing definitions of telehealth, which makes it difficult to determine the current level of involvement by occupational therapists providing mental health services through this method. Some definitions limit telehealth to the provision of formal assessment and intervention completed in real time through video conferencing. Within this definition, occupational therapists do not have a major role in the provision of telehealth mental health services. However, descriptions of telehealth have recently broadened to include a wide range of technologies. The AOTA (2017) includes email, cell phone text messaging, teleconferencing with colleagues, video games, and chat rooms. With this broadened definition, occupational therapists routinely use telehealth because it is quite common for occupational therapists to use these tools, especially for providing reinforcement and reminders.

The Risks of Technology

Schurgin O'Keeffe and Clarke-Pearson (2011) discuss several benefits of social media, including increased socialization and communication, enhanced learning opportunities, and the ability to access health information. However, they also express several concerns regarding risks, particularly for young people. These risks include cyberbullying and online harassment, sexting, and privacy concerns.

Matthews et al. (2017) conducted a study exploring the interplay between symptoms of bipolar disorders and use of technology. They found that the people in the study with bipolar disorder showed an increased vulnerability to online exploitation and increased acting on impulses such as online spending. However, they concluded that "technology acts as a double-edged sword for people with bipolar, in that it can both worsen symptoms of the condition as well as enable recovery toward emotional stability" (p. 299).

Recent news reporting shows rising alarm regarding the dangers of tech addiction (also called *cyber addiction* or *internet addiction*) and dependence on social media. The Tech Addiction website links over 30 research articles, going back to 2004, addressing a wide range of mental health concerns and psychological vulnerability (Tech Addiction, 2018). There are also several recent popular books discussing what some people see as a crisis in overdependence on technology and its wide-ranging effects (Alter, 2017; Twenge, 2017). Even leaders of technology industries are now calling for restraint and further research (Richtel, 2012). In addition, there is a growing awareness that technologies are being used to manipulate the feelings and thoughts of millions of people for a wide range of covert reasons. Considering that occupational therapists work regularly with digital occupations, it is an important area of investigation for the profession.

THE NATURAL ENVIRONMENT

The natural environment has widespread appeal and is seen by many people as a critical element of mental health. As stated by Corazon, Schilhab, and Stigsdotter (2011), "A growing body of interdisciplinary research shows that natural environments, which are experienced as aesthetically pleasing and unthreatening, automatically affect our nervous system, our emotions and our cognition and hereby support general health processes" (p. 162). Moreover, the power and vastness of the nature inspires spiritual reflection and a personal sense of connection to the world at large.

Although the *Framework* acknowledges that the natural world as part of the physical environment falls within the domain of occupational therapy, there is no rationale provided for how nature effects or is integrated into practice (AOTA, 2014). Nevertheless, it can be implied, based on literature presented here and in other sources, that nature can and should be one of the environments in which to conduct occupational therapy. The *Framework* states that "all aspects of the domain, including occupations, client factors, performance skills, performance patterns, and context and environment, are of equal value, and together they interact to affect the client's occupational identity, health, well-being, and participation in life" (AOTA, 2014, p. S4). The premise put forth in this section is that the natural world is a powerful vehicle or vessel to create meaningful connections between occupations, client factors, performance skills, and performance patterns, as well as the other contexts and environments.

The Natural World in Populated Areas

Because elements of nature seem to be particularly important in developing a healthful environment, there has been an increased interest in combining the natural world with the built environment. For some individuals, the natural environment is crucial in establishing a meditative or reflective state of mind. However, as previously discussed, people are increasingly reliant on electronic media for recreation and communication, creating an alienation from the natural world. This is a particular concern with the development of children and young adults because this lack of exposure to the natural world, named "nature deficit" by Louv (2008, 2012), may be linked to reported rises in such disorders as attention deficit and depression.

Occupational therapy programs that include experiences in nature can address a wide range of physical, emotional, and social problems. For example, an occupational therapist in private practice founded a program in the San Francisco Bay Area called *Outdoor Kids Occupational Therapy*. This program combines "nature play" with occupational therapy and operates 10-week outdoor sessions for children in small groups. A unique aspect of this program is that it uses a peer play model, which includes children without known diagnoses with children who have a range of diagnoses, vulnerabilities, or symptoms. This model not only addresses deficits, but it also uses nature as a preventative measure and a method to enhance inclusion and tolerance for all. (See Suggested Resources for the website.)

Green space is a term used to denote the presence of vegetation and other natural elements, usually within an urban environment. Research has shown that neighborhoods that have high-quality green space have lower levels of psychosocial stress (Cox et al., 2017; Roe et al., 2013; Sugiyama, Francis, Middleton, Owen, & Giles-Corti, 2010). A related term is *Green Care*, which is the application of nature for therapeutic purposes. Cutcliffe and Travale (2016) identified "four principal theoretical propositions that appear to underpin the contemporary practice of Green Care. These are: Connectedness; Contact with Nature; Benefits of Exercise; and Occupation/Work as Therapeutic" (p. 143). Something as simple as a walk on the beach or in a park may provide relaxation and stress reduction and be a mechanism for the development of healthy hobbies and leisure pursuits. Although it is extremely important for neighborhoods, particularly urban ones, to provide for access to nature, it is also important to assess the mental health benefits of incorporating natural elements into people's homes and everyday living routines.

Animals and Plants

Social and Psychological Value

Animals and plants are often used by occupational therapists to facilitate nurturing and a sense of connectedness. An outcome study of a therapeutic gardening program concluded that "[p]articipants felt significantly more energetic after engaging in horticultural activities. Participants demonstrated markedly higher levels of involvement and spontaneity in gardening sessions than they did during other recreation periods at the center" (Smidl, Mitchell, & Creighton, 2017, p. 383). A case study by Zimolag and Krupa (2010) suggests that pet ownership can enable community reintegration by fostering a sense of belonging and acceptance. There has also been extensive research on the effect of animal engagement in improving affect, decreasing anxiety, and even reducing blood pressure. However, the studies do not definitely conclude the mechanisms involved in producing such results. One area of potential study that is especially pertinent for occupational therapists is the role of tactile sensory input. Figure 6-3 is an example of the potential calming and nurturing effects of interaction with an animal.

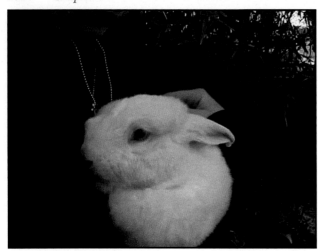

Figure 6-3. The soft fur of a rabbit providing comfort.

Responsibility and Productive Roles

Occupational therapists also help service users develop roles and responsibilities of daily living using plant- and animal-based modalities. Care of plants increases responsibility and organization because tasks need to be completed at set intervals of time. Moreover, while indoor and outdoor gardening activities can enhance the beauty of the environment, they can also provide a healthy, cost-effective food source. Allen, Kellegrew, and Jaffe (2000) concluded that pet ownership can be a meaningful and significant occupation, and studies on the use of animals in conjunction with occupational therapy have demonstrated improved social interaction.

A study using the Photovoice methodology conducted with at-risk youth showed that participants who were engaged in a rescue animal training program had an increased desire to better themselves and make better choices (Williams & Metz, 2014).

Animal-Assisted Therapy

A common form of animal-assisted therapy is visitation of specially trained animals in institutional settings such as hospitals, prisons, and skilled nursing facilities. However, there is also a growing interest in developing programs using animals as a primary therapeutic modality, such as hippotherapy, also known as *equine therapy*. Studies about the effect of using horses have primarily been limited to the neuromuscular benefits for children with cerebral palsy and the benefits for children with autism and intellectual disabilities. The potential benefits for people with mental illness are unknown.

A growing field of interest for service users, practitioners, and researchers is the use of companion or service animals for people with mental illness. The qualifications and definitions of companion animals versus service animals varies depending on geographic locale. Therefore, practitioners are urged to explore the legal requirements

of their own communities. The American Psychiatric Association (APA; 2016) specifically supports the use of therapy dogs for people with mental illness and suggests that they may be particularly effective for people with depression and posttraumatic stress disorder.

Precautions

Animals and plants should not be viewed as a panacea for all dysfunction, nor are they a replacement for comprehensive occupational therapy. Plants and animals may provide a mechanism for achieving or enhancing therapeutic outcomes, but occupational therapists must use their professional judgment and skill in activity and environmental analysis to determine the specific uses, benefits, and risks for particular individuals. Included in such an analysis is the determination of personal and cultural attitudes, as well as assessment of any potential risk of infection, injury, or allergic reactions.

Adventure and Wilderness

Incorporating natural elements into a built environment, whether in the home or neighborhood, is not only healthy, it is a practical approach for positively affecting many people's daily lives. However, it is also important to examine the healing benefits of nature outside of the built environment. Matise and Price-Howard (2017) suggest that the term *ecotherapy* be used to represent a variety of practices that are based on the connection between humans and nature. Other terms used in the literature related to therapeutic techniques include the previously mentioned *Green Care* and *outdoor play*, as well as the more intense aspects of the nature intervention spectrum, namely *adventure* and *wilderness*.

Adventure and wilderness experiences can be profound and transformative. For some people, the experience helps overcome any number of behavioral health issues. With or without current diagnoses or symptoms, the experiences are beneficial in preventing emotional distress, enhancing one's sense of place in the world, developing a spiritual awareness, encouraging potential bonding and trust building with a surrogate family, and providing new skills. Figure 6-4 shows a group of outdoor adventurers braving the elements to experience the Sierra Nevada mountains and the giant redwoods. Case Illustration 6-2 shares the personal story of a young man's wilderness experiences and highlights the need, power, and benefits of such experiences.

Clough, Houge Mackenzie, Mallabon, and Brymer (2016) stated that there is a "relative absence of adventure activities in mainstream health and well-being discourses and in large-scale governmental health initiatives. However, recent research has demonstrated that even the most extreme adventurous physical activities are linked to enhanced psychological health and well-being outcomes" (p. 963). Therapeutic wilderness programs, also known as *outdoor behavioral health programs*, have been shown to be successful in meeting a variety of treatment goals, especially with adolescents who have not benefited from traditional approaches (Fernee, Gabrielsen, Andersen, & Mesel, 2017; Roberts, Stroud, Hoag, & Massey, 2017). However, in the United States, these programs are rarely covered by health care insurance adequately, if at all, and they are prohibitively expensive for most families.

There is a paucity of literature on the current or potential role of occupational therapy in adventure or wilderness therapy. However, Jeffery and Wilson (2017) provide a persuasive argument for the inclusion of occupational therapists:

> Occupational therapists are well positioned to influence the development of adventure therapy as a specialist approach in mental health work. The two fields share skills and knowledge regarding selection of activity to meet therapy goals and activity adaptation and modification; however, occupational therapists have specific training to the level where they are more adept at these skills, and integrate them into most of their practice. Adventure therapy and occupational therapy also share views regarding the importance of the environment, and purposefully select or modify the environment to meet individual needs. Here again, occupational therapists are trained in this more extensively than other disciplines using adventure therapy so occupational therapists can claim expertise in these areas. (p. 37)

However, based on their research, Jeffery and Wilson (2017) suggest that occupational therapists wishing to pursue adventure therapy have additional training in the related practice, activities, and process. This additional training may include skill development in particular activities such as rock climbing, first aid, and survival skills.

ENVIRONMENTAL ASSESSMENT AND INTERVENTION

The most obvious environmental role of the occupational therapist is related to architectural barriers and adapting the physical environment for increased accessibility. Occupational therapists also address the cognitive and sensory components of occupational performance through such tools as the Allen Cognitive Levels Screen (Allen et al., 2007) to determine what kind of structure and environmental cues are needed to engage the client in task completion and Brown and Dunn's (2002) Adolescent/ Adult Sensory Profile Assessment to determine with the client the optimum environment for his or her sensory processing preferences. Recent studies have demonstrated that there may be an association between certain mental health conditions, such as depression and anxiety, and sensory over-responsiveness. Kinnealey, Koenig, and Smith (2011)

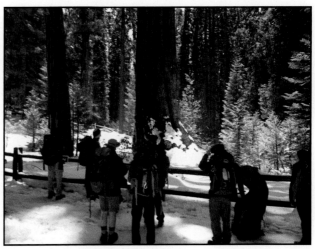

Figure 6-4. Adventurers in the mountains.

state that people who are over-responsive to environmental stimuli "describe their daily experience as irritating, overwhelming, disorganizing, and distracting. They spend an inordinate amount of time coping with their responses to environmental stimuli, a situation that leaves them feeling exhausted and frequently isolated" (p. 320). Such experiences have an obvious impact on one's ability to engage in occupation; therefore, sensory sensitivity should be identified as early as possible in assessment and addressed in all recommended environmental adaptations.

Occupational therapists have made important contributions to the understanding and evaluation of the physical, cognitive, and sensory aspects of the environment that affect occupational performance. Attention to the influence of the larger sociocultural context, inclusive of political-economic factors, on the occupational engagement of communities and populations is emerging. The political activities of daily living reasoning tool (Pollard, Kronenberg, & Sakallariou, 2008) and the Participatory Occupational Justice Framework (Whiteford & Townsend, 2011) offer conceptual frameworks and tools to guide the therapist in the assessment and analysis of environments that account for the interests and goals of multifaceted societal entities. Wilcock (2006) describes an occupation-focused eco-sustainable community development approach to assessment and intervention to promote policies and community-wide action that support participation in ecologically sustainable occupations. Further research needs to be done on addressing the environment in its totality. Specifically, studies are needed that focus on the interrelatedness of the social and physical environments, with the cultural, personal, temporal, and virtual contexts, and the role of occupational therapists in enabling occupation within these environments and contexts.

Environmental Analysis and Adaptation

Occupational therapists tend to be creative problem solvers and be action (doing) oriented. They also are highly

CASE ILLUSTRATION 6-2: JONAH'S WILDERNESS EXPERIENCES

I've had lots of different nature and wilderness experiences, I guess starting as a child when I got to go camping and hiking. After taking some really wrong turns as a teenager, my parents sent me to a therapeutic wilderness program. I resented being forced into this, but I was not willing to change on my own, and looking back I was at far more risk than I realized and didn't have any hope for the future. I was doing all sorts of things to fit in, including drugs and vandalism, but just ended up feeling worse and hurting myself. Being forcefully disconnected from your toxic environment can be life-changing; I know it saved my life. Wilderness and hard manual labor can help improve your self-esteem in some extraordinary ways; just being able to go through major physical obstacles in a beautiful wild landscape takes the focus off your immediate emotional or mental struggles and makes you feel good about yourself. Eventually, people can learn to acclimate to do this for themselves for their own health and growth without being told to do so.

The wilderness is a place where you have the opportunity to feel every emotion, good and bad. Survival situations can really help overcome negative emotions and toxic vibes. One thing that I realized about myself is that I'm an adrenaline junkie, but now I know that I can have those experiences without being destructive. Rock climbing is a perfect example; yes, it can be dangerous, but it is mostly healthy and socially acceptable. Also, once you start feeling better about yourself, you are more likely to learn safety skills and take precautions.

The mandated therapeutic wilderness program helped break a vicious cycle and put me on a new path, but I think my follow-up wilderness experiences really shaped who I am today. I volunteered and then got hired for work in the wilderness. Programs that are not entirely based on therapy or the idea that there is something wrong with the "troubled child" help you grow in very different ways. The most important thing that I want to relay to therapists, from my personal point of view, is don't always focus on the negatives. My experience with various kinds of therapy was important and probably necessary for me, but just talking about drugs and alcohol all the time and how we're all so troubled and have huge problems and are different from "normal" people can be very overwhelming, and sometimes is a total cop-out. I would also advise therapists and therapy programs to focus on young people: young adults in their twenties, teenagers, and even preteens. Get them help before self-destructive patterns are too ingrained or get them into trouble that alters their whole lives.

I think the best kind of wilderness experiences bring together all different kinds of people. If you put together a bunch of addicts, they can bring out the worst in each other, just like prison can make you a better criminal. Everybody has got some problems, but I think having people with identified problems (addiction, mental illness) work side by side with people who are viewed by society as intelligent, healthy, driven, "normal" people for a season in the wilderness would be ideal. I know that's a really tall order and most people won't get that chance, but that's what saved me, or at least redirected me. After I got to do this, I just felt a whole new understanding of people as humans that make mistakes (sometimes REALLY big ones).

I still, to this day, struggle a lot with identity issues because I am so used to being a chameleon and adapting to my surroundings. So, I try to surround myself with positive people. I now work for the National Park Service with a great crew of people and have a girlfriend who loves the wilderness as much as I do. I have a wonderful life.

Discussion

Jonah's personal story highlights several therapeutic benefits of wilderness: the effect of hard work and beautiful scenery on self-esteem, how overcoming physical obstacles can heal emotional wounds, and how having successful experiences can provide lifelong health benefits. Moreover, Jonah's advice to therapists should be well heeded. Prevention and early intervention with a strengths-based focus and positive role modeling are the basis for successful long-term outcomes.

---

trained in observation and occupational analysis. In addition, occupational therapy philosophy is consistent with client-centered practice and a recovery perspective. This constellation of traits makes occupational therapists the ideal collaborative partners to analyze and adapt environments with a service user to facilitate the recovery process.

TABLE 6-2. ENVIRONMENTAL ANALYSIS AND ADAPTATION

CONTEXT AND ENVIRONMENT	ENVIRONMENTAL ANALYSIS (OBSERVATIONS)	RECOMMENDED ADAPTATION(S) (INTERVENTIONS)
Cultural	• Bare walls with stains and cracks • No evidence of artifacts that represent a culture identity or diversity	• Plan with client(s) additions of art or other artifacts that represent a specific cultural group and/or demonstrate sensitivity to potential diversity. • Provide opportunities for multi-model cultural expression, space for celebrations and rituals.
Personal	• Apartment shows little personal representation, with the exception of collection of cookbooks • Grooming and hygiene items are minimal and/or outdated	• Organize cookbooks for increased display and accessibility. • Consider with client(s) adding other items that represent personal investment. (e.g., decorations and space/equipment for hobbies). • Create grooming kit with client(s) to be stored on bathroom shelf.
Physical	• Several pieces of furniture are poor ergonomic fit for client(s) • Underutilized outside space • Poor ventilation	• Adapt furniture heights. • Consider with client(s) increased use of natural objects (e.g., plants) and outside furniture. • Instruct client(s) on use of existing vents and fans. • Consider adding security screen door.
Social	• Limited space for interaction • No observed incorporation of social roles and routines	• Change furniture placement to facilitate interaction. • Support the development of meaningful roles as well as healthy social routines and habits. Provide cueing as needed.
Temporal	• Previous tenants left child-sized table/chairs • Cartoon sheets used as curtain • Prior year calendar on corner wall	• Add relevant, meaningful, and age-appropriate artwork, decorations, and furniture. • Add current calendar and large display clock in prominent site. • Add seasonal displays as appropriate and desired.
Virtual	• No computer or gaming console visible	• Provide computer access as well as training and supervision as needed to ensure personal safety.

Table 6-2 provides examples of specific observations within each context and environment as defined by the *Framework*, as well as recommendations for adaptation. This table represents an individual service user or client; however, a client may also be a family, population, or organization (AOTA, 2014). The format presented in this table can easily be used with a variety of populations and settings. For example, the format of this table was used as the basis for an occupational therapy consultation with the staff of a recently opened board and care home and a wellness drop-in center.

SUMMARY

This chapter addresses the built, virtual, and natural environments and describes the significant roles that occupational therapy has in all these environments. At this time in history, there are multiple societal and technological upheavals that require not only occupational therapists, but all global citizens to voice concerns and act to protect healthy environments for all.

REFERENCES

Allen, C. K., Austin, S. L., David, S. K., Earhart, C. A., McCraith, D. B., & Riska-Williams, L. (2007). *Allen Cognitive Level Screen 5 (ACLS-5), Large Allen Cognitive Level Screen 5 (LACLS-5)*. Camarillo, CA: ACLS and LACLS Committee.

Allen, J. M., Kellegrew, D. H., & Jaffe, D. (2000). The experience of pet ownership as meaningful occupation. *Canadian Journal of Occupational Therapy, 6*, 271-278.

Alter, A. (2017). *Irresistible: The rise of addictive technology and the business of keeping us hooked*. New York, NY: Penguin Books.

American Occupational Therapy Association. (2014). Occupational therapy practice framework: Domain and process (3rd ed.). *American Journal of Occupational Therapy, 68*(Suppl. 1), S1-S48. doi:10.5014/ajot.2014.682006

American Occupational Therapy Association. (2015). Complex environmental modifications. *American Journal of Occupational Therapy, 69*(Suppl. 3), 1-7. doi:10.5014/ajot.2015.696S01

American Occupational Therapy Association. (2017). *The American Occupational Therapy Association Advisory Opinion for the Ethics Commission: Telehealth*. Retrieved from https://www.aota.org/~/media/Corporate/Files/Practice/Ethics/Advisory/telehealth-advisory.pdf

American Psychiatric Association. (2016, December). *Therapy dogs: Helping improve lives of people with mental illness [Web log post]*. Retrieved from https://www.psychiatry.org/news-room/apa-blogs/apa-blog/2016/12/therapy-dogs-helping-improve-lives-of-people-with-mental-illness/

Brown, C. E., & Dunn, W. (2002). *Adolescent/Adult Sensory Profile*. New York, NY: Pearson Clinical.

Canadian Association of Occupational Therapists. (2009). *Position statement: Universal design and occupational therapy*. Ottawa, Canada: Author.

Clough, P., Houge Mackenzie, S., Mallabon, L., & Brymer, E. (2016). Adventurous physical activity environments: A mainstream intervention for mental health. *Sports Med, 46*, 963-968.

Corazon, S. S., Schilhab, T. S., & Stigsdotter, U. K. (2011, December). Developing the therapeutic potential of embodied cognition and metaphors in nature-base therapy lessons from theory to practice. *Journal of Adventure Education & Outdoor Learning, 11*(2), 161-171.

Cox, D., Shanahan, D., Hudson, H., Plummer, K., Siriwardena, G., Fuller, R., ... Gaston, K. (2017). Doses of neighborhood nature: The benefits for mental health of living with nature. *BioScience, 67*, 147-155.

Cutcliffe, J. R., & Travale, R. (2016). Unearthing the theoretical underpinnings of "Green Care" in mental health and substance misuse care: Theoretical underpinnings and contemporary clinical examples. *Issues in Mental Health Nursing, 37*(3), 137-147. doi:10.3109/01612840.2015.1119220

Fernee, C. R., Gabrielsen, L. E., Andersen, A. J., & Mesel, T. (2017). Unpacking the black box of wilderness therapy: A realist synthesis. *Qualitative Health Research, 27*(1), 114-129.

Fritz, H., & Cutchin, M. P. (2017). Changing neighborhoods and occupations: Experiences of older African-Americans in Detroit. *Journal of Occupational Science, 24*(2), 140-151. doi:10.1080/14427591.2016.1269296

García-Lizana, F., & Muñoz-Mayorga, I. (2010). What about telepsychiatry? A systematic review. *The Primary Care Companion to the Journal of Clinical Psychiatry, 12*(2), 19. doi:10.4088/PCC.09m00831whi

Harrison, M., Angarola, R., Forsyth, K., & Irvine, L. (2016). Defining the environment to support occupational therapy intervention in mental health practice. *British Journal of Occupational Therapy, 79*(1), 57-59.

Iwama, M. K. (2006). *The Kawa Model: Culturally relevant occupational therapy*. Edinburgh, Scotland: Elsevier.

Jeffery, H., & Wilson, L. (2017). New Zealand occupational therapists use of adventure therapy in mental health practice. *New Zealand Journal of Occupational Therapy, 64*(1), 32-38.

Joines, S. (2009). Enhancing quality of life through universal design. *NeuroRehabilitation, 25*, 155-167.

Kinnealey, M., Koenig, K. P., & Smith, S. (2011). Relationships between sensory modulation and social supports and health-related quality of life. *American Journal of Occupational Therapy, 65*, 320-327.

Law, M., & Mills, L. (1998). Client-centered occupational therapy. In M. Law (Ed.), *Client-centered occupational therapy*. Thorofare, NJ: SLACK Incorporated.

Louv, R. (2008). *Last child in the woods: Saving our children from nature deficit disorder*. Chapel Hill, NC: Algonquin Books of North Carolina.

Louv, R. (2012). *The Nature Principle: Reconnecting with life in a virtual age*. Chapel Hill, NC: Algonquin Books of North Carolina.

Matise, M., & Price-Howard, K. (2017). Ecotherapy: An alternative treatment modality for veterans. *Counselor, 18*(4), p. 29-33.

Matthews, M., Murnane, E., Snyder, J., Guha, S., Chang, P., Doherty, G., & Gay, G. (2017). The double-edged sword: A mixed methods study of the interplay between bipolar disorder and technology use. *Computers in Human Behavior, 75*, 288-300.

McIntyre, E. (2018). *Hoarding and cluttering behaviors in persons with a primary diagnosis of psychosis*. The POTAC Newsletter, Winter 2018, 1-2. Retrieved from https://www.potac.org/newsletter/archives

National Disability Authority. (n.d.). *What is universal design*. Retrieved from http://universaldesign.ie/What-is-Universal-Design/

Polatajko, H. J., Townsend, E. A., & Craik, J. (2007). Canadian Model of Occupational Performance and Engagement (CMOP-E). In E. A. Townsend & H. J. Polatajko (Eds.), *Enabling occupation II: Advancing an occupational therapy vision of health, well-being, & justice through occupation* (pp. 22-36). Ottawa, ON: CAOT Publications ACE.

Pollard, N., Kronenberg, F., & Sakellariou, D. (2008). A political practice of occupational therapy. In N. Pollard, D. Sakellariou, & F. Kronenberg (Eds.), *A political practice of occupational therapy* (pp. 3-19). Edinburgh, Scotland: Elsevier.

Richtel, M. (2012, July 23). Silicon Valley says step away from the device. *The New York Times*. Retrieved from https://www.nytimes.com/2012/07/24/technology/silicon-valley-worries-about-addiction-to-devices.html

Rigby, P., & Kirsh, B. (2016). Person-Environment-Occupation Model applied to mental health. In T. Krupa, B. Kirsh, D. Pitts, & E. Fossey (Eds.), *Bruce & Borg's psychosocial frames of reference*. Thorofare, NJ: SLACK Incorporated.

Roberts, S. D., Stroud, D., Hoag, M. J., & Massey, K. E. (2017). Outdoor behavioral health care: A longitudinal assessment of young adult outcomes. *Journal of Counseling & Development, 95*, 45-55.

Roe, J. J., Thompson, C. W., Aspinall, P. A., Brewer, M. J., Duff, E. I., Miller, D., ... Clow, A. (2013). Green space and stress: Evidence from cortisol measures in deprived urban communities. *International Journal of Environmental Research and Public Health, 10*, 4086-4103.

Rushford, N., & Thomas, K. (2016). Occupational stewardship: Advancing a vision of occupational justice and sustainability. *Journal of Occupational Science, 23*(3), 295-307. doi:10.1080/14427591.2016.1174954

Schurgin O'Keeffe, G., & Clarke-Pearson, K. (2011). The impact of social media on children, adolescents, and families. *Pediatrics, 127*(4), 800-804. doi:10.1542/peds.2011-0054

Simó Algado, S., & Townsend, E. A. (2015). Eco-social occupational therapy. *British Journal of Occupational Therapy, 78*(3) 182-186.

Smidl, S., Mitchell, D. M., & Creighton, C. L. (2017). Outcomes of a therapeutic gardening program in a mental health recovery center. *Occupational Therapy in Mental Health, 33*(4), 374-385. doi:10.1080/0164212X.2017.1314207

Standnyk, R., Townsend, E., & Wilcock, A. (2010). Occupational justice. In C. H. Christiansen & E. S. Townsend (Eds.), *Introduction to occupation: The art and science of living* (pp. 329-358). Upper Saddle River, NJ: Pearson.

Sugiyama, T., Francis, J., Middleton, N. J., Owen, N., & Giles-Corti, B. (2010). Associations between recreational walking and attractiveness, size, and proximity of neighborhood open spaces. *American Journal of Public Health, 100*, 1752-1757.

Sumsion, T. (Ed.). (2006). *Client-centered practice in occupational therapy: A guide to implementation* (2nd ed.). Edinburgh, Scotland: Churchill Livingstone.

Tech Addiction. (2018). *Internet addiction statistics.* Retrieved from http://www.techaddiction.ca/internet_addiction_statistics.html

Tipple, A. G., & Speak, S. (2005). Definitions of homelessness in developing countries. *Habitat International, 29*(2), 337-352.

Twenge, J. M. (2017). *iGen: Why today's super-connected kids are growing up less rebellious, more tolerant, less happy—and completely unprepared for adulthood and what that means for the rest of us.* New York, NY: Simon & Schuster.

Weiner, S. (2018, February). Addressing the escalating psychiatrist shortage. *AAMC News.* Retrieved from https://news.aamc.org/patient-care/article/addressing-escalating-psychiatrist-shortage/

Whiteford, G., & Townsend, E. (2011). Participatory occupational justice framework (POJF) 2010: Enabling occupational participation and inclusion. In F. Kronenberg, N. Pollard, & D. Sakellariou (Eds.), *Occupational therapies without borders: Towards an ecology of occupation-based practices* (Vol. 2, pp. 65-84). Edinburgh, Scotland: Elsevier.

Wilcock, A. (2006). *An occupational perspective of health* (2nd ed.). Thorofare, NJ: SLACK Incorporated.

Williams, R. L., & Metz, A. E. (2014). Examining the meaning of training animals: A Photovoice study with at-risk youth. *Occupational Therapy in Mental Health, 30*, 337-357.

World Federation of Occupational Therapists. (2012a). *Position statement: Environmental sustainability, sustainable practice within occupational therapy.* Retrieved from http://www.wfot.org/ResourceCentre/tabid/132/did/500/Default.aspx

World Federation of Occupational Therapists. (2012b). *Position statement: Universal design.* Retrieved from http://www.wfot.org/ResourceCentre/tabid/132/did/504/Default.aspx

World Health Organization. (2018). *International classification of functioning, disability and health (ICF).* Retrieved from http://www.who.int/classifications/icf/en/

Young, D. (2013, March). Universal design and livable communities. *Home & Community Health Special Interest Section Quarterly, 20*(1), 1-4.

Zimolag, U., & Krupa, T. (2010). The occupation of pet ownership as an enabler of community integration in serious mental illness: A single exploratory case study. *Occupational Therapy in Mental Health, 26*, 176-196.

SUGGESTED RESOURCES

Kawa Model: http://www.kawamodel.com
Outdoor Kids: Occupational Therapy: https://www.outdoorkidsot.com
Tech Addiction: http://www.techaddiction.ca

Personal and Social Identity

Anne MacRae, PhD, OTR/L, BCMH, FAOTA

The decision to combine personal and social identity into one chapter was intentional. It is the position of this author that individual—hence human—rights and choices must always be respected. However, it is also important to understand the connection between individuals and others. This inherent connection is captured by the African philosophy of *ubuntu*, which is often translated as "a person is a person through other persons" (Gade, 2011, p. 303). Recently, the worldview of *ubuntu* has been applied to programs addressing poverty and social protections (Metz, 2016); social accountability in health care (Green-Thompson, McInerney, & Woollard, 2017); and collective occupations, occupational therapy, and occupational science (Ramugondo & Kronenberg, 2015).

For the purposes of this chapter, the emphasis is on the interwoven nature of persons with a focus on social supports and barriers. The complexity of this topic cannot be fully covered within a single chapter. Indeed, the whole profession is struggling with philosophical challenges and evolving to encompass new ideas of the meaning of occupational therapy. Gerlach, Teachman, Laliberte-Rudman, Aldrich, and Huot (2018) propose that occupational therapy needs to move beyond perspectives or models that individualize occupation and further develop critical perspectives for a social and transformative occupational therapy practice, as well as education and research.

STIGMA

Stigma is a constellation of negative and unjust beliefs, typically based on superficial generalizations, that often results in blatant prejudice and discrimination. Keusch, Wilentz, and Kleinman (2006) eloquently defined *stigma* as a "cultural disease that marks its victims as morally tainted" (p. 526).

Although any group of people with shared traits may be stigmatized, people with mental illness experience pervasive stigma. A study conducted by Jenkins and Carpenter-Song (2009) concluded that "96% of participants reported an awareness of stigma that permeated their daily life" (p. 520). Stigma appears to be especially prevalent in the United States and Western Europe, where it is estimated that a majority of people have stigmatizing attitudes regarding mental illness (Corrigan, Markowitz, & Watson, 2004). Other countries appear to have a lower prevalence of stigmatizing attitudes, but it is unclear whether this represents a genuine difference or is due to poor reporting or difficulty categorizing cultural variations (Angermeyer et al., 2016). Although degrees of stigmatizing attitudes are variable, stigma exists worldwide, and this powerful and hurtful phenomenon is also a local community and personal experience. In order to understand and hence combat the stigma of mental illness, it is important to recognize the various forms of stigma.

MacRae, A. (Ed.). *Cara and MacRae's Psychosocial Occupational Therapy: An Evolving Practice, Fourth Edition* (pp 109-121).
© 2019 Taylor & Francis Group.

Self-Stigma

Due to the pervasiveness of stigma regarding mental illness, many people internalize negative beliefs, resulting in poor self-esteem and significant struggles in achieving recovery goals (Watson, Corrigan, Larson, & Sells, 2007). The shame of having a mental illness, brought about by rampant stigma, also prevents many people from seeking help because of fear of labeling. Shame, hopelessness, and despair are generally recognized as contributing factors to suicidality, and, according to the National Alliance on Mental Illness (n.d.), 90% of people who die by suicide experienced a mental illness. However, it also should be noted that there are many contributing factors to self-stigma and not all people will internalize societal stigma. Instead, some resilient people with lived experience have galvanized their anger regarding these attitudes into action, to have their voices heard and create change. This is the cornerstone of the recovery movement. (See Chapter 1 for further discussion.)

Concurrent Stigmas

Stigma and resulting discrimination can be focused on any aspect of identity, including cultural, religious, or secular affiliations, as well as lifestyles, gender identification, sexual preferences, or even body type. People with mental illness who are also identified with other stigmatized populations may experience even more significant problems with social inclusion, self-acceptance, and decreased ability to meet recovery goals. Among the most egregious examples of concurrent stigma are those involving mental illness with gender or racial identity. *Minority stress theory* purports that health disparities are increased because of discrimination endured by minorities, but there needs to be further research on the increased health risks when multiple (or concurrent) stigmas exist (McConnell, Janulis, Phillips, Truong, & Birkett, 2018). Minority stress theory is based on the concept of persistent *microaggressions*, a term defined by Sue et al. (2007) as "daily exchanges that send denigrating messages to individuals belonging to a racial minority group" (p. 273). Subsequent literature has also included the lesbian, gay, bisexual, transgender (LGBT) community. Balsam, Molina, Beadnell, Simoni, and Walters (2011) state that "[l]esbian, gay, and bisexual individuals who are also racial/ethnic minorities (LGBT-POC) are a multiply marginalized population subject to microaggressions associated with both racism and heterosexism" (p. 163).

Discrimination against the LGBT community and people of color unfortunately sometimes results in violence, which obviously poses an immediate health risk but can also be detrimental to long-term physical and mental health. However, there is also a range of ubiquitously found, subtle, but still potentially damaging concurrent stigmas, especially when one of the stigmas is mental illness. For example, in the United States, the practice of body shaming is common. It is well documented in the literature that people with mental illness have a higher-than-average rate of obesity and therefore experience a "double stigma" (Mizock, 2012).

There are a number of factors that increase the rate of obesity in people with mental illness, including side effects of psychotropic medication, poor eating habits, and sedentary lifestyle. Healthy living strategies are an important part of psych rehab, but interventions that focus on losing weight have met with mixed results and may increase self-stigma. Mizock (2012) recommends using a size acceptance approach "for individuals in recovery from mental illnesses to promote health at every size" (p. 86).

Community and Relational Stigma

Some forms of stigma are subtle and may even appear to be benign, but they can still be damaging. Well-meaning but misguided attempts to protect the individual with mental illness may instead be preventing him or her from achieving recovery goals. For example, the parents of an adult child with mental illness may insist that the individual remain at home with them rather than find an apartment. Another example is a family doctor who tells a patient with mental illness that he or she will never be able to hold a job. Although some people with mental illness do indeed struggle with independent living or gainful employment, the cornerstone of the recovery movement is hope, and every person has a right to aspire to lofty goals, even if it means the right to fail. Moreover, constantly being told what one cannot do feeds into the self-stigma of a "less worthy" person and thereby actually does decrease the motivation and ability to achieve goals.

Institutional Stigma

The most overwhelming and insidious form of stigma is *structural discrimination*. Corrigan et al. (2004) state:

> Structural, or institutional, discrimination includes the policies of private and governmental institutions that intentionally restrict the opportunities of people with mental illness. It also includes major institutions' policies that are not intended to discriminate but whose consequences nevertheless hinder the options of people with mental illness. (p. 481)

Institutional stigmatizing policies are often introduced with the stated goal of "protecting the community." Safety is, of course, a primary concern of governments and extends not only to communities, but also to people with mental illness themselves. (See Chapter 2 on psychiatric institutions and hospitals.) However, too often these policies are formed by ignorance and fear, are not well researched, and are arbitrarily administered. In addition to safety issues, restrictions of rights, particularly if there is a criminal history, can affect the ability to vote and be hired in certain types of employment and can restrict housing opportunities.

Stigma Reduction

All that is necessary for the triumph of evil is that good men do nothing. —Edmund Burke (Irish political philosopher, 1729-1797)

One of the most common questions I receive when conducting workshops on stigma is, "Who can fix this?" My answer is always a version of, "Everybody is responsible." Box 7-1 is a summary of my advice in these workshops.

Personal Responsibility

As previously implied, people with personal (lived) experience of mental illness have the potential for being the most effective change agents in their communities. One of the most powerful tools that service users can use for stigma reduction is sharing their own personal stories. However, there are many factors that influence an individual's ability or willingness to disclose his or her sometimes-painful past. He or she may be afraid of rejection or humiliation, may lack the necessary skills, may still be experiencing florid symptoms, or may not have the insight to understand how his or her stories matter. Only the individual can decide if and when his or her stories can be shared with others. Moreover, regardless of recovery or health status, not everyone has the temperament or desire to be a public speaker. Other methods of sharing include the following:

- Written stories/poetry/song writing
- Personal artwork/group murals
- Poster presentations
- Photography/video
- Website postings
- Short plays or skits

Using creative, expressive, and skill-based modalities, occupational therapists are in an ideal position to help service users become advocates, in essence finding their voices.

Organizational Responsibility

Clinics and wellness centers provide the structure and services to assist individuals in enhancing personal visibility and perceived social value. However, the responsibility doesn't end there. There are many ways that agencies can engage in stigma reduction through public relations, collaboration, and community education. Specific activities in each of these three spheres of action are listed in Table 7-1.

BOX 7-1. WHO IS RESPONSIBLE FOR STIGMA REDUCTION? (EVERYBODY!)

- Individuals with mental illness as well as their families and friends.
  Avoid Shame. Don't Isolate!
- Individuals and families without a known history of mental illness.
  Be Brave. Speak Up!
- All local, state, and global agencies dedicated to mental health.
  Be Proactive and Effective. Reach Out!
- All other government and community entities.
  Be Inclusive and Productive. Collaborate!

DIMENSIONS OF IDENTITY

The expressed desire of service users is to be seen as complex human beings with mixed desires, interests, roles, strengths, and beliefs. Figure 7-1 reflects these feelings in a poster titled "This Is Me," developed by service users in conjunction with occupational therapists in a project of the community mental health services of Malta.

Having a diagnosis of mental illness, or any other illness or disability, becomes a part of one's identity, but being labeled with a diagnosis, as if that is synonymous with one's personal identity, is demeaning. This message is powerfully conveyed in a short video clip created by young people titled "Removing the Labels." (See Suggested Resources for link.) Much attention has been paid to using more sensitive descriptive language, such as identifying someone as a "person with schizophrenia" rather than "a schizophrenic." However, the new terms, although perhaps more sensitive, still do not recognize the many facets of the human experience and are not sufficient to identify or combat the underlying reasons for the stigma and prejudice felt by people with mental illness.

Personal Choices and Attributes

Personal identity is certainly not limited to the presence or absence of a diagnosis. Throughout history, people have attempted to individuate their personas through choices of clothes, makeup, and body art. Freedom to make such choices is affected by cultural and societal norms and may not seem like a choice at all because the actions may be illegal or may be the cause of significant shunning or marginalization.

TABLE 7-1. ORGANIZATIONAL ACTIVITIES FOR STIGMA REDUCTION	
PUBLIC RELATIONS	• Develop a working relationship with local media (newspaper, radio, TV). • Advertise services through media and distribute flyers in the community. • Submit editorial commentaries on related issues (worldwide or local). • Sponsor display booths at community events (e.g., county fair, local festivals). • Publish success stories related to fiscal management, received grants, new programs, expanded services and outcome data.
COLLABORATION	• Develop and follow through with communication protocols between various clinical services and wellness services. • Appoint representatives to serve on related agency boards in the community. • Create interagency tasks forces on specific and timely topics (e.g., prisoner releases, emerging or changing drug problems, homelessness). • Develop mechanisms for information sharing and role clarification among various community groups (e.g., family services, interfaith councils, tribal councils, transportation services, schools, police department). • Volunteer to help other organizations with their fundraisers and special events.
COMMUNITY EDUCATION	• Offer workshops or trainings that are open to the community. • Conduct informational sessions at local organizations (e.g., benevolent and business associations). • Keep up to date on accurate national data related to mental health and use existing recognized sources to educate the community. • Write and disseminate your own information sheets (e.g., flyers, brochures, tips, resources). • Develop a community ambassador program for peer specialists to conduct outreach and ongoing education.

Some choices may be purposefully selected to ensure acceptance in a segment of society, whereas other choices seem to have the intent of pushing people away, as a rebellion, or to isolate from society, perhaps forming a self-fulfilling prophecy predicting rejection. Although these affectations are often a typical sign of a developmental stage, sometimes they do not fall into the age-stage range of typical behavior and may create serious obstacles for engaging in desired occupations. This is particularly true regarding employment opportunities because employers can set standards of deportment as long as the rules are equally applied. These standards may include not allowing visible tattoos, body piercings, or certain types of garb.

Affiliation with recognized lifestyles is another way that people create both a personal and social identity. For example, one may be identified as a techie or gamer based on actions and interests involving computers. Conversely, there are those who overtly reject technology and adopt a lifestyle of self-sufficiency by living off the grid.

Still other lifestyle affiliations have definite negative connotations and consequences. The most prominent of these is gang membership. Although joining a gang does provide a sense of belonging and protection, there is a link between gang membership and a wide range of criminal enterprises.

Family

Understanding the nature of relationships is pivotal in understanding a person and in helping the service user maintain both physical and mental health. As discussed in Chapter 1, family members can be the most valuable social support for people with mental illness or those who are in current or potential psychological distress. For example, a focus group of participants in recovery reflecting on family involvement elicited the following comments:

- "The best thing my parents did when I told them I had a mental illness was to go out and learn as much as they could about my diagnosis and the medications I was taking. They also helped find a good psychiatrist and therapist, and they did research on self-help groups and things like that. I think they knew more about my illness than I did!"
- "My entire family has been my biggest supports and advocates. They read up on everything but didn't go overboard with their knowledge. They helped me

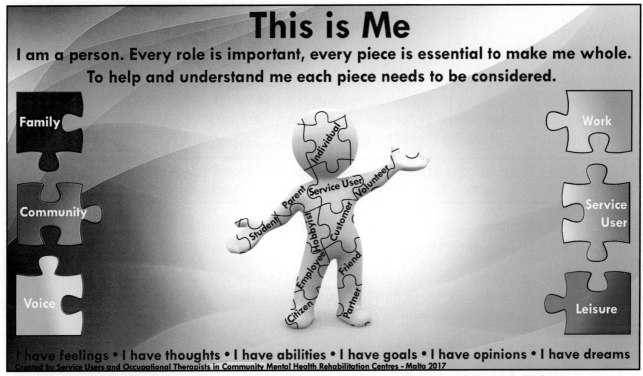

Figure 7-1. This Is Me. (Reprinted with permission from the Mental Health Service Users and Occupational Therapists of Malta.)

make it okay to be around company, they went with me places when I was afraid to go alone, but they didn't smother me. They were awesome. They still are."

Unfortunately, many people who develop mental illness do not have the benefit of supportive family. The same focus group that provided the previous statements also elicited these comments:

- "When I was first diagnosed with major depression, my family was afraid to talk about it to me. If I said anything, they sort of started talking about something else."

- "I had no family near me when I was at my worst. I was sort of glad because I would have been embarrassed and they wouldn't have known how to act. I did send them brochures and literature on my diagnosis, but they never responded or even mentioned that they had received them. I don't know if they read them or not."

Occupational Therapy and Identity Issues

Many approaches and techniques used in occupational therapy address identity issues, including self-esteem building, communication skills, and the interpersonal strategies outlined in Chapter 4. However, a related and specific skill set of occupational therapy is addressing roles and habits. Critics of role theory in occupational therapy voice concern that the aim of developing expected roles produces conformity and does not recognize the individual's freedom of choice (Bonsall, 2009; Jackson, 1998). However, facilitating role development has been an important theoretical underpinning of occupational therapy since Mary Reilly's introduction of the occupational behavior frame of reference (1966) and Ann Mosey's subsequent work on the role acquisition frame of reference (1986). The introduction of the *role checklist* by Frances Oakley provided a reliable assessment of current and emerging roles (Oakley, Kielhofner, Barris, & Reichler, 1986). This tool is still in use today and is considered to be a nonmedical, strengths-based assessment to engage people in exploring opportunities for occupational engagement (Krupa, Kirsh, Pitts, & Fossey, 2016).

Role development and identity is an especially important focus for people with mental illness because of the frequency of poorly developed or maladaptive roles, as well as the self-esteem issues that result from the lack of productivity, acceptance, and inclusion. The role checklist, as well as other role-related assessments and interventions, has been used extensively in vocational and substance abuse programs and with a variety of diagnostic groups.

It is also common for occupational therapists to design their own instruments that cover roles and related areas. For example, the self-developed Roles and Habits worksheet is particularly successful in helping people increase awareness of their daily functions and occupations. It is also a starting point for developing meaningful goals. An example of a completed Roles and Habits worksheet that was transcribed from a verbal interview is shown in Figure 7-2. The instructions and questions on this form could be conducted as a verbal interview as in this figure,

---

Roles and Habits

Name: <u>Kathy</u>   Date: <u>April 4, 2018</u>

To help plan the best treatment with you, it is important for the occupational therapist to understand the things that you do in your daily life that you feel are successful and things that are causing you problems. Looking at roles and habits is one way of exploring what is meaningful or harmful to your well being. (If you need more room to write, use the back of the page).

> **ROLES** are responsibilities and actions that you choose to do or are expected of you and help identify who you are in the community. Examples: Mother, friend, employee, student, group member, roommate.

What roles do you currently have in your home or community? **I'm a single mother and I'm a client here. I don't do much else.**

Are there roles that you had in the past that are gone? **Yes, I used to work and go to school. (Employee and student). But I can't handle any of that right now. I guess my role as daughter is also gone since my mom died—I miss her a lot.**

Are there roles that you would like to have in the future? **I think about going back to school and getting a good job but then I get overwhelmed and don't know where to start.**

Which roles are most important or meaningful to you? **Being a good mother—I really don't think I am, but I want to be.**

> **HABITS** are things that you do very frequently, often without thinking about it. Habits can be healthy or unhealthy. Examples: A daily walk, smoking cigarettes, going to the gym, mealtime with family, checking locks in the house, "cracking" knuckles, going to self help meetings.

Which habits do you think help you stay productive and healthy (that are "good for you")? **Hmmm—I guess that's my problem! (Laughter). Is making dinner a "habit"? I think having regular meals is healthy.**

Which habits may be damaging to your health and productivity? **Well obviously the booze—that's what got me here and almost lost me my kid.**

Are there habits that you would like to develop? **I like what you said about self help groups being a habit. It would be a good habit for me to go to AA.**

Are there habits that you would like to try and break? **The drinking again—I think I should quit smoking too. Oh—and yelling too much.**

Figure 7-2. Completed Roles and Habits worksheet.

but many people, depending on learning style, literacy, and needed processing time, benefit from having a written form in addition to, or instead of, verbal questions. These kinds of worksheets can be administered individually with the therapist or given to the service user to complete at home to be discussed in a subsequent meeting. They also can be the prime activity in a group setting and followed up with peer group sharing.

SPIRITUALITY AND RELIGION

One of the most intricate and potentially controversial manifestations of both personal and social identity is the expression of religion and spirituality. In very simplistic terms, *religion* is organized and social, whereas *spirituality* is a deeply personal consideration. There is also a complex

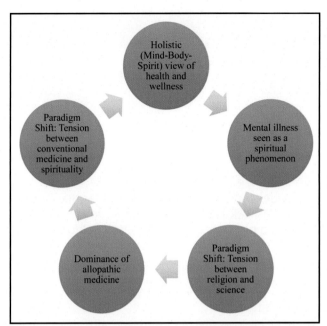

Figure 7-3. The relationship between religious/spiritual beliefs and beliefs about mental illness.

relationship between spiritual beliefs and beliefs about mental illness that has gone through many changes over the years (Figure 7-3).

In general, health care providers, especially in the United States, do not feel qualified to discuss religion in practice settings and are uncomfortable doing so. There are some very good reasons for this, including overstepping one's therapeutic boundaries and scope of practice. It violates ethical principles to use one's position of power (as a health care provider) to misrepresent one's expertise or proselytize one's own beliefs. There is also significant and legitimate concern in the behavioral health community about vulnerable populations being exploited by fringe and cult groups under the umbrella of religious freedom.

However, the compartmentalizing of religious beliefs to be outside of behavioral health services is not consistent with the holistic and person-centered approach espoused by the occupational therapy profession, as well as every major behavioral health organization. "Given the important role that spirituality and religion play for many people in the experiences of coping with health and illness, it seems odd that such important elements are in the margins" of diagnosis and behavioral health care (Chandler, 2012, p. 577). Furthermore, service users themselves have identified overt and subliminal messages that it is not acceptable to talk about their religious beliefs in therapeutic settings, further devaluing a significant part of identity (Macmin & Foskett, 2004). Behavioral health interventions that address religious issues are often best provided in collaboration with the faith-based community, as discussed in Chapter 3 on community behavioral health services. Clearly, this is an

area requiring refined definitions, theoretically consistent interventions, and interdisciplinary research.

Spirituality, rather than religion, appears to be a more comfortable fit for service providers because it does not imply adherence to a particular dogma. A dynamic interpretation of spirituality is provided in Box 7-2. Using this broad interpretation, recovery and spirituality have many shared values, beliefs, and practices, including the following:

- Meaning making and purpose
- Inclusion and acceptance
- Hope and healing
- Focus and clarity
- Love and forgiveness
- Structure and function

Ritual and Traditions

Incorporating the elements of spirituality and recovery provided in Box 7-2 often takes the form of rituals and traditions. Traditions are usually carried down through generations to create a social bond and identity. However, new traditions can be consciously created to fill a void. Rituals are specific and may be part of a greater tradition. They can be personal (unique) or part of shared social experience. In mental health settings, the term *ritual*, although accurately descriptive, should be used with caution because of a possible association with ritualistic trauma.

Rituals and traditions are very consistent with the modalities used in occupational therapy because they are organized ways of providing comfort and structure to daily living. They often use material objects (icons) as symbolic representation of spirituality and cultural identity (e.g., artwork, prayer beads), and they are a means to creatively express and share group identity (e.g., dances, songs, festivals). Spiritual rituals and traditions include personal practices, community building, and seasonal celebrations (Table 7-2).

TABLE 7-2. SPIRITUAL RITUALS AND TRADITIONS

PERSONAL PRACTICES *Honoring and Nurturing Inner Strength*	• Meditation and mindfulness • Yoga • Prayer • Relaxation
COMMUNITY BUILDING *Honoring and Nurturing the Social Connection*	• Religious services and feasts, communal meals (e.g., Shabbat), group pilgrimages • Rites of passage (e.g., baptism, confirmation, Bar and Bat Mitzvah) • Many faith-based groups provide community services, such as soup kitchens and homeless shelters, as well as social services; religious organizations also assist displaced persons, such as the Jesuit Refugee Services and the Hebrew Immigrant Aid Society • Charity and service are often strongly encouraged to demonstrate faith (e.g., Mormon mission trip) or perform other outreach services
SEASONAL CELEBRATIONS *Honoring the Connection With Nature*	• Summer: Solstice celebrations, saint's days • Autumn: Equinox, Halloween, All Hallows Eve, All Saints and All Souls, Day of the Dead, harvest feasts, Thanksgiving • Winter: Solstice, Yule, solar/secular and religious New Year, Christmas (Christian), Chanukah (Jewish), Ashura (Muslim), Bodhi Day (Buddhist) • Spring: Equinox, cleansing, rebirth, renewal, Easter

TRAUMA

The Substance Abuse and Mental Health Services Administration (SAMHSA, 2014) defines trauma as:

> Individual trauma results from an event, series of events, or set of circumstances that is experienced by an individual as physically or emotionally harmful or threatening and that has lasting adverse effects on the individual's functioning and physical, social, emotional, or spiritual well-being. (p. 7)

An awareness of the relationship between traumatic events and the development and severity of mental illness has long been recognized, but according to recent data, the link was dramatically underestimated. A study called the *Adverse Childhood Experience Study* was conducted from 1995 to 1997 by Kaiser Permanente Health Maintenance Organization and the Centers for Disease Control and Prevention. (See Suggested Resources for the website.) The results of this study showed both a high incidence of adverse experiences and a strong correlation between adverse childhood experiences and subsequent physical and mental health problems. This landmark study formed the basis for a plethora of subsequent studies that further advanced our understanding of the effects of trauma and helped develop the basis for the trauma informed approach, also known as *trauma-informed care* (TIC). SAMHSA (2014) identifies six key principles of a trauma-informed approach:

1. Safety
2. Trustworthiness and transparency
3. Peer support
4. Collaboration and mutuality
5. Empowerment, voice, and choice
6. Cultural, historical, and gender issues

These broad-based principles are designed to be used across multiple settings and adapted to the situation and environment. They are not specific or prescribed interventions, nor a "cookbook" approach. Rather, these guiding principles are meant to be incorporated in all interactions within the therapeutic milieu.

The complex relationship between symptoms and traumatic events, as well as strategies for healing, is graphically depicted in Figure 7-4. Table 7-3 elaborates on the range of potential physical, behavioral, cognitive, emotional, and psychological effects of trauma. Although traumatic experiences affect all areas of health and wellness, the relationship to mental illness is overwhelming. SAMHSA (2014) and the National Council for Behavioral Health (n.d.) have concluded that over 90% of people diagnosed with mental illness or seeking help for psychosocial distress have experienced recent or past traumatic events.

It is important to understand that the experience of trauma is unique to the individual, with some experiences being subtle and others being catastrophic. Considering the almost universal incidence of trauma for people with mental illness and the wide range of possible adverse effects, it

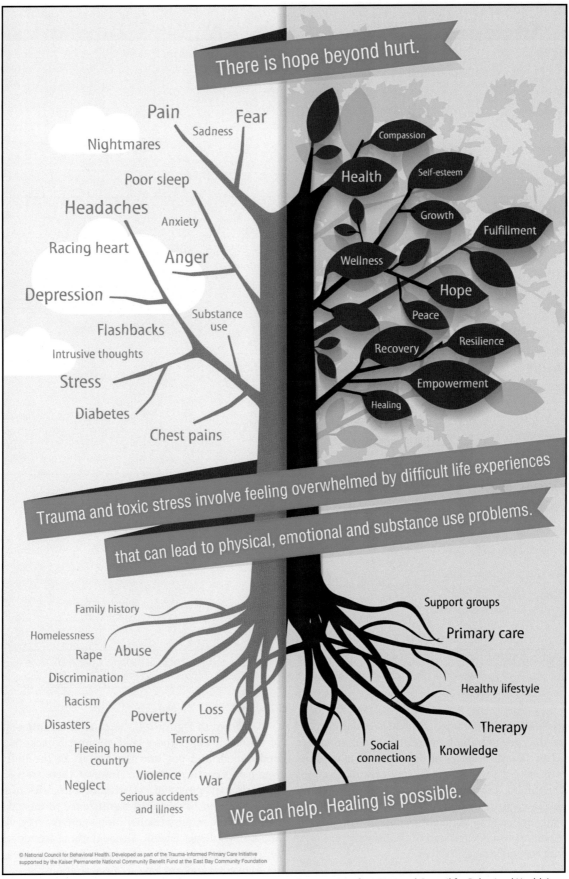

Figure 7-4. Trauma Tree: There Is Hope Beyond Hurt. (Reprinted with permission from National Council for Behavioral Health.)

TABLE 7-3. POTENTIAL EFFECTS OF TRAUMA

PHYSICAL	<ul><li>Excessive alertness, looking for signs of danger</li><li>Easily startled</li><li>Fatigue</li><li>Disturbed sleep</li><li>General aches and pains</li><li>Muscle tension</li><li>Digestive issues</li><li>Heart palpitations</li></ul>
BEHAVIORAL	<ul><li>Social withdrawal and isolation</li><li>Loss of interest in normal activities</li><li>Irritability, aggression, verbal or physical outbursts</li><li>Self-injurious behaviors</li><li>Substance abuse</li><li>Reenactments of trauma</li><li>Self-care neglect or impairment</li><li>Avoidance of places or activities</li></ul>
COGNITIVE	<ul><li>Intrusive thoughts and/or memories of the event</li><li>Visual images of the event</li><li>Nightmares</li><li>Poor concentration and memory</li><li>Disorientation</li><li>Confusion</li></ul>
EMOTIONAL AND PSYCHOLOGICAL	<ul><li>Shock, denial, or disbelief</li><li>Fear, anxiety, and panic</li><li>Numbness, disconnectedness, and detachment</li><li>Feeling sad, hopeless, helpless</li><li>Depression</li><li>Guilt, shame, self-blame</li><li>Anger and irritability</li><li>Mood swings</li><li>Loss of sense of self or sense of meaning</li></ul>

Adapted from McNamara, K., & Sovyak, P. (2017, October). *Trauma-informed care and occupational therapy: A perfect fit.* Workshop session presented at the meeting of the Occupational Therapy Association of California (OTAC), Sacramento, CA.

is not possible to cover the topic adequately in one chapter. Therefore, the issue of trauma and related interventions are addressed in several chapters of this book. Furthermore, readers are invited to review the many case illustrations included in this book through the lens of trauma awareness. Although the majority of these case illustrations were not intentionally designed to highlight trauma, it will be obvious that trauma is an integral part of the life experiences of people with mental illness.

As shown in Figure 7-4, there are many different types of traumatic experiences, and all must be acknowledged, understood, and put into the context of the individuals who have experienced them. However, there are a few particularly damaging and catastrophic categories of trauma that appear to have special significance to mental health and therefore require further discussion: poverty, violence, and human displacement. Although these are addressed as separate entities in the following subsections, they sometimes overlap and can have a causal relationship.

Poverty

There are several types of poverty, each one with differing causes and outcomes and with varying degrees of associated stress and trauma:

- *Relative poverty* is defined as income or resources in relation to the average. It is concerned with the absence of the material needs to participate fully in accepted daily life but also may represent a perception of "doing without" as can happen even in affluent countries.

- *Situational poverty* is a temporary condition when a person falls below the poverty line because of an outside event. Resultant trauma is usually due to the nature of the event rather than the loss of income or financial support. For example, if the situational poverty is due to natural disaster, loss or death of the household provider, or sudden loss of a job, the related stress could be considered traumatic. If the financial setback is understood to be temporary or is due to a conscious choice, such as going to college, the related stress is less likely to be traumatic.

- *Generational poverty* exists for at least two generations and is often associated with a decrease in independent and productive living skills, limited education, and poor coping skills. The likelihood of life events being considered traumatic is increased at least in part due to a decreased sense of hope and locus of control.

- *Absolute poverty* is the lack of sufficient resources for basic human needs (i.e., food, water, shelter). The acute deprivation can cause suffering and premature death. Although people in absolute poverty can be found anywhere in the world, the condition is most often associated with impoverished nations and areas with multiple stressors, such as war and displacement.

Being in poverty is usually not a single factor condition but rather representative of *social exclusion*, a term originally used in Europe but now found in literature and policies throughout the world. Social exclusion involves the lack of or denial of resources, rights, or goods and services and the inability to participate in the normal relationships and activities. It is a combination of linked problems such as unemployment, poor skills, low incomes, poor housing, high crime environments, bad health, and family breakdown. Considering that social inclusion is a primary goal of occupational therapy, there is an obvious role for occupational therapists to address poverty in practice. However, given the enormity of the issues of social exclusion, many disciplines and agencies must be involved, preferably in collaboration, to make effective changes.

Violence

The most obvious arena for experiencing violence is in war zones. However, everyone, military or civilian, on either side of the conflict can experience significant trauma. Occupational therapists, particularly in the United States, have focused on interventions for active military service members and veterans. Acute stress disorder, traumatic brain injury, and posttraumatic stress disorder in returning soldiers have received attention in the media. What is not discussed is the occupational disruption or deprivation experienced during deployment, which can indeed reach the threshold of trauma. Service members are apart from families and friends for more than 6 months at a time, and many have been away for much longer. This distance greatly impacts a soldier's role as a spouse, parent, caregiver, friend, and son or daughter. These roles become blurred and many times lead to feelings of anxiety and depression. The United States Army has specified Combat Stress Control Units that include occupational therapists to address all mental health issues on site.

Criminal activity, gang violence, and random acts of gun violence, particularly as in mass shootings, have traumatized thousands of people to varying degrees. Although there has been extensive media attention and some attempts at addressing underlying problems, to date there is not a comprehensive interdisciplinary action plan to address violence. Longitudinal studies are needed to determine the full extent of harm caused by these traumas, especially the lasting impact on health, wellness, and function.

Other forms of violence often seen in conjunction with the presentation of mental health symptoms are domestic violence or intimate partner violence and sexual assault. These traumatic incidents are sometimes difficult to address because they fall within both the health domain and the justice domain, and traditionally these are considered separate areas of study and practice (Walker & Logan, 2018). The American Occupational Therapy Association (2017) has framed these forms of violence as occupational injustices that are clearly within the realm of occupational therapy services and has extensively documented the daily living activities, sleep patterns, and social participation that are disrupted by intimate violence.

Violence is not solely limited to physical acts. Psychological and emotional abuse are forms of violence that can be particularly detrimental to mental health (Centers for Disease Control and Prevention, 2017). As shown in the results of the Adverse Childhood Experience Study, child abuse of all forms has devastating long-term physical and mental health consequences. (See Suggested Resources for the website.)

It is not uncommon to find intimidation, coercion, and exploitation within intimate relationships, but these emotionally violent tactics are also used to control people who may be vulnerable. Examples include people dominated by cult and cult-like charismatic leaders as well as people, particularly women, who have been deceived and then controlled in human trafficking and sexual slavery operations.

Human Displacement

> The displacement of people refers to the forced movement of people from their locality or environment and occupational activities. It is a form of social change caused by a number of factors, the most common being armed conflict. Natural disasters, famine, development and economic changes may also be a cause of displacement. (United Nations Educational, Scientific and Cultural Organization, n.d.)

There is significant evidence that human displacement can cause myriad mental health problems and psychosocial distress. Thela, Tomita, Maharaj, Mhlongo, and Burns (2017) conducted a study of refugees and migrants in Africa and found that the "prevalence of mental distress was high: 49.4% anxiety, 54.6% depression, and 24.9% post-traumatic stress symptoms" (p. 715). Services for displaced persons are not well coordinated and certainly not sufficient to meet the overwhelming need. Creative funding and service delivery models need to be further developed worldwide, in addition to the expansion of collaborative partnerships with governments, nongovernmental organizations, and faith-based organizations.

Trauma-Informed Approach in Occupational Therapy

The six principles of a trauma-informed approach previously discussed are consistent with the client-centered, recovery-oriented approach now used in occupational therapy, especially in mental health services. Furthermore, the symptoms and behaviors that are the potential effects of trauma, as outlined in Table 7-3, are also consistent with the *Occupational Therapy Practice Framework* (American Occupational Therapy Association, 2014). In other words, an argument could be made that the services currently offered by occupational therapists, many of which are described in this chapter and throughout this book, are consistent with TIC. However, a key element that is missing is conscious and universal application of trauma-informed principles, which can only occur if there is a robust body of occupational therapy scholarship to support the applications of these principles. To date, no specific scholarly literature on the role of occupational therapy in TIC could be found.

Another key issue in occupational therapists becoming trauma informed is increasing trauma awareness. The Suggested Resources listed at the end of this chapter are provided to increase awareness and broaden one's understanding of the possible causes and effects of trauma. It is also highly recommended that occupational therapists familiarize themselves with the writings of Dr. Judith Herman, especially her preeminent book, *Trauma and Recovery: The Aftermath of Violence—From Domestic Abuse to Political Terror* (2015). Although there is a tremendous amount of information now available, one also has to consider the emotional readiness to accept it. This is especially true when the traumatic events are far removed from the experiences of the majority of service providers. Examples would include torture, enslavement, and witnessing mass murder, as well as surviving terrifying natural disasters, especially with loss of family, friends, and homes. Considering the universality of trauma and the vulnerability of those we serve in occupational therapy, it is essential for occupational therapists to have their own emotional support and resilience to continue the work.

SUMMARY AND RECOMMENDATIONS

This chapter ambitiously attempts to cover the complex interaction between personal and social identity while also exploring the significant obstacles of stigma and trauma. Although the problems facing people with mental illness as well as the general population can appear to be overwhelming, there are glimmers of hopeful resiliency and creative solutions being attempted.

Occupational therapists are urged to increase involvement in social and occupational justice practice, research, and education; advocate for all people at risk or in distress; and conduct outreach to organizations and other disciplines to highlight the value of occupational therapy in addressing occupational injustices.

ACKNOWLEDGEMENTS

Material for the family subsection was gathered in focus groups conducted by Carol Underwood. Material related to trauma experienced by military service members was provided by Robinette J. Amaker, PhD, OTR/L, CHT, FAOTA; Anne Pas Burke, EdD, OTR/L, FAOTA; Cecilia Najera, MOT, OTR, CPT, SP; and Mary Vining Radomski, PhD, OTR/L, FAOTA. Resources for the section on trauma were provided in part by Kelly McNamara, OTR/L, and Patrice Sovyak, OTR/L.

REFERENCES

American Occupational Therapy Association. (2014). Occupational therapy practice framework: Domain and process (3rd ed.). *American Journal of Occupational Therapy, 68*(Suppl. 1), S1-S48. doi:10.5014/ajot.2014.682006

American Occupational Therapy Association. (2017). Occupational therapy services for individuals who have experienced domestic violence. *American Journal of Occupational Therapy, 71*(Suppl. 2), 1-13. doi:10.5014/ajot.2017.716S10

Angermeyer, M. C., Carta, M. G., Matschinger, H., Miller, A., Refaï, T., Schomerus, G., & Toumi, M. (2016). Cultural differences in stigma surrounding schizophrenia: Comparison between Central Europe and North Africa. *British Journal of Psychiatry, 208*, 389-397. doi:10.1192/bjp.bp.114.154260

Balsam, K. F., Molina, Y., Beadnell, B., Simoni, J. & Walters, K. (2011). Measuring multiple minority stress: The LGBT People of Color Microaggressions Scale. *Cultural Diversity & Ethnic Minority Psychology, 17*(2), 163-174. doi:10.1037/a0023244

Bonsall, A. (2009, October). *Revisiting role theory in occupational science*. Paper presented at the Eight Annual Research Conference, Society for the Study of Occupations, New Haven, CT.

Centers for Disease Control and Prevention. (2017). *Intimate partner violence: Definitions*. Retrieved from http://www.cdc.gov/violenceprevention/intimatepartnerviolence/definitions.html

Chandler, E. (2012). Religious and spiritual issues in DSM-5: Matters of the mind and searching of the soul. *Issues in Mental Health Nursing, 33*(9), 577-582. doi:10.3109/01612840.2012.704130

Corrigan, P. W., Markowitz, F. E., & Watson, A. C. (2004). Structural levels of mental illness: Stigma and discrimination. *Schizophrenia Bulletin, 30*(3), 481-491.

Gade, C. (2011). The historical development of the written discourses on ubuntu. *South African Journal of Philosophy, 30*(3), 303-329.

Gerlach, A. J., Teachman, G., Laliberte-Rudman, D., Aldrich, R. M., & Huot, S. (2018). Expanding beyond individualism: Engaging critical perspectives on occupation. *Scandinavian Journal of Occupational Therapy, 25*(1), 35-43.

Green-Thompson, L. P., McInerney, P., & Woollard, B. (2017). The social accountability of doctors: A relationship based framework for understanding emergent community concepts of caring. *BMC Health Services Research, 17*(269), 1-7. doi:10.1186/s12913-017-2239-7

Herman, J. (2015). *Trauma and recovery: The aftermath of violence—from domestic abuse to political terror*. New York, NY: Basic Books.

Jenkins, J. H., & Carpenter-Song, E. (2009). Awareness of stigma among persons with schizophrenia: Marking the contexts of lived experience. *Journal of Nervous and Mental Disease, 197*(7), 520-529.

Jackson, J. (1998). Contemporary criticism of role theory. *Journal of Occupational Science, 5*(2), 49-55.

Keusch G. T., Wilentz, J., & Kleinman, A. (2006). Stigma and global health: Developing a research agenda. *Lancet, 367*(9509), 525-527.

Krupa, T., Kirsh, B., Pitts, D., & Fossey, E. (2016). *Bruce and Borg's psychosocial frames of reference: Theories, models, and approaches for occupation-based practice* (4th ed.). Thorofare, NJ: SLACK Incorporated.

Macmin, L., & Foskett, J. (2004). "Don't be afraid to tell." The spiritual and religious experience of mental health service users in Somerset. *Mental Health, Religion & Culture, 7*(1), 23-40.

McConnell, E. A., Janulis, P., Phillips, G. 2nd, Truong, R., & Birkett, M. (2018). Multiple minority stress and LGBT community resilience among sexual minority men. *Psychology of Sexual Orientation and Gender Diversity, 5*(1), 1-12. doi:10.1037/sgd0000265

Metz, T. (2016). Recent philosophical approaches to social protection: From capability to Ubuntu. *Global Social Policy, 16*(2), 132-150.

Mizock, L. (2012). The double stigma of obesity and serious mental illnesses: Promoting health and recovery. *Stigma and Health, 1*(S), 86-91.

Mosey, A. (1986). *Psychosocial components of occupational therapy*. New York, NY: Raven Press.

National Alliance on Mental Illness. (n.d.). *Risk of suicide*. Retrieved from https://www.nami.org/learn-more/mental-health-conditions/related-conditions/suicide

National Council for Behavioral Health. (n.d.). *Trauma-informed care*. Retrieved from https://www.thenationalcouncil.org/areas-of-expertise/trauma-informed-behavioral- healthcare/

Oakley, F., Kielhofner, G., Barris, R., & Reichler, R. (1986). The role checklist: Development and empirical assessment of reliability. *Occupational Therapy Journal of Research, 6*, 151-170.

Ramugondo, E. L., & Kronenberg, F. (2015). Explaining collective occupations from a human relations perspective: Bridging the individual collective dichotomy. *Journal of Occupational Science, 22*(1), 3-16. doi:10.1080/14427591.2013.781920

Reilly, M. (1966). The challenge of the future to an occupational therapist. *American Journal of Occupational Therapy, 20*(5), 221-225.

Substance Abuse and Mental Health Services Administration. (2014). *SAMHSA's concept of trauma and guidance for a trauma-informed approach*. Rockville, MD: Author.

Sue, D. W., Capodilupo, C. M., Torino, G. C., Bucceri, J. M., Holder, A. M., Nadal, K. L., & Esquilin, M. (2007). Racial microaggressions in everyday life: Implications for clinical practice. *American Psychologist, 62*(4), 271-286.

Thela, L., Tomita, A., Maharaj, V., Mhlongo, M., & Burns, J. K. (2017). Counting the cost of Afrophobia: Post-migration adaptation and mental health challenges of African refugees in South Africa. *Transcultural Psychiatry, 54*(5-6), 715-732. doi:10.1177/1363461517745472

United Nations Educational, Scientific and Cultural Organization. (n.d.). *Displaced person/displacement*. Retrieved from http://www.unesco.org/new/en/social-and-human-sciences/themes/international-migration/glossary/displaced-person-displacement

Walker, R., & Logan, T. K. (2018). Health and rural context among victims of partner abuse: Does justice matter? *Journal of Interpersonal Violence, 33*(1), 64-82.

Watson, A. C., Corrigan, P., Larson, J. E., & Sells, M. (2007). Self-stigma in people with mental illness. *Schizophrenia Bulletin, 33*(6), 1312-1318.

SUGGESTED RESOURCES

CDC: Adverse Childhood Experiences (ACE): https://www.cdc.gov/violenceprevention/acestudy/index.html

Healthy Place for Your Mental Health: What Is Stigma?: https://www.healthyplace.com/stigma/stand-up-for-mental-health/what-is-stigma

LGBTQ and OT: https://www.LGBTQ-OT.com

National Consortium of Torture Treatment Programs: http://www.ncttp.org

Occupational Opportunities for Refugees & Asylum Seekers Inc.: http://www.oofras.com

Removing the Labels: https://www.youtube.com/watch?v=5JCFBXCHdcQ&feature=youtu.be

The Case of Trauma and Recovery, Psychological Insight and Political Understanding, with Judith Herman: https://www.uctv.tv/shows/The-Case-of-Trauma-and-Recovery-Psychological-Insight-and-Political-Understanding-with-Judith-Herman-Conversations-with-History-6233

UNHCR: The United Nations Refugee Agency: http://www.unhcr.org/en

Cultural Identity and Context

*Anne MacRae, PhD, OTR/L, BCMH, FAOTA
and Tiffany (Debra) Boggis, MBA, OTR/L*

The *Occupational Therapy Practice Framework* defines the context of *culture* as "customs, beliefs, activity patterns, behavioral standards, and expectations accepted by the society of which the client is a member" (American Occupational Therapy Association [AOTA], 2014, p. S28). However, it should be noted that many other definitions of culture specifically include values and beliefs, which the *Occupational Therapy Practice Framework* identifies as *client factors*, separate from the contextual concept of culture. Values and beliefs can be highly personal and individual, but they can also be deeply intertwined with one's culture and are therefore discussed in this chapter.

Although the AOTA definition provides parameters for culturally responsive care, it lacks an explanation of the purpose of culture, which is to create meaning, develop or enhance personal and role identity, and provide structure and organization to our daily lives. The World Federation of Occupational Therapy (2010) states that "every person is unique in the way they combine the dynamic interplay between cultural, social, psychological, biological, financial, political and spiritual elements in their personal occupational performance and participation in society" (para. 5). The World Federation of Occupational Therapy's *Guiding Principles on Diversity and Culture* provides a resource for practitioners, educators, and researchers to discuss and explore strategies for culturally competent and inclusive practice (Kinébanian & Stomph, 2009).

CULTURAL IDENTITY

The significance of cultural identity cannot be overstated because it influences all aspects of daily life as well as the process of how societies are organized and governed. Cultural identity plays a major role, both positive and negative, in psychological well-being and is particularly important when addressing issues such as stigma and one's view of mental illness (Shefer et al., 2012). Cultural identity may include nationality, ethnicity, religion, social class, generation, and locality, among others, but it is personalized for each individual. One cannot assume, for example, that one who hails from an Irish, White, Christian, and middle-class background and resides in the United States self-identifies with the mainstream values of each of these cultural affiliations. In occupational therapy, understanding of cultural identity is vital because of the profession's focus on roles and habits as well as community inclusion, which are directly or indirectly influenced by culture.

The Language of Identity

Terminology used to identify cultural groups inherently runs the risk of superficial labeling and stereotyping. There is also an unfortunate tendency to use the language of cultural identity in a derogatory and mean-spirited fashion. Of course, this kind of insensitivity is offensive and

MacRae, A. (Ed.). *Cara and MacRae's Psychosocial Occupational Therapy:
An Evolving Practice, Fourth Edition* (pp 123-136).
© 2019 Taylor & Francis Group.

unacceptable; however, the designation of which terms they might be is more difficult than one might think. There are geographical, generational, situational, and personal differences in one's choice of terms. For example, depending on a person's age and where he or she grew up, one might identify him- or herself as Negro, Black, African American, or person of color. Another example is how to designate people who speak Spanish as their primary language or people who originate from Spanish-speaking countries. In the eastern United States, the term *Hispanic* is most commonly used (geographical difference), whereas in the West, the term *Latino* or *Latina* (gender difference) is more common. As another example, in Canada the preferred term for indigenous people is *First Nation*. To some people, the designation of *tribal* is considered archaic and offensive. However, in many parts of the United States, the word *tribal* is used with pride (regional difference). There are still tribal councils that have political authority on reservations and tribal ceremonies that are conducted, sometimes for members of the group only, other times for the larger community. The designation *Indian* to mean Native American (rather than East Indian) is usually considered to be derogatory, especially in some Caucasian cultures. However, tribal political activists use the term frequently. Some tribal members report that the term *Native American* is an artificial distinction coined to assuage the guilt of White liberals (personal difference). There is also quite a bit of debate going on among American Indian groups about the value of being identified only by one's tribe or nation (e.g., Mohawk, Pomo). Although this is probably more precise and acknowledges the differences between the groups, it can also weaken their unity when addressing political and social issues (situational difference).

Culturally sensitive, or what is commonly called *politically correct*, terminology is an attempt to eliminate or reduce bias and stereotypes. However, it does nothing to solve the underlying problem of why is stigma developed in the first place. Attitudinal differences may not be significantly affected by a change in terminology. Sometimes the concern about not offending anyone becomes so complicated that conversation simply shuts down. That is the worst possible scenario for culturally informed health care.

Racial and Ethnic Identity

One common method of cultural identification is race or ethnicity. This is partially because there are usually easily recognized and observable features. However, research using race or ethnicity as designated populations of studies is discouraged unless there is a very specific, usually biologic, rationale. The reason for this caution is that, all too often, faulty conclusions have been drawn from otherwise well-designed research. It is now thought that behaviors and social consequences are much more affected by socioeconomic status and education than they are by race or ethnicity. Many references in the literature suggest

that the concept and definitions of culture are too limited and need to be broadened to include a global multinational, postethnic perspective. Some even suggest that human beings are evolving past the need for limited ethnic identity (Rifkin, 2009). However, this position is somewhat countermanded by a dramatic rise for further information on one's genetic origins as indicated by the proliferations of ancestry and DNA identification websites. It appears to be an innate desire of human beings to know where we come from, which has led to a great increase in queries not only about genetic ancestry, but also the geographical paths of our ancestors. This quest is poignantly demonstrated at the Ellis Island Immigration Museum in New York City, which has had over 30 million visitors since 1990. (See Suggested Resources for the website.)

Despite the limitations of ethnic identity, it continues to be a powerful force for both individuals and groups. Ethnic identity provides a structure and richness to the internal aspects of culture, such as values and beliefs, but also helps us celebrate the wonderful diversity of the external aspects of culture, such as food, clothing, music, art, and rituals. Case Illustration 8-1 describes a wellness center activity that is primarily designed to celebrate ethnic identification.

The Complexity of Cultural Identification

Identification of culture with ethnicity alone does not represent the many interrelated facets of culture, such as gender, socioeconomics, age, and geographic location. Cultural identity may also be linked to chosen or inherent lifestyles based on personal choice, religious affiliation, disability, or sexual orientation; thus, care must be taken to not assume that an individual will always represent or agree with all aspects of a designated ethnic culture. One of the hallmark traits of culture is that it is dynamic, and so are the individuals within a culture.

In our complex society influenced by many events, some people may feel cultureless, whereas others identify themselves as members of several cultures (e.g., African American, gay, Christian, occupational therapist). This polyculturalism gives rise to a situation where some people feel cultural conflicts within themselves, let alone with the various communities in which he or she must interact. The significance of either a lack of cultural identity or a conflicted cultural identity is profound. Stress, guilt, poor self-esteem and self-concept, and lack of support are all contributing factors to poor health. Case Illustration 8-2 highlights a lack of cultural identity, but the incidence of cultural conflict within an individual is also extremely common. For example, a woman who has immigrated to the United States from a country with a traditional Islamic culture may want to be a part of the working and social world of American women but feels conflicted about her role. She may also lose the emotional support of her family

CASE ILLUSTRATION 8-1: JUNETEENTH AT THE WELLNESS CENTER

Yvonne is an occupational therapist who provides groups, consultation, and program development for a peer-operated wellness center. The center membership is highly diverse, but approximately 40% of the participants identify themselves as African American or Black. Through many informal conversations, it became clear to Yvonne that many of these group members did not have a strong understanding of their ethnic history but were curious about it. Yvonne suggested that they could research and plan a Juneteenth celebration. An initial presentation was brought to the center's steering committee by peer representatives. They explained that the holiday historically commemorated the June 1865 announcement of the abolition of slavery in Texas, but it is now a special day of observance celebrating the emancipation of African American slaves in the United States. Following this presentation, funding for a Juneteenth celebration at the wellness center was unanimously approved, and a planning committee comprising diverse peers at the center was formed.

After extensive internet research, the group decided to host a day of education and Juneteenth barbeque open to the community. Yvonne offered to help prepare for this event through activities in the occupational therapy groups. Menu planning, shopping, budgeting, and cooking were conducted in the living skills group. The communication and social skills group took responsibility for choosing and practicing several traditional songs as well as practicing reading parts of the Emancipation Proclamation and parts of speeches from Dr. Martin Luther King Jr. and other civil rights activists. Flyers and decorations were created in the workshop (arts and crafts) group. It was also decided to have demonstrations of various crafts known to have been used by slaves on Southern plantations. The workshop participants divided into subgroups to prepare and practice demonstrations of rake knitting, coil pottery, and gourd drum making.

Discussion

This event is an ideal way to instill a sense of pride and belonging to many participants through a celebration of ethnic heritage. It also contributes to cultural awareness by educating peers and members of the community. Although the occupational therapist was heavily involved in the preparation of the event, it was a peer-driven effort that enhanced the sense of ownership, belonging, and accomplishment.

CASE ILLUSTRATION 8-2: THE CULTURELESS WORLD OF JASON

Jason is a 23-year-old man who self-identifies as White but doesn't actually know his genetic or ethnic background. His upbringing was fairly chaotic, with little structure and few ties to the community. Jason's father left the family years ago, and his mother often expressed anger at all the "unfair" things in her life. Jason's upbringing was virtually devoid of cultural traditions or even acknowledgement. He once asked his mother about her background and she simply said she was a "mutt" and didn't know anything about her family history and didn't care.

Discussion

Individuals are free to choose which aspects of their birth-related culture(s) they choose to honor, but some people don't have that opportunity. In Jason's situation, his dysfunctional upbringing caused the thread of his heritage to be lost because elements of cultural identity are typically passed down through the generations.

Sometimes in such situations, resentment toward attention paid to cultural groups or celebrations can fester. The cultureless individual may feel marginalized or displaced. In the worst case scenario, Jason may be vulnerable to the exploitation of hate groups, such as White supremacists, who take advantage of young peoples' emotional state or lack of identity.

for choices they view as rebellious. Another example is a young man from a fundamentalist Christian family coming to grips with an emerging homosexual identity. For some individuals, acknowledging an identity as a gay man would mean a conscious rejection of familial or religious culture. Unless other support networks are available, the individual may feel cultureless or disconnected from any group. For others, especially those who continue to cherish some parts of their cultural upbringing, there are unresolved conflicts regarding morals, lifestyle, and acceptance that can lead to guilt, shame, and poor self-esteem.

Polyculturalism can also develop due to geographical migrations. For example, a *third culture kid* (TCK) is defined as having "spent a significant part of his or her developmental years outside of the parents' culture" (Walters & Auton-Cuff, 2009, p. 755). Research has shown that TCKs (self-reported preferred term) often have difficulty in identifying with any culture and miss a sense of belonging, but also "TCKs consider themselves to be different from their home country kids because they are more open minded, exposed to different cultures, know more about the world, and they are more aware of their cultural differences" (McGregor, Renu, & Deepa, 2013, p. 122). However, it should be noted that research conducted with TCKs has primarily been confined to children who have migrated due to their parents' employment postings (e.g., diplomatic service or multinational corporations), and these children may be considered privileged in many ways. Therefore, the results of these studies are not transferable to children, such as refugees, who migrated due to poverty, oppression, or war.

As society becomes more polycultural, there must be greater sophistication in how cultures are identified. It is clear that the concept of culture has often been used to marginalize and stereotype certain groups of people. However, simply choosing to not recognize differences in people is a form of *cultural blindness*, that is, "the incapacity to comprehend how specific situations may be seen by individuals belonging to another culture due to a strict alignment with the viewpoints, outlooks, and morals of one's own culture" (Nugent, 2013, para. 1). Some theorists have identified cultural blindness as one stage along a progressive continuum as one advances toward a heightened level of cultural competence. Theorists have proposed models of cultural competency development, yet no single model is universally agreed upon. Variations in cultural competency terminology and its characteristics, as well as various models of cultural competency development, are explored in the next section.

CULTURAL COMPETENCE

Cultural competency has been defined in many different ways, and it has provoked considerable controversy over its assumption and effects. Culturally competent terminology in health care policy has been found to be ambiguous, making it difficult to assess intended health outcomes, especially for marginalized populations (Grant, Parry, & Guerin, 2013). More recent terminology has emerged to help capture some of the nuances that may or may not be implied in the term *cultural competency*. These include the terms *cultural humility, cultural responsiveness, cultural capability,* and *cultural agility,* among others, which have been used in various contexts.

Perhaps the most subtle and difficult aspect to change is cultural blindness. Many well-meaning people feel that "everybody is the same" and differences should not be acknowledged. Unfortunately, what this often means is "I will accept you looking different if you think and act like me." Cultural blindness takes many forms, including some public officials who support the dismantlement of equalization policies and laws. Although such melding and equalization may someday become reality, it seems that we have a long way to go to embrace the world's diversity. As long as racism and discrimination exist, a concerted effort to understand—not ignore—differences is needed.

All definitions of cultural competence go beyond the simple acquisition of knowledge and skills to discuss the necessity for interpersonal skills and attitudes, such as self-reflection, flexibility, acceptance of differences, and lifelong learning. The ability to understand different cultural values and viewpoints and integrate these into therapeutic interventions is necessary for service users to have a meaningful therapeutic experience.

The development of cultural competency is a dynamic process that occurs throughout one's lifespan. Hammer (2009, 2012) describes the Intercultural Development Continuum (IDC), adapted from Bennett's (1993) original formulation of the Developmental Model of Intercultural Sensitivity. The IDC provides a developmental continuum to understand how people tend to think and feel about diversity, progressing from a lesser to a more complex perception and experience of cultural differences. Five specific orientations that range from monocultural to more intercultural or global mindsets are described. Those who have a more intercultural mindset have a greater capability to respond effectively to cultural differences. The first two orientations are monocultural in nature and include *denial*, defined as an indifference to or ignorance of cultural difference, and *polarization*, characterized by either a negative evaluation of cultures different than one's own (i.e., defense) or a perception that other cultures are better than one's own (i.e., reversal). *Minimization* is a transitional phase in which there is recognition of superficial differences, such as food and dress preferences, while similarities of human beings are emphasized. The final two orientations are intercultural in nature. An intercultural mindset includes the *acceptance* stage, at which point difference is recognized and appreciated. The final stage, *adaptation*, is characterized by the development of empathy to take on another's point of view and ability to adapt behaviors to accommodate for the differences.

The IDC provided the framework for developing the Intercultural Development Inventory, which is an assessment designed to identify and build cultural competence in individuals and organizations. (See Suggested Resources for online access.) Gaining an understanding and appreciation of commonalities between one's culture and those of others is helpful to avoid negatively judging cultures in terms of "us" and "them," indicative of a monocultural perspective.

It allows for tolerance of other cultures, characteristic of a minimization worldview. Development of an in-depth understanding of how one's own culture differs from other cultures as well as alternative culture-specific knowledge lays the foundation for acceptance and fosters the ability to make ethical judgments that take into consideration other cultural values as well as one's own. A more thorough recognition and appreciation of cultural differences pave the way to shift cultural perspectives and to adapt intervention in consideration of cultural differences, characteristic of an adaptation orientation.

Guidelines for culturally competent occupational therapy began to emerge in the literature in the early 1990s (Dillard et al., 1992) and continue to be a topic of discussion in the current literature (Balcazar, Suarez-Balcazar, & Taylor-Ritzler, 2009; Castro, Dahlin-Ivanoff, & Martensson, 2016). Indeed, one study using a literature review of rehabilitation professions found that "studies on cultural competence occur most frequently in occupational therapy" (Grandpierre et al., 2018, p. 1).

Critiques of Cultural Competence Models

Some argue that cultural competence schemas are overly focused on individual attitudes and, therefore, minimize the devastating effects of institutional racism and oppression (Abrams & Molo, 2009). Other critiques focus on the inherent risk of *cultural relativism*, the acceptance of the cultural beliefs and practices of others rather than judging behavior through one's own cultural norms. Although cultural relativism has provided a nonjudgmental framework for accessing and attempting to understand the life world experiences of others, it presents moral and ethical dilemmas, especially in regard to human rights. For example, if all behavior is viewed through a nonjudgmental cultural lens, then how does an individual or society determine right from wrong?

Some critiques of cultural competence or even cultural acceptance unfortunately mirror the ebbs and flows of reactive social movements and politics. At the current time, we are witnessing an increase in nationalism, especially in Europe and the United States, which is causing increased tension and intractable posturing along the cultural spectrum. Perhaps these words, widely attributed to Aristotle, can provide a roadmap for negotiating and hopefully resolving these dilemmas: "It is the mark of an educated mind to be able to entertain a thought without accepting it."

CULTURE AND HEALTH CARE

Recently, there's been an effort to understand health and illness in a cultural context and to research the role of traditional medicine as well as complementary and alternative medicine in providing adequate health care for the world's population. The literature is inconsistent in the use of the terms *traditional, alternative,* and *complementary*; therefore, some definitions are in order. Traditional (also referred to as *conventional*) medicine simply means the tradition or approach that is primarily used within one's culture. In the dominant culture of the United States, allopathic or Western medicine is traditional (also called the *medical model*), whereas in India, the traditional medical system is Ayurvedic. This ancient health care system (approximately 4,000 years old) is primarily based on using elements of nature, including diet and herbs.

Alternative practices are health care techniques and approaches that are not typically viewed as compatible with Western medicine but may or may not be viable health care options (instead of Western medicine). Complementary health care practices are those that can be used in conjunction with Western medicine but fall outside of the traditional domain of the allopathic system. Whether a particular practice should be considered alternative or complementary often depends on the attitudes and knowledge of the health care provider and the client rather than on any inherent quality of the practice. There are several alternative and complementary practices that have become so popular that they are now considered somewhat mainstream. These include chiropractic; acupuncture; homeopathy; and various bodywork, movement, and massage techniques, as well as the use of diet and herbs. Some of these practices have ancient cultural histories, whereas others are more recent. As our population changes, the mixture of these beliefs becomes profound.

The various terms used in describing health care practices are understandably confusing, especially as new acronyms and definitions are introduced. For example, in many documents prior to the mid-1990s, the term *complementary and alternative medicine* was commonly used. The World Health Organization (WHO) modified the term to *traditional and complementary medicine* (T&CM) and continues to use this term in official documents. However, more recently, the National Center for Complementary and Integrative Health (2016), which is part of the National Institute of Health, recommends using the term *complementary health approaches and integrative health* and further defines the term *integrative health* to mean the incorporation of complementary health approaches into conventional health care. AOTA has also adopted the terminology of the National Center for Complementary and Integrative Health (AOTA, 2017). Regardless of the choice of terminology, it is becoming more common to find physicians and other health care providers willing to work in conjunction with an alternative/complementary practitioner and, perhaps most important, willing to work with service users for health promotion and awareness. This pluralistic wellness model is both client oriented and holistic, and consumers and health professionals alike are beginning to nurture this trend. In their research, Ibeneme, Eni,

Ezuma, and Fortwengel (2017) found that personal health care decisions are determined by many factors, including past experiences, family and traditions, and cultural and professional knowledge. Therefore, they concluded that "no medical system has been shown to address all of these elements; hence, the need for collaboration, acceptance, and partnership between all systems of care in cultural communities" (p. 18).

People in Western society tend to be either very skeptical of complementary/alternative techniques or uncritically embracing of nonallopathic approaches. The WHO is addressing this gap through the WHO T&CM strategy document (2013), which aims to assist countries to develop national policies for evaluation and regulation of T&CM practices, create an evidence base, determine the safety of practices, and ensure the affordability and availability of T&CM throughout the world. As stated in this document:

> Many countries now recognize the need to develop a cohesive and integrative approach to health care that allows governments, health care practitioners and, most importantly, those who use health care services, to access T&CM in a safe, respectful, cost-efficient and effective manner. (WHO, 2013, p. 7)

Given that the majority of people throughout the world now use some form of nonallopathic treatment either in isolation or in conjunction with Western medicine (WHO, 2013), occupational therapists are likely to encounter unfamiliar practices in their work and may misinterpret their observations. For example, moxibustion and cupping are healing rituals based on the traditional Chinese medicine principles of heat and cold. These techniques, as well as the Vietnamese ritual of coining (rubbing the body with a coin for the treatment of colds and flu), tend to leave marks on the body that have been misconstrued as evidence of abuse. Although these practices, like many others, can be potentially dangerous if administered incorrectly, they have been in use for a long time, and there is ample evidence that when properly administered, such techniques do no permanent harm and may have positive psychological as well as physical effects. In order for occupational therapists to provide the optimal interventions for their clients, it is imperative that clinicians continue to expand their knowledge base of T&CM and to determine its importance in the individual service user's life.

There has also been extensive debate regarding the actual use of complementary health care techniques by occupational therapists. Many practitioners have chosen to specialize with further training in a number of complementary practices, and some have incorporated them into their occupational therapy practice. In response to this trend, AOTA (2017) determined that "evidence-based [complementary health approaches and integrative health] may be used as preparatory methods, tasks, occupations, and activities when supporting active engagement and participation in meaningful occupations" (p. 3).

Culture and Mental Health

Cultural awareness is necessary for the delivery of all quality health care, but it has particular significance for the mental health field because of the very nature of practice. Concepts of normal and abnormal behavior are the basis for psychiatric diagnosis. Normality, however, can differ cross-culturally. What is normal to one can be abnormal to another. Because the concept of normality is undoubtedly value laden, the issue of culture must be addressed not only in the treatment process, but also in the assessment and diagnostic process. There have been efforts to identify manifestations of mental illness unique to a particular cultural group. One example is *ataque de nervios*, which is a sense of being out of control, where the person may exhibit verbal or physical aggression, uncontrollable crying, shouting, and sometimes fainting and dissociative experiences. This condition is commonly recognized among the Caribbean Latino population, as well as other Latino groups around the world. Another culture-bound syndrome is *shenjing shuairuo*. This condition, found in China and among other traditional Chinese populations, is characterized by fatigue, irritability, and various physical complaints, including headaches and stomachaches. Individuals who experience either of these culture-bound syndromes may or may not also meet the existing psychiatric criteria for an anxiety or mood disorder. However, the conditions are unique, and it cannot be assumed that they are synonymous with the Western view of psychopathology. Whether or not a practitioner acknowledges these syndromes as distinct conditions, it is important to understand the perspective of the service user because he or she may use these terms to explain his or her experiences.

CULTURE AND OCCUPATIONAL THERAPY

Every profession comes with inherent biases, as does the profession of occupational therapy. The culturally competent therapist must take care to recognize the cultural biases inherent in the theory, philosophy, and models of occupational therapy practice. Therapists are encouraged to be acutely aware of one's own cultural identity and that of the unique people whom they serve in order to discern the appropriateness and applicability of the documented ideals of the profession (Watson, 2006). This level of cultural competence requires *cultural humility*, which is defined by Hammell (2013) as "an approach to redressing power imbalances in client-therapist relationships by incorporating critical self-evaluation and recognizing that cultural differences lie not within clients but within client-therapist relationships" (p. 224). Hammell (2013) further states that "[c]ultural humility is advocated as an approach to theoretical development and in efforts to counter professional

Eurocentrism, ethnocentrism, and intellectual colonialism" (p. 224).

The word *occupation*, itself, may have a negative connotation to a client who has experienced life under the occupation of an oppressive governmental regime. The seven core values embraced by the AOTA (2015) include *altruism, equality, freedom, justice, dignity, truth*, and *prudence*. These values may not be interpreted in the same way by all cultures. The profession of occupational therapy historically derives its philosophy grounded in Western thought, embracing social norms of individualism, autonomy, independence, self-determination, and notions of mastery over nature and the environment. Other cultures may embrace alternative values of collectivism, interdependence, hierarchy, multiple truths, and balance with nature.

As world demographics continue to shift toward a diverse society and occupational therapy strives to be increasingly client driven, it is necessary that every occupational therapist develop a myriad of interventions that can acknowledge, honor, and address the complex cultural backgrounds of service users. Choices of occupations, including styles and approaches to activities of daily living, work habits, hobbies, and recreation, as well as the practice of rituals and traditions, are all representative of one's culture and must be individually tailored to the client or client group. Throughout this book, the illustrations and examples are designed to represent the diversity of occupational therapy service users. An aware occupational therapist creatively addresses culture with interventions; however, culturally appropriate assessment provides different challenges.

Culturally Relevant Occupational Therapy Assessment

The cultural sensitivity of standardized assessments continues to be a controversial subject, and many formal evaluation tools have such significant bias that their use with culturally diverse populations is questionable. Even the informal tools and interview protocols commonly used in occupational therapy rarely adequately address the cultural background of the client. Table 8-1 provides a format for a culturally based interview and observation. This structure allows the therapist to understand the client's values and beliefs as well as cultural style, in addition to the personal meaning of the individual's culture. As discussed in Chapter 4, observation is also a critical component of any occupational therapy evaluation, but perhaps especially so in mental health settings for a variety of reasons, which are further discussed in the subsequent section on communication.

Western values are reflected in many of the profession's models of practice, such as the Canadian Model of Occupational Performance and the Model of Human Occupation. Although these models and their related assessments are extremely valuable, especially for client-centered

goal setting, their focus on the individual as the central agent to effect change in the environment and occupational performance can be limiting in a cross-cultural situation. The Kawa Model (Iwama, 2006a) arose from a Japanese or Eastern social context that focuses on the harmony between the individual and the collective wider environment. Identification of an optimal model to guide the occupational therapy process with any given client is not dependent on the country where services are provided or the service user's country of origin. The Kawa Model has been used successfully in various contexts, including a mental health setting in the United Kingdom with clients of Caucasian and Asian backgrounds (Lim, 2006) and in Canada with a client of Guatemalan origin (Iwama, 2006b). It is the responsibility of the therapist to determine which model, or adaptation thereof, is the best fit given the cultural identity and cultural contexts relevant to the client.

CULTURAL VARIANTS IN SERVICE DELIVERY

In order to provide truly culturally competent occupational therapy services, it is essential that the provider continually attend to all aspects of culture. In other words, the occupational therapist must not only perform culturally sensitive assessments, but also provide interventions informed by culture. Furthermore, cultural sensitivity must also be demonstrated in environmental modifications, discharge planning, and referrals. Among the most significant variants are communication styles, values and social relationships, and time sense.

Communication Styles

Both nonverbal and verbal communication can vary in style, and this is at least partially culturally determined. In some parts of the United States, there is a strong value placed on direct, assertive communication. Sometimes, this value is taken to the point where all other styles of communication are considered to be pathologic. However, there are many cultures where either aggressive or passive communication styles are the norm and American-style communication is either not respected or considered offensive. Occupational therapists must sometimes adjust their style to the service user's style and adjust expectations. This becomes particularly difficult when the demands of the environment do not match the cultural background of the individual, which is highlighted in Case Illustration 8-3.

Communication is often thought of merely in terms of language. Although this is a critical component of communication, it is not the sum total, nor in many cases is it even the most important or reliable means of communication. Nonverbal communication, including body language and gestures, often carries more meaning and is more readily

TABLE 8-1. CROSS-CULTURAL INITIAL INTERVIEW AND OBSERVATION

Name: _____

Setting (Context): _____

CULTURAL IDENTITY	OBSERVATIONS
Where were you born?	Apparent cultural identity (e.g., features, dress, icons)
How long have you lived here?	
Do you identify with a specific culture? (*or* Do you feel more like a part of the culture in which you live or a different culture?)	
Do you identify with a specific religion?	

COMMUNICATION	OBSERVATIONS
What is your preferred language?	Comments on use of silence and nonverbal communication
If you had something important to discuss with your family, how would you approach them?	Communication style (e.g., passive, assertive, aggressive)

TIME SENSE	OBSERVATIONS

Do you use a device to tell time (e.g., watch, phone, computer)?	Arriving at scheduled appointment
	   Early _
	   On time _
	   Late _

Do you use a schedule or date book (electronic or paper)?	
Do you usually arrive early, late, or right on time to planned events?	
Is that pattern typical in your family or community?	

SOCIAL AND SPATIAL ORGANIZATION	OBSERVATIONS
What are some activities you enjoy? (*or* What are your hobbies? *or* What do you like to do during your free time?)	Touch (e.g., startles or withdraws when touched, accepts touch/touches others with or without difficulty)
What are your roles? (*or* What is your role [or obligations] in your family/community?)	Degree of comfort with space/distance in conversations

HEALTH/LOCUS OF CONTROL
What is good health to you?
Is there anything in your heritage/background that affects your approach to being well/healthy?
What do you think is going to make you or keep you well? (*or* What is going to keep you from getting well?)

SUMMARY

CASE ILLUSTRATION 8-3: THE PASSIVITY OF OI LING

Oi Ling is a 19-year-old college student being treated for major depression in an interdisciplinary outpatient treatment program. One of the regular weekly groups is on the topic of assertive communication. The social worker and the occupational therapist who co-lead the group encourage her to speak up and coach her in both nonverbal and verbal techniques for assertive communication. The clinical documentation reflects little change in Oi Ling's demeanor or affect.

Discussion

Although passivity may be a symptom of depression, many cultures value silence and expect people, especially women, to be quiet and deferential, particularly to their elders. It is up to the team and Oi Ling together to decide whether this group is appropriate for her. If her home or community environment does not value an assertive Westernized style of communication, there is little benefit to be derived from participation in this group, and it is very unlikely that any meaningful change will occur. The social worker and occupational therapist should avoid pathologizing behavior that is acceptable in the context of Oi Ling's life.

On the other hand, if Oi Ling needs to function within a school, work, or community environment that expects assertiveness, an open discussion about the topic should be pursued. The leaders of an assertive communication group need to assess the relevance of the topic in all clients' lives and help them identify what, if any, benefits would be gained from participating in the group. If Oi Ling sees the lack of assertiveness as a problem in her daily life, then participation is appropriate. However, the group leaders need to be aware that Oi Ling may be experiencing polyculturalism (i.e., living in two cultural worlds) and may need to develop further strategies for dealing with inherent conflicts.

understandable. However, this is assuming that one knows the meaning of the nonverbal communication for a particular culture. Even when people are competent linguists, misunderstandings can and do occur because of poorly understood nonverbal communication. For example, the thumbs-up gesture is commonly used in the United States to signify a job well done, whereas in some Middle Eastern cultures, it could have a derogatory meaning. In Western cultures, eye contact is generally expected in social interaction. Alternatively, in some Asian cultures that place a high value on hierarchical relationships, steady eye contact is considered inappropriate or disrespectful, especially in interactions with those considered to be in position of authority, such as a health professional.

Occupational therapists by tradition are doers and do not overly rely on verbal communication. However, all practitioners require practice in using and accurately reading nonverbal messages, as well as understanding the context of verbal language. Table 8-2 provides several clinical examples highlighting the linguistic challenges between a therapist and a service user.

Obviously, people who do not share a common language or dialect will have serious limitations in communication. It is certainly in the best interest of the professional to be fluent in more than one language. (In large, culturally diverse urban areas, linguistic ability often becomes a factor in hiring policies.) However, it is not sufficient to simply know the words or the grammar because all language occurs within a cultural context. This leads to a practice dilemma for monolingual therapists. Words are often used interchangeably, but they are really very different. A trained interpreter takes into account the cultural meanings of the words and applies them to the concepts of the other language and culture. Taking the time to learn other languages may be more than individual occupational therapists can realistically be expected to do. However, occupational therapists should strive to become cultural interpreters themselves or learn to work closely with interpreters so as not to miss the nuances of the languages encountered. Case Illustration 8-4 shows how the use of terms can have different meanings depending on context. Additionally, the therapist can collaborate with these specialists and the organization within which the therapy service resides to ensure linguistic access to written home therapy programs, educational materials, survey instruments, and signage to the clinic area in languages and terminology that is responsive to the clients' cultures and literacy levels. It should not be assumed that all service users are literate even in their native language. Use of demonstration and visual representations may be viable methods to incorporate into therapeutic interventions. Box 8-1 lists guidelines for cross-cultural communication that can be used in any clinical or community environment.

Values and Social Relationships

Closely tied to communication is the process of relationship development, the values and attitudes regarding relationships, and the concept of social space. How one interacts with others is largely environmentally and culturally

TABLE 8-2. COMMUNICATION IN CONTEXT

SERVICE USER	EXAMPLE	COMMENT
Individuals who are monolingual are often treated in settings that do not routinely use their primary language.	A Spanish-speaking person being treated in an English-speaking clinic	The use of translators/interpreters is highly recommended but cannot take the place of direct clinician interaction with the client for building rapport; therefore, nonverbal communication is essential.
Individuals who may be bi- or multilingual may be treated in a setting that does not routinely use their primary language.	A Cantonese-speaking person known to have learned English as an adult and uses English when needed in routine community tasks	During times of stress, such as might occur during interactions with any authority figures (e.g., health care providers or police), it is typical for an individual to revert to the use of primary language and have difficulty with recently acquired language.
Individuals may speak the same primary language as the health care provider but use a colloquial form of the language not shared by the clinician.	An African American urban youth may have difficulty explaining personal experiences in terms understandable to the clinician and may resent the expectation to use "standard" English.	It is NOT acceptable for the clinician to attempt to use the colloquial form of the language if it is not part of his or her cultural identity. Rather than building rapport, this attempt will more likely be seen as ridicule.
Individuals may have limited or nonexistent language usage secondary to a perceived social climate.	Situations that may induce fear, suspicion, or paranoia, such as a recent arrest, political refugee status, or other concerns for personal safety	Clinicians need to take care not to over-pathologize behavior that, in fact, may be appropriate to the context.

CASE ILLUSTRATION 8-4: THE OCCUPATIONAL THERAPIST AND CULTURAL INTERPRETATION

Mary is an American occupational therapist working in Central America. She knows some Spanish, but not the indigenous dialect spoken here. Several of her clients insist on calling her "doctor." Each time, she feels an ethical responsibility to correct them, stating, "No, I'm the occupational therapist, not the doctor." The clients look puzzled but drop the subject.

Discussion

It could be that the clients don't know the role of the various health professionals, but more likely the problem lies in the literal translation of the language. In most countries throughout the world, there is a word (or words) for *healer* that often gets translated as *doctor*. The culture may not have the rigid regulations (e.g., years of schooling, licenses) that Americans assume entitles one to be called "doctor," but they do understand and respect the role of healers. These individuals would not feel comfortable using their native word for healer (e.g., *curandera*, *santeria*, *shaman*) because clearly the occupational therapist is not one of them.

determined. Embedded in one's culture are beliefs and attitudes regarding spirituality, family structure, gender roles, and health care. All of these affect relationships, choice of activity, and preferred environment.

Proxemics, a term coined by E. T. Hall (1966), is an aspect of culture that refers to people's use and comfort with personal and social space. For example, in some cultures it is acceptable and expected to touch frequently and to stand very close together in a conversation. However, in other cultures, this closeness would feel intrusive. Therapists must be aware of the cultural value of proxemics in their clients and adjust their interactions accordingly.

Box 8-1. Guidelines for Cross-Cultural Communication

- There are times when using a cultural or ethnic term is necessary for the preciseness of a particular topic in conversation. However, sometimes the use of qualifiers is its own form of bias. In a client-centered practice, it is important to not define a person by a label (e.g., Black, Latino).
- Make an attempt to identify a person as he or she wants to be identified, keeping in mind the generational, geographic, situational, and personal differences affecting choice of terms. (Do not make assumptions—ask!)
- Be sensitive to different cultural standards of speech, including rate of speech (fast or slow), acceptable volume, use of silence, appropriate response time, and order of speakers (amount of deference, acceptance of interruptions, or simultaneous multiple speakers).
- Be aware of use of time and acknowledgment of relationships. Clients may need to establish a social relationship prior to a professional relationship, which may not be viewed as productive time by the therapist.
- Be aware of posture and body language. Familiarize yourself with culturally acceptable use of eye contact, proximity of speakers, and hand gestures.

It may not be possible to have advanced knowledge of this particular cultural trait, but an occupational therapist with strong observation skills will take cues from the client and adapt to his or her sense of proximity. In mental health service, this becomes difficult because there are many space-related behaviors that are part of psychopathology. For example, someone who is experiencing paranoia or who has sensory processing problems may not want to have anyone near, let alone touching, him or her. Conversely, a person with a brain injury or psychotic disorder may lose sense of personal boundaries and act impulsively with touch. He or she will often not be able to pick up the subtle social cues that the behavior is inappropriate or is uncomfortable for another person. Each situation is unique, but the occupational therapist who has an understanding of cultural traits such as proxemics will be less likely to overpathologize behavior simply because it is different from his or her own.

Cultural values regarding relationships and space vary tremendously and must be taken into account when planning any aspect of intervention. For example, grooming in European-American culture is considered a private activity usually undertaken in the morning in one's bedroom or bathroom. However, in some cultures, such as among Latina women, grooming can be a very social activity, where helping each other with hair styles and makeup is considered highly desirable (Dillard et al., 1992). It is the responsibility of occupational therapists to educate themselves about the particular values and relationship styles of the cultural groups who may be the recipients of occupational therapy services. The degree of privacy is only one of several important values that must be considered in occupational therapy practice. Table 8-3 lists other common cultural values and provides examples and suggestions for the practitioner.

Time Sense

Although the importance of temporality has long been recognized in the occupational therapy literature, it must be acknowledged that particularly in the profession's early writings, the view of temporality was firmly embedded in Western society's concept of time. This view of temporality does not take into account the vastly different time sense or perception that is partially mediated in individuals by their culture. Some cultures value a future orientation, whereas others are firmly grounded in the present or past.

People in poverty tend to have a present sense of time, meaning that the day-to-day issues or crises must take priority over future plans; therefore, goal setting may be difficult or unrealistic for a person who may not know where the next meal is coming from. Because health care providers will typically be in a higher socioeconomic bracket than many of their clients, it is critical that an awareness of the effects of poverty on time sense be developed. This increased awareness will help occupational therapists negotiate realistic and manageable goals for their clients in poverty.

Hall (1976) suggests that the perception of time is not an inborn trait but rather determined by the culture or society. He classified time sense as being either *monochronic* (M-time) or *polychronic* (P-time). M-time societies view time as linear and rely on implicit or explicit scheduling. People in M-time societies also tend to view time as a commodity, as a thing that can be saved or lost, spent or wasted, or squandered or managed (Peloquin, 1991). However, P-time cultures do not share the same time values. P-time tends to be cyclical and unscheduled, typically a natural rhythm where several things can happen at once and not be controlled by human beings.

TABLE 8-3. CULTURAL VALUES

CULTURAL VALUE	COMMENTS AND SUGGESTIONS
Formality	Specific knowledge of a particular culture's value of formality will help clinicians decide how to introduce themselves, plan for treatment, address the client, and explain their role. For example, in some societies, it is expected to arrange appointments with another family member and be granted permission to proceed, whereas in others, the informality of arriving without notice is perfectly acceptable. Some cultures expect the use of formal titles, whereas others would see this type of communication as cold and distant.
Individuality	The emphasis in American culture and health care is to meet the needs of the individual. However, many cultures around the world value the needs and health of the family, or even the whole community, above the individual. When planning treatment, the occupational therapist should be cognizant of who else, besides the individual client, should be involved. It may include immediate or extended family as well as other members of the community.
Independence	Independence is highly valued in Western, particularly dominant American, culture. It is also highly emphasized within the professional culture of occupational therapy. However, in many cultures, caregiving is a strong and noble value, and there is no shame in having to be cared for. For some cultures, wanting a client to be independent is seen as selfish because family members would not be taking their expected responsibility to care for the person.
Locus of control	Many people around the world believe that what happens to them is out of their control, that either a greater spiritual power is in control or "things just happen." People with an external locus of control may not be willing to make a large investment (emotionally, financially, or otherwise) to change the course of their health. Occupational therapists tend to hold the value of internal locus of control and usually attempt to empower their clients to take responsibility for and control of their lives. The downside of this approach is that clients may feel guilt, shame, denial, or personal responsibility for their illness.
Authority	Respect for authority is common in many cultures. As occupational therapy moves more toward a client-centered approach, it is important to consider that many clients expect the therapist to be the expert and to know what's best for them. They may not feel comfortable in expressing their personal goals.

Working with a service user with a different time sense is one of the most frustrating aspects of working cross-culturally. Part of the frustration stems from not being aware that different time senses even exist. A culturally competent therapist first determines if the client's time sense is culturally different from what would be expected in the treatment setting or dominant culture. Otherwise, it is possible to erroneously assume a pathology or dysfunction that does not exist within the individual's cultural world. Case Illustration 8-5 shows how a culturally different time sense may affect the ability to delivery services.

In order for occupational therapists to provide culturally competent treatment to a diverse population, it is essential that the profession's beliefs about time be explored. Occupational therapy originally developed in an M-time society. Specifically, the middle- and upper-class values of the northeastern United States at the turn of the century greatly affected the development of occupational therapy as a profession. However, in today's multicultural environment, and with the growth of the profession around the world, occupational therapists must adapt to include, or at least recognize, the values of other societies. There are many implications for treatment when the therapist has a different time sense from the person receiving services. The demands for productivity in the workplace incorrectly equates the quantity of therapy with quality of intervention. The challenge for all health care providers is to somehow reconcile the pressure for productivity with the multicultural and individual perspectives and needs of service users.

CASE ILLUSTRATION 8-5: MR. MALIU'S PERCEPTION OF TIME

Mr. Maliu recently arrived in the United States from a small village in Samoa. He now lives with his brother's family, who arranged for his migration because they felt that he could receive better care in the United States for his longstanding mental illness. His brother arranged for an initial assessment at a county mental health office that also operates a day treatment center on site. Mr. Maliu arrived 2 hours late for his initial appointment and was asked to reschedule for another time. He was considerably late for the second appointment as well; however, the interviewing team, consisting of a psychiatrist, social worker, and occupational therapist, was able to accommodate him. He was accepted into the program but told that he would have to arrive on time to remain in the treatment group. He immediately established a pattern of late arrival to the group. Therefore, the treatment team is considering discharging him and referring him to outreach case management only. The conclusion of the treatment team is that he is perhaps too ill to benefit from the program at this time. Furthermore, his behavior is disruptive to the rest of the group.

Discussion

Time-related behaviors such as those displayed by Mr. Maliu may be due to symptoms of serious mental illness such as disorganization, disorientation, or avolition. However, care must be taken to avoid pathologizing behaviors that may be culturally appropriate. First and foremost, an understanding of the meaning of time to the client is essential to determine whether Mr. Maliu's behavior is related to his illness. If it is determined that his time sense is consistent with his cultural background and lifestyle, the treatment team has several options. It may indeed be in the client's and the group's best interest for him to receive individual treatment or case management initially. However, another approach would be to involve the family in a discussion of the norms, expectations, and benefits of group participation. If the client and his family saw the group treatment as desirable, then strategies such as telephone reminders and schedules or pairing him with a travel partner from the group could be developed to help Mr. Maliu adapt to the environment's expected time sense. Still another option open to the team is to simply let Mr. Maliu attend the program with late arrival. Clients are often more tolerant of flexible time schedules than professionals, and his late arrival may not be as disruptive as the team assumes.

SUMMARY

Cultural identity is a complex phenomenon partially based on race or ethnicity, but also influenced by myriad different factors. Furthermore, all aspects of the occupational therapy process must be tailored to address cultural nuances, with special attention to cultural variants such as communication styles, values and beliefs, and time sense.

REFERENCES

Abrams, L. S., & Molo, J. A. (2009). Critical race theory and the cultural competence dilemma in social work education. *Journal of Social Work Education, 45*(2), 245-261.

American Occupational Therapy Association. (2014). Occupational therapy practice framework: Domain and process (3rd ed.). *American Journal of Occupational Therapy, 68,* S1-S51.

American Occupational Therapy Association. (2015). Occupational therapy code of ethics (2015). *American Journal of Occupational Therapy, 69*(3), S1-S8.

American Occupational Therapy Association. (2017). Occupational therapy and complementary health approaches and integrative health. *American Journal of Occupational Therapy, 71*(Suppl. 2), 7112410020. doi:10.5014/ajot.2017. 716S08

Balcazar, F. E., Suarez-Balcazar, Y., & Taylor-Ritzler, T. (2009). Cultural competence: Development of a conceptual framework. *Disability and Rehabilitation, 31*(14), 1153-1160.

Bennett, M. J. (1993). Towards ethnorelatism: A developmental model of intercultural sensitivity. In R. M. Paige (Ed.), *Education for the intercultural experience* (pp. 21-72). Yarmouth, ME: Intercultural Press.

Castro, D., Dahlin-Ivanoff, S., & Mårtensson, L. (2016). Development of a cultural awareness scale for occupational therapy students in Latin America: A qualitative Delphi study. *Occupational Therapy International, 23*(2), 196-205.

Dillard, M., Andonian, L., Flores, O., Lai, L., MacRae, A., & Shakir, M. (1992). Culturally competent occupational therapy in a diversely populated mental health setting. *American Journal of Occupational Therapy, 46*(8), 721-726.

Grandpierre, V., Milloy, V., Sikora, L., Fitzpatrick, E., Thomas, R., & Potter, B. (2018). Barriers and facilitators to cultural competence in rehabilitation services: A scoping review. *BMC Health Services Research, 18*(23), 1-14.

Grant, J., Parry, Y., & Guerin, P. (2013). An investigation of culturally competent terminology in healthcare policy finds ambiguity and lack of definition. *Australian and New Zealand Journal of Public Health, 37,* 250-256. doi:10.1111/1753-6405.12067

Hall, E. T. (1966). *The hidden dimension.* Garden City, NY: Doubleday.

Hall, E. T. (1976). *Beyond culture.* Garden City, NY: Anchor/Doubleday.

Hammell, K. R. (2013). Occupation, well-being, and culture: Theory and cultural humility. *Canadian Journal of Occupational Therapy, 80*(4), 224-234. doi:10.1177/0008417413500465

Hammer, M. R. (2009). The Intercultural Development Inventory. In M. A. Moodian (Ed.), *Contemporary leadership and intercultural competence* (pp. 203-217). Thousand Oaks, CA: Sage.

Hammer, M. R. (2012). The Intercultural Development Inventory: A new frontier in assessment and development of intercultural competence. In M. Vande Berg, R. M. Paige, & K. H. Lou (Eds.), *Student learning abroad* (pp. 115-136). Sterling, VA: Stylus Publishing.

Ibeneme, S., Eni, G., Ezuma, A., & Fortwengel, G. (2017). Roads to health in developing countries: Understanding the intersection of culture and healing. *Current Therapeutic Research, 86,* 13-18.

Iwama, M. K. (2006a). *The Kawa Model: Culturally relevant occupational therapy.* Edinburgh, Scotland: Elsevier.

Iwama, M. K. (2006b). The Kawa Model as a window into client occupational therapy contexts: The case of Pedro Mendez. In M. K. Iwama (Ed.), *The Kawa Model: Culturally relevant occupational therapy* (pp. 180-184). Edinburgh, Scotland: Elsevier.

Kinébanian, A., & Stomph, M. (2009). Guiding principles on diversity and culture. *World Federation of Occupational Therapy (WFOT).* Retrieved from http://www.wfot.org/ResourceCentre/tabid/132/did/306/Default.aspx

Lim, K. H. (2006). The Kawa Model in mental health contexts: Two cases from the UK. In M. K. Iwama (Ed.), *The Kawa Model: Culturally relevant occupational therapy* (pp. 197-205). Edinburgh, Scotland: Elsevier.

McGregor, B., Renu, G., & Deepa, S. (2013). The perceptions of third culture kids of being different to children of their home country. *International Journal of Nursing Education, 5*(2), 122-126.

National Center for Complementary and Integrative Health. (2016). *Complementary, alternative, or integrative health: What's in a name?* Retrieved from https://nccih.nih.gov/health/integrative-health

Nugent, P. (2013). Cultural blindness. *Psychology Dictionary.* Retrieved from https://psychologydictionary.org/cultural-blindness

Peloquin, S. M. (1991). Time as commodity: Reflections and implications. *American Journal of Occupational Therapy, 45*(2), 147-154.

Rifkin, J. (2009). *The Empathic civilization: The race to global consciousness in a world in crisis.* New York, NY: Penguin Books.

Shefer, G., Rose, D., Nellums, L., Thornicroft, G., Henderson, C., & Evans-Lacko, S. (2012). 'Our community is the worst': The influence of cultural beliefs on stigma relationships with family and help-seeking in three ethnic communities in London. *International Journal of Social Psychiatry, 59*(6), 536-544.

Walters, K., & Auton-Cuff, F. (2009). A story to tell: the identity development of women growing up as third culture kids. *Mental Health, Religion & Culture, 12*(7), 755-772.

Watson, R. (2006). Being before doing: The cultural identity (essence) of occupational therapy. *Australian Occupational Therapy Journal, 53*(3), 151-158.

World Federation of Occupational Therapy. (2010). *Position statement: Diversity and culture.* Retrieved from http://www.wfot.org/ResourceCentre.aspx

World Health Organization. (2013). *Traditional Medical Strategy 2014-2023.* Retrieved from http://apps.who.int/iris/bitstream/handle/10665/92455/9789241506090_eng.pdf;jsessionid=E3AD2DE901C52D0D16FF4B928221842C?sequence=1

SUGGESTED RESOURCES

Academic Collaborative for Integrative Health: http://integrativehealth.org

The History of Ellis Island: http://www.history.com/topics/ellis-island

Intercultural Development Inventory: https://idiinventory.com

Kawa Model: http://www.kawamodel.com

National Center for Complementary and Integrative Health: https://nccih.nih.gov

National Center for Cultural Competence: https://nccc.georgetown.edu

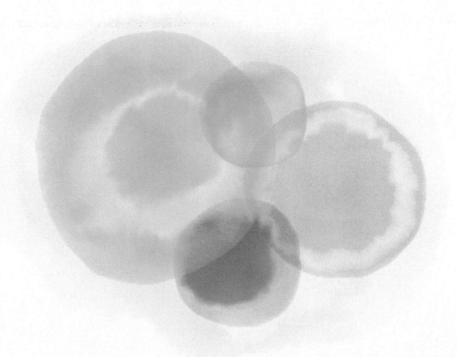

SECTION III

Mental Health Across the Lifespan

Mental Health of Infants
Attachment Through the Lifespan

Elizabeth Cara, PhD, OTR/L, MFT

Fieldwork students Benedict and Daneisha worked with emotionally disturbed teenagers in a special education program that included a program in early intervention. In this program, they realized how important psychosocial occupational therapy is, no matter which setting or age. While working with infants, Daneisha learned that you treat the entire family, not just infants. Both students illustrated why it is important to learn about attachment and how it infuses all of our work with infants, their caregivers, and the family system. Research in attachment theory has illustrated the influence of children's earliest experiences on their later development and has also shown that attachment disturbances are the root of many children's and adults' disorders.

Research in attachment relationships has shown the connections of early attachments to one's self-regulation, sense of self, and sense of later relationships. There has been an explosion of information about attachment theory and how it affects people throughout their lives, and attachment theory has spawned much research that is now occurring in many clinical programs. The attachment ideas include many theoretical frameworks and disciplines. Therefore, knowledge of attachment theory and research is important in clinical practice not only in early intervention, but in middle childhood, adolescence, and adulthood. Indeed, the research and popularity of attachment theory dictate that occupational therapists who work with all populations and in all settings have some knowledge of this exciting theory and practice.

HISTORY OF ATTACHMENT

John Bowlby was a psychoanalyst in England who, in the mid-20th century, first proposed in a series of seminal papers and books (1973, 1988a, 1988b) how infants developed into social and interactional human beings. It was no accident that Bowlby became interested in how infants manage their emotional and psychological world and focused on the infant-caregiver dyad because he himself had been raised by a nanny who left the family's employment when he was 7 years old. He was bereft after her loss and later realized that he possibly was more attached to his nanny than to his rather formal British parents (Bowlby, 2002).

Bowlby was influenced by contemporary psychological practice in England based on the theory of object relations, or how infants developed into self-contained emotionally and psychologically healthy young people and adults who felt self-worth, related to others, and adequately functioned in society. His beliefs about the reason for infants' ties to their mothers was different from the predominant psychoanalytic beliefs at the time that infants bonded with their caregivers because they were associated with the pleasure that accompanies being fed and satiated (Cassidy, 2016). He believed that the relationship was biologically based on the proximity of the infant to the mother, which guaranteed protection and the continuation of the species.

MacRae, A. (Ed.). *Cara and MacRae's Psychosocial Occupational Therapy:*
An Evolving Practice, Fourth Edition (pp 139-156).
© 2019 Taylor & Francis Group.

CASE ILLUSTRATION 9-1: JOEY AND HIS MOM—AN ATTACHMENT SYSTEM

Joey was 4 months old and had just woken up. He was wet and needed to be changed. His mother was in the room but not near him. He started to fidget, but she did not respond. He began to cry, and soon his mother was gazing at him, talking to him in a soothing manner, and lifting him to change him. His crying decreased and then stopped. As soon as he was changed, he and his mother cooed and gazed at each other.

Discussion

Joey and his mother demonstrated attachment behavior in a system that is evolutionary and also can be found in nonhuman primates.

He spoke of the *attachment system*, a behavioral concept from ethology (the study of primates in their environments and how they are influenced by their environment) and evolutionary theory (how "species-specific system behaviors" lead to certain predictable outcomes and contribute to survival and reproductive fitness [Cassidy, 2016]) involving "inherent motivation." In the attachment system, proximity seeking is activated when an infant receives information that a goal, the desired distance from the mother, is exceeded. The system remains activated until the goal is achieved. For example, an infant may sense that a caregiver is distracted and not tuned in when the infant needs to be soothed. Therefore, the infant may reach for the caregiver or fidget or begin to cry. Then, the caregiver will hopefully read the infant's signals that he or she needs soothing, give attention, and provide a response in tune with the infant's needs. Having received a satisfactory response, the infant will be soothed, and the proximity-seeking behavior will be terminated. The attachment system will then be deactivated. This system, if working as it should, represents behavioral homeostasis. The story of Joey in Case Illustration 9-1 demonstrates these principles.

Bowlby developed his theory of attachment based on psychoanalytic, evolutionary, and ethological ideas influenced by professionals from these different fields (Cassidy & Shaver, 2016). He particularly was influenced by Rene Spitz's film, *Grief: A Peril in Infancy* (1947); James Robertson's film, *A Two-Year-Old Goes to Hospital*; Harry Harlow's films of the effects of maternal deprivation on monkeys; and the films of Robert Hinde. This interdisciplinary perspective was important because research in ethology is naturalistic, and people are observed in their environments. Thus, Bowlby was aware of many rich observational studies that occurred during the 1930s and 1940s of the ill effects of prolonged institutionalization and mother-figure changes in early life on individual development.

During World War II, the Germans frequently bombed London. In order to protect their children, many parents sent their infants and toddlers out of London to nurseries in the countryside where loving people, some professional nurses and therapists, cared for the infants and toddlers. Psychoanalysts were observing these infants and children.

These observations led to scientific research of present and real attachment (ethological research) interactions instead of reconstructing them from an adult perspective (psychoanalytic research), as had been the case previously.

Bowlby was also commissioned to investigate the factors that led to juvenile delinquency. He concluded via case study combined with statistical methods that delinquency was generated partly by parents' inconsistent, absent, or abusive behavior (Cassidy, Jones, & Shaver, 2013). (True to the context of that decade, mothers were studied, but male partner abusive behavior was also researched.)

Bowlby was appointed a special consultant to the World Health Organization in 1950 to contribute to a United Nations study of the needs of homeless children. He described this as a golden opportunity because he was able to read and discuss the literature with many other researchers, and he employed a social worker, James Robertson, who had trained with Anna Freud at her nurseries and who used video to observe infants and children during separation. The result of his work was a report in a monograph titled *Maternal Care and Mental Health*. He found that the evidence "regarding the adverse influences on personality development of inadequate maternal care during early childhood and ... the acute distress of children who find themselves separated from those they know and love [was] ... far from negligible" (Bowlby, 1988a, p. 21; 1988b).

An American psychologist, Mary Ainsworth, later collaborated with Bowlby, and she developed a formal research method to research situations where infants and toddlers were separated from their caregivers and then reunited with them. This famous research study, called the *Strange Situation* (Salter Ainsworth & Bell, 1970), operationalized Bowlby's concepts about attachment and spawned many future studies of attachment in several different countries with many different age groups (Mesman, Van IJzendoorn, & Sagi-Schwartz, 2016). As stated by Slade and Aber (1992):

[A]ttachment theory offers a set of testable hypotheses about the nature of development and ... offers a means of systematically evaluating a variety of modes of clinical interventions ... clearly [it] provides a new framework for observing preverbal and early representational processes and making

TABLE 9-1. PHASES OF ATTACHMENT

CHRONOLOGICAL AGE	DEVELOPMENTAL BEHAVIOR
Birth to 2 to 3 months	Preference for attachment figure
2 to 3 months to 7 months	Discrimination for attachment figure
7 months to 3+ years	More active physical proximity seeking; internal working models develop; functions of system appear (maintenance of proximity, having a safe haven, developing a secure base from which to explore; stages of emotions in response to separation
3+ years	Goal-directed partnership; aware of other's perspective; joint activities and plans; psychological proximity seeking

valid inferences about the child's subjective experience on the basis of these observables. (p. 180)

Bowlby suggested that the earliest years of life are critical for later development. Attachment theory provides a reasonable explanation of how an attachment bond is formed, how attachment behaviors are developed and used in parenting or caregiving, and how a sense of self in relationships and interactional patterns is developed. Attachment theory provides the biological and evolutionary component of how an infant develops psychologically and becomes a healthy adult, positing attachment behaviors as evolutionarily adaptive for survival. Attachment theory and Ainsworth's later research studies delineate the types of attachments and attachment behaviors that are optimal for the infant-parent dyad and that predict later functioning in the relationships and social world. More contemporary attachment theorists focus less on the dyad and more on multi-caregiver relationships, as well as how attachment bonds affect children, adolescents, and adults and their relationships and adaptive functioning in response to traumatic and adverse environments or events.

WHAT IS ATTACHMENT EXACTLY?

Attachment theory states that the infant is predisposed at birth to form a selective attachment relationship with one or a few caretaking adults (Ainsworth, 1967, 1977; Bowlby, 1973, 1988a, 1988b; Bretherton & Waters, 1985; Salter Ainsworth & Bell, 1970; Slade & Aber, 1992; Sroufe & Waters, 1977). Over the course of the phylogenic development, human and nonhuman primates evolved built-in behavioral systems that enabled attachment to occur. These systems are called *attachment behaviors.*

The pattern of attachment consistent with healthy development is that of secure attachment, in which the individual is confident that his parent (or parent-figure) will be available, responsive, and

helpful should he encounter adverse or frightening situations. With this assurance, he feels bold in his explorations of the world and also competent in dealing with it. (Bowlby, 1988b, p. 167)

The attachment behaviors are those verbal gestures such as crying, cooing, laughing, and other language and those nonverbal gestures such as taking initiative, reaching, looking, smiling, approaching, and turn taking (Atkinson et al., 2008). They are behaviors that indicate showing affection, seeking comfort, cooperating, asking for help, exploring, controlling, and reuniting with caregivers (Champagne, 2011). The type of attachment cannot be inferred from any particular behavior but must be considered according to patterns and context.

The biological goal of the attachment behavioral system is proximity to the caregiver. This establishes what Ainsworth later called the *feeling of security, felt security,* or *psychological goal.* The system is a goal-corrected feedback system; when the infant is feeling secure and safe by virtue of proximity to the caregiver, the need to signal the mother, or the attachment behavioral system, is deactivated. The infant is then free to explore his or her environment. When the infant needs comfort, when there is a perception of the mother being distant or she really is distant, the attachment behavioral system is activated in the form of attachment behaviors, such as crying, crawling, and so on.

PHASES OF ATTACHMENT

There are developmental phases in attachment throughout the lifespan (Simpson & Belsky, 2016), but particularly in infancy and toddlerhood. See Table 9-1 for age-appropriate phases and behavior; also see Case Illustration 9-2.

Emotions and cognitions are associated with attachment. Many emotions arise during the formation, maintenance, disruption, and renewal of attachment bonds. Positive emotions are associated with attachment, and

CASE ILLUSTRATION 9-2: A MOTHERS' GET-TOGETHER—DEVELOPMENTAL AND ATTACHMENT BEHAVIORS IN ATTACHMENT SYSTEMS

A new mothers' group met each week at the local café. They met each week with their children, but the primary purpose was to provide a social outlet to young mothers. Jackie's daughter was 2.5 months, Alexandra's daughter was 2 months, Consuela's son was 6 months, and Uyen's son was 2 years and her daughter was 3.5 years. Jackie's and Alexandra's daughters occasionally gestured and made noises, and they responded happily to any member who attended to them. Consuela's son would not stop reaching unless Consuela responded with a verbal or nonverbal affirmation. When Uyen got up to get another latte, her son became distressed, looked for her, and began to cry, whereas her daughter watched her and continued to play contentedly with her toys.

Discussion

Each child demonstrated different attachment behavior according to different stages of development.

---

negative emotions are associated with loss of attachment. The cognitive components are mental representations of the self, the attachment figure, and the environment, and they are based on actual experiences of the infant (Cassidy, 2016). These components act in a dynamic balance and infants develop *internal working models* (IWMs) of self and others in relationship. These IWMs will then guide the developing individual throughout life.

INTERNAL WORKING MODELS

IWMs are representations of past interactions and allow predicting future experience (Cassidy et al., 2013; Slade & Aber, 1992). An infant's sense of secure self and perception as self-as-worthy are derived from the attachment interaction with caregivers. If the infant comes to expect security and comfort through the caregiver's availability, the infant will internalize these expectations as scripts and stories or, in other words, form internal mental representations of the availability of others and the worthiness of self. If the infant comes to expect that caregivers will be unavailable and/or rejecting, then IWMs or beliefs about the self, others, and relationships will be insecure and not worthy.

Infants rely on these IWMs to make decisions about how to behave in specific situations with specific persons. Thus, IWMs will influence later sense of self, interactions, and relationships and, most importantly, one's ability to parent or develop satisfactory attachment behaviors and patterns with one's own infants.

IWMs have a "central role in adaptive human development to supportive interpersonal relationships" (Bretherton & Munholland, 2016). Importantly for occupational therapists, Bowlby was influenced by Piaget when he described IWMs as *sensorimotor-affective representations* that become increasingly complex and mentally flexible and enable simple short-term predictions and later reflection on current,

past, and future relationships. He considered these representations as being developed through the senses (in early infancy), and the end result was "mental model building" (in toddlerhood, childhood, and adulthood). Bowlby elaborated on the importance of the senses in the formation of IWMs:

> Every situation we meet with in life is construed in terms of the representational models we have of the world about us and of ourselves. Information reaching us through our sense organs is selected and interpreted in terms of those models. ... On how we interpret and evaluate each situation ... turns also how we feel. (Bowlby, 1980, cited in Bretherton & Munholland, 2008, p. 103)

> Starting ... towards the end of his first year and probably especially actively during his second and third when he acquires the powerful and extraordinary gift of language, a child is busy constructing working models of how the physical world may be expected to behave, how his mother and other significant persons may be expected to behave, how he himself may be expected to behave, and how each interacts with the other. (Bowlby, 1969/1982, cited in Bretherton & Munholland, 2016, p. 103)

In summary, IWMs are the mental representations originally developed in attachment relationships that, through the senses, become more cognitively complex as the infant develops. The mental models are of the interactions that an infant has with his or her caregiver and will dictate how the infant, child, or adult feels and behaves about him- or herself, about others in the environment, and in romantic attachments. The IWMs will influence cognitive development and how the infants, children, and later adults will parent their own children. The IWMs are a person's psychological and social building blocks that enable secure, healthy development.

TABLE 9-2. THE STRANGE SITUATION	
SEQUENTIAL STEP	**SITUATION**
1.	Mother, infant, researcher enter room
2.	Researcher leaves; mother and infant alone
3.	Stranger (researcher) joins mother and infant
4.	Infant and stranger alone; mother leaves
5.	Stranger leaves; mother returns
6.	Infant alone; mother leaves
7.	Stranger returns
8.	Mother returns; stranger leaves

Adapted from McLeod, S. (2018). *Mary Ainsworth.* Retrieved from http://www.simplypsychology.org/mary-ainsworth.html; Salter Ainsworth, M. D., & Bell, S. M. (1970). Attachment, exploration and separation: Illustrated by the behavior of one-year-olds in a strange situation. *Child Development, 41*(1), 49-67.

CATEGORIES OF ATTACHMENT: EVIDENCE BASE OF ATTACHMENT

Mary Ainsworth expanded research on the identification of how infants and, later, children and adults actually are attached in an experiment known as the *Strange Situation* (Salter Ainsworth & Bell, 1970). The research is presented in detail here because it is the evidence for the existence of attachment styles and is known universally, as well as being a model for infant research.

The Strange Situation

The aim of this experiment was to assess separation and stranger anxiety and the reaction of the infant when reunited with a caregiver. In the original experiment, all of the caregivers were the infants' mothers. The assessment took place in a room with a one-way mirror so that observers could watch the behavior of fifty-six 12- to 18-month-old infants with their parent or with a stranger. There were eight situations, each of which was 3 minutes long. Table 9-2 lists the eight situations.

The room was set up so that there were three chairs: at one end, a baby's chair filled with toys; at another end, the mother's chair; and at the other end near the door, the stranger's chair. The baby was free to roam (and its locomotion and location marked) in a triangle of space demarcated by the three chairs.

The 3-minute episodes were designed in the following ways:

- In episode #1, the researcher and a mother with her baby enter the room.

- In episode #2, the mother put the baby down, then sat in her chair unless her baby sought her attention.

- In episode #3, the stranger entered and sat for 1 minute, then spoke for 1 minute with the mother, then approached the baby, showing him or her a toy.

- In episode #4, if the baby happily engaged in play, then the stranger did not participate; if the baby was not active, the stranger attempted to engage him or her; if the baby was distressed, the stranger attempted comfort; or the situation was terminated if the baby was inconsolable.

- In episode #5, the mother entered and stopped at the door so that her baby could organize a response to her; the stranger left, and, when baby was happily playing, the mother left again, but this time waved and said, "Bye-bye."

- In episode #6, the baby was left alone to play, but the situation was terminated if the baby was in distress.

- In episode #7, the stranger entered with the same script as in episode #4.

- In episode #8, the mother returned, the stranger left, and reunion behavior took place.

Methods

Two observers, independent of each other, observed the situation. In the first subsample, another person took notes, and in the second subsample, the observer was recorded. Then, the researchers took frequency counts of the occurrence of certain behaviors and coded for classes of behaviors using a 7-point scale. The classes of behaviors were those that we consider attachment behaviors and are listed in Table 9-3.

TABLE 9-3. BEHAVIORS OBSERVED IN THE STRANGE SITUATION

CATEGORIES OF BEHAVIORS	EXAMPLES OF BEHAVIORS
Proximity and contact seeking	Approaching, clambering up, reaching, leaning, directed cries
Contact maintaining	Embracing, clinging, holding on, clutching, vocal protest
Proximity and interaction avoiding	In a situation that ordinarily elicits greeting, ignoring, looking, turning, or moving away
Contact and interaction resisting	Attempts to push away, angry screaming, throw self or toys, kicking, pouting, cranky, fussing, or petulance
Searching	Following mother to door, opening or banging door, looking at or going to mother's chair

Adapted from Salter Ainsworth, M. D., & Bell, S. M. (1970). Attachment, exploration and separation: Illustrated by the behavior of one-year-olds in a strange situation. *Child Development, 41*(1), 49-67.

CASE ILLUSTRATION 9-3: FATHER AND SON—AN ATTACHMENT SYSTEM AT RISK

Michael, an early interventionist, observed a father playing with his son. Michael noticed that the father was not quite comfortable with playing and did not understand reciprocal behavior or his son's gestures. Dad would sometimes not engage in play, even though his son reached for him, and sometimes when his son reached for his toy, his father would grab it and show him how to play with it, then press it into his hand and say, "Now you do it." His son would throw the toy and turn his head, and Dad would become exasperated.

Discussion

Dad was not yet attuned to his son's behavior and did not know how to play with his son. He presented conflicting behavior that was not responsive or overly responsive, and his son reacted with avoidance. If this behavior developed into a pattern, his son would be at risk for an insecure-avoidant attachment.

Results

From the results of the Strange Situation procedure, the researchers determined that there were three general attachment styles: (1) secure, (2) ambivalent (*contact resistant*; also later named *anxious-ambivalent* or *resistant*), and (3) defensive (*proximity avoidant*; also later named *anxious-avoidant* or *avoidant*). Observations were as follows:

- In a secure attachment, the infant used the caregiver as a secure base from which to explore; in a resistant attachment, the infant cried more and explored less; and in an avoidant attachment, the infant was accepting of comfort from both the caregiver and the stranger equally.
- Separation anxiety: In a secure attachment, the infant was appropriately distressed when the caregiver left; in a resistant attachment, the infant was intensely distressed; and in an avoidant attachment, the infant was not at all distressed.

- Stranger anxiety: In a secure attachment, when the caregiver was present, the infant was friendly, but when the caregiver was not present, the infant avoided the stranger. In a resistant attachment, the infant feared and avoided the stranger; and in an avoidant attachment, the infant was okay with the stranger or displayed normal play behavior with the stranger.
- Reunion behavior: In a secure attachment, the infant was happy and positive with the caregiver; in a resistant attachment, the infant resisted or pushed the caregiver away; and in an avoidant attachment, the infant was not interested in the caregiver.

The researchers concluded that the three attachment styles were determined by the caregivers' behavior. Case Illustration 9-3 describes the at-risk relationship of a father and son.

Later, a student of Ainsworth's, Mary Main, along with her colleagues, researched adults' patterns. These experiments provided evidence for Bowlby's original hypothesis that early attachment is related to later behaviors. Research

TABLE 9-4. PATTERNS OF ATTACHMENT

PATTERN	STRATEGIES
Secure	Reciprocal (proximity seeking or attachment and exploration) interactions: Caregiver provides warm, attuned, responsive caring and infant straightforward in eliciting protection and free to explore = positive expectations, trust, healthy selves, and relationships
Insecure-Resistant[a] Anxious/Ambivalent (originally Ambivalent)	Inconsistent interactions: Caregiver provides demanding, erratic caring and infants maximize behavior, resist soothing, comforting = negative expectations, distrust, depleted selves, and erratic relationships
Insecure-Avoidant[a] Anxious/Avoidant (originally Defensive)	Unresponsive interactions: Caregiver provides unresponsive or overstimulating caring, less contact and infants minimize behavior, avoid soothing and comforting = negative expectations, distrust, overly reliant selves, and empty relationships
Disorganized	Unsafe interactions: Caregiver provides disorganized, bizarre, off-cue caring and infants disorganized, fearful, coercive behavior = negative expectations, distrust, incoherent selves, and fear relationships
Disinhibited	Indiscriminate interactions: Caregiver provides no care and infants unable to selectively bond = negative expectations, incoherent, erratic selves, and socially indiscriminate relationships
Inhibited	Failure to attach: Caregiver provides no care and infants unable to bond, withdrawn = negative expectations, incoherent selves, no relationships

[a]The styles were renamed over time.

Adapted from Berlin, L. J., Ziv, Y., Amaya-Jackson, L., & Greenberg, M. T. (Eds.). (2005). *Enhancing early attachments: Theory, research, intervention, and policy*. New York, NY: Guilford; Brandell, J., & Ringel, S. (2007). *Attachment and dynamic practice: An integrative guide for social workers and other clinicians*. New York, NY: Columbia University Press; Karen, R. (1994). *Becoming attached: Unfolding the mystery of the infant mother bond and its impact on later life*. New York, NY: Warner Books; McLeod, S. (2018). *Mary Ainsworth*. Retrieved from http://www.simplypsychology.org/mary-ainsworth.html; Salter Ainsworth, M. D., & Bell, S. M. (1970). Attachment, exploration and separation: Illustrated by the behavior of one-year-olds in a strange situation. *Child Development, 41*(1), 49-67; Simpson, J. A., & Belsky, J. (2016). Attachment theory within a modern evolutionary framework. In J. Cassidy & P. R. Shaver (Eds.), *Handbook of attachment: Theory, research, and clinical applications* (3rd ed., pp. 91-116). New York, NY: Guilford.

continues that explores which attachment patterns in adults predict attachment patterns in their children and in romance and intimate partner attachment (Cassidy & Shaver, 2016) and the effects of attachment styles on various populations, including schizophrenia (Harder, 2014), anorexia (Delvecchio, DiRiso, Salcuni, Lis, & George, 2014), depression (Diamond, Reis, Diamond, Siqueland, & Isaacs, 2002), and pain and chronic illness.

THE PATTERNS OF ATTACHMENT

Bowlby's theory and Ainsworth's research initiated rich studies of attachment in all ages (Cassidy & Shaver, 2016). Generally, with more research, more styles have been delineated (Table 9-4). Attachment concepts have permeated other fields, and the significance of the attachment system and attachment behaviors is universally recognized.

CROSS-CULTURAL STUDIES

Ainsworth (1967) first developed her classification system of attachment in Uganda, and her later study in the United States (1977) replicated the earlier one. Her first study established some important principles of attachment and raised some important cross-cultural issues, including (1) the universality of the infant-mother attachment and classification system, (2) the crucial role of maternal sensitivity as an antecedent to attachment, and (3) the contextual dimension of attachment, such as having multiple caregivers. Thus, attachment theory posits that in all Western countries, infants become attached to one or more specific caregivers (the *universality hypothesis*), the majority of infants are securely attached in Western cultures (the *normativity hypothesis*), secure attachment depends on the caregivers' sensitive and consistent responses (the *sensitivity hypothesis*), and attachment security yields differences in children's abilities to regulate their emotions; develop healthy relationships with peers, teachers, and later romantic partners; and develop cognitive competence (the competence hypothesis; Mesman et al., 2016).

There have been cross-cultural studies in other non-Western countries, including Kenya, Nigeria, Mali, Botswana, Zambia, and South Africa, in both urban and hunter-gatherer societies. These studies have confirmed the maternal sensitivity and universality hypotheses and that sensitive caregiver responses lead to independence rather than dependence. In China, where interdependence is considered a major social difference from Western societies and a social policy of only one child per family exists, studies also confirmed the universality hypothesis (Cassidy et al., 2013).

Studies of attachment in Japan present different results. Japan itself can be considered a challenge to attachment research due to alternative ideas of relatedness. Specifically, in Japan there is a concept called *amae*, which describes the attachment bond as inherently psychologically dependent, unlike the claims of attachment in Western society (Mesman et al., 2016; Young-Bruehl & Bethelard, 2002). Therefore, it is difficult to evaluate attachment in Japan, but this different cultural idea provides a unique opportunity to further expand on the attachment concept.

Overall, "the evidence for the cross-cultural validity of attachment theory is impressive and the universality hypothesis appears to be supported most strongly. The cross-cultural studies … support Bowlby's … idea that attachment is indeed a universal phenomenon, and an evolutionary explanation seems to be warranted" (Cassidy et al., 2013, p. 897). However, the sensitivity and competence hypotheses are less supported, with the most important disconfirming evidence being the Japanese studies. The three attachment categories are universal and found in every culture studied; however, the strategies are contextually different and naturally adaptive. There appears to be pressure toward general selection of a secure attachment in all cultures studied. Other cultures have confirmed that there are multi-caregiving societies, so attention in the future should be paid to social networks of caregiving.

To summarize, three hypotheses regarding attachment that have been supported by cross-cultural research are as follows: (1) secure attachment is the most prevalent one in all cultures and is viewed as the most desirable by all, (2) maternal sensitivity does influence infant attachment patterns, and (3) secure attachment predicts cognitive and social competence (Cassidy et al., 2013).

ATTACHMENT AND AFFECT REGULATION

An explanation of attachment that relates directly to occupational therapists is the fact that attachment allows the ability to develop self-regulation and coping skills. An understanding of attachment and how it relates to affect regulation will position the occupational therapy practitioner to attend to attachment behavior in settings where infants and toddlers are treated. The quality of attachment is important for infants and children to develop organizing and self-regulating patterns of behavior (Cassidy & Shaver, 2016) and ultimately prosocial behavior (Narvaez & Gleason, 2012). Infants develop the ability to organize emotions and to regulate their emotions within the caregiver-infant dyad.

> A securely attached child is able to use the caregiver as a safe haven when in distress (i.e., return of positive mood), and the child is then able to return to exploration of the environment. Furthermore, it is hypothesized that securely attached children internalize effective ways to cope with stress and are consequently resilient when coping with problems, even in the absence of the caregiver. (Kerns, 2008, p. 375)

Although it is hypothesized that there is a strong correlation between quality of attachment and regulation, there are few studies of emotional regulation in childhood. However, the field of neurobiology holds promise for explaining how emotional regulation develops.

Interpersonal Neurobiology

From birth, the developing relationship between infants and their parents help them to regulate arousal, excitement, or discomfort. It has been suggested that attachment theory is really a regulatory theory, one that reflects the plastic, experience-dependent nature of the brain (Papousek, 2011; Schore, 2000, 2010, 2016). Recent advances in the neurosciences and neuroimaging are beginning to reveal how parent-child relationships carried out during life's daily activities and based in the earliest attachment processes are influencing brain structure and physiology. These structural and functional changes in the brain influence self-regulation and interpersonal relationships throughout life (Cozolino, 2006; Schore, 2000, 2010, 2016; Siegel, 2012).

Neglect and trauma cause the person who is neglected or traumatized by consistent parental misattunement or separation to be in a constant state of hyperarousal with an inability to regulate emotions (Corbin, 2007; Creeden, 2009). Early stress and trauma disturb sleep and rest and also interfere with the amygdala, the brain structure responsible for symbolic memory, both implicit (unconscious) and explicit (available to consciousness).

ATTACHMENT AND TRAUMA

Attachment theorists suggest that abuse and particularly neglect lead to problems in attachment and later pathology. In particular, problems in attachment lead to *reactive attachment disorder* (RAD) or *disinhibited social engagement disorder* (DSED) as defined in the *Diagnostic and Statistical Manual of Mental Disorders, 5th edition* (American Psychiatric Association, 2013). In RAD, one may be inhibited or withdrawn and unable to form attachments with any one person. In DSED, one may be disinhibited or forming attachments with any person indiscriminately, regardless of attachment history (American Psychiatric Association, 2013). However, it has been suggested that both may be more fluid, and perhaps this behavior is adaptive in institutions (Hardy, 2007).

Foster Care and Institutionalization

Institutionalized children face many obstacles to healthy attachment. In the United States, in 2016 there were at least 437,465 children in foster care (Adoption and Foster Care Analysis and Reporting System, 2017), and usually they are separated from caregivers due to neglect or abuse during the period when developing attachment bonds is most important, that is, from age 0 to 3 years (Dozier & Rutter, 2016). Approximately 15% of children who are removed are placed in group homes where there may be up to 11 children. Research has established that such group care has a deleterious effect on the healthy development of children. Many also stay in foster care for longer than 2 years, and approximately half of those are reunited with their birth families. Of that half, 28% return to foster care within 3 years. Typically, experiences prior to foster care are depriving, neglectful, or abusive. Outside of the United States, many infants and toddlers have lengthy stays in institutions and also face neglect and abuse and miss opportunities to develop attachment bonds (Dozier & Rutter, 2016).

Adoption

Occupational therapy practitioners treat adopted infants and children and their families, and knowledge of the challenges that adopted children and families face may enable better practice. Some children are adopted either from the foster care system (domestic adoption) or from foreign institutions (international adoption). Those who are adopted within 1 year of age may be quicker to develop attachment bonds with adoptive parents than those adopted after 1 year of age. Although children may be adopted and provided with loving caregivers, there are still difficulties that could occur depending on the vulnerabilities of the child and the state of mind of the caregivers who adopt. Those adopted from institutions have higher rates of disorganized attachments and indiscriminate attachment behaviors, and, whether from foster care or an institution, children with insecure attachment often elicit rejecting behaviors from new caregivers.

Although statistics about children from foster care and institutions can be discouraging, there is some good news that a large number of adopted children do not display the same patterns of insecure or disorganized attachment, and even those with severe neglect and abuse may dramatically catch up with their healthy peers. Those who do not develop maladaptive attachments may be more resilient temperamentally, may be less vulnerable (e.g., they were not born of a substance abusing parent), and may have been institutionalized for less than 6 months. The children may have been placed with caregivers who have secure attachments and who are able to understand the multiple attachment problems that their children bring, and foster parents may display a strong commitment to their adopted children (Dozier & Rutter, 2016).

As will be described later in this chapter, interventions may be crafted to support parents to understand and respond to their children's attachment signals and to assist in regulating emotions and rest and sleep. As well, interventions can aid children with RAD and DSED and attachment problems to understand appropriate behavior and to become more sensitive to others, as well as to understand their own arousal needs and ways of dealing with them.

Children Who Are Atypical

Research with mixed results has been conducted on attachment in relationships with an infant or child who has a disability. Children with autism, both preschool age and older, can develop attachments despite social interaction deficits; however, they are more insecure attachments than those in children with typical development or with other developmental disorders (Rutgers, Bakermans-Kranenburg, van Ijzendoorn, & van Berckelaer-Onnes, 2004; Rutgers et al., 2007). There is also a higher percentage of disorganized attachment. However, attachment may be more secure in those with higher mental functions. Although these studies indicated that there is a higher percentage of insecure attachments, the parents did not report more stress than is usually associated with parenting a child with autism disorders.

CLINICAL PROGRAMS THAT FOCUS ON ATTACHMENT

Since the previous edition of this text, rigorous evidence has documented the lasting positive effects of intervention programs (Berlin, Zeanah, & Lieberman, 2016). The area of intervention that is most successful consists of intervening with the internal working models of the caregiver or with parenting behaviors. Also, it is important for the practitioner to serve as a secure base for the parent. Although occupational therapy practitioners may not be working directly on attachment behaviors, they could serve as models of secure attachment in gaining trust with parents, as well as models of behavior that will facilitate or strengthen internal working models of secure attachment. Examples include supporting parents with an empathic approach and in all of their stressful daily activities or promoting routines and rituals that indicate care and respect in a consistent manner in all interactions or sessions. They could also intervene in parental behaviors by suggesting how parents could behave with their infants or children in play or care activities such as feeding and toileting.

The successful program's treatment strategies include one or more of three therapeutic tasks: (1) targeting the parents' IWMs, (2) targeting the parenting behavior, and (3) developing or modeling a treating professional-parent relationship (Berlin et al., 2016). In the first task, the intervener helps the caregiver gain insight into his or her own internal models of self and other, with the goal of helping the parent recognize how the past strategies interfere with current interactions. In the second task, the intervener helps the caregiver develop a capacity for reflection on interactions with their child. Thus, the parent can interpret the child's behavior differently. The parent learns that there are two primary parenting tasks: to provide closeness as a response to the child's attachment needs and autonomy as a response to the child's exploration needs. In the third strategy, the parent learns that there could be a caring and mutual supportive relationship; therefore, new attachments can develop, and the parent can then develop a different attachment relationship with his or her child. Research has supported various intense programs that last longer than 1 year or are of a 10- to 20-week duration, as well as brief, three- to four-session programs.

Child-Parent Psychotherapy

In child-parent psychotherapy, the patient is the infant-parent dyad, and the clients are most often impoverished and traumatized families. Based on infant-parent psychotherapy, developed by Selma Fraiberg (1980, 1982), child-parent psychotherapy is a manualized intervention for toddlers between birth and 5 years that incorporates the goals of improving caregivers' capacity for insight, reflection, and an empathic relationship and adds a focus on caregivers' current stressful lives and cultural values (Berlin et al., 2016). Often the therapists are masters- and PhD-level students who are trained rigorously in the interventions. The programs usually include weekly interventions that take place in the home or program playroom. Some are long term, over 1 year or more, and begin when caregivers are pregnant. Others are briefer but just as intense and focus on didactic sessions regarding the caregivers' parenting skills

and understanding of attachment and attachment behaviors, their own and their children's.

Video-Feedback Intervention to Promote Positive Parenting

A short-term program that includes four to six sessions of 90 minutes each targeted to parents is the Video-Feedback Intervention to Promote Positive Parenting (Juffer et al., as cited in Berlin et al., 2016). This program uses video of in-home interactions between caregivers and children. Essentially, such programs provide here-and-now graphic feedback reviewed with interveners that enables parents to see how their behaviors influence their children and are able to modify them accordingly to promote positive attachment behaviors and reciprocal interaction. An adaptation of the program emphasizes positive discipline for those children who show behavioral problems. Although occupational therapists will not necessarily use video-feedback of their sessions, they can access some strategies to use with caregivers to promote attachment behaviors.

Attachment and Biobehavioral Catch-Up

This program is for children who have experienced early adversity, and it is often used with foster parents. Trained parent-coaches make 10 visits weekly that last 1 hour. Each session focuses on a specific topic and incudes the parent-child dyad and a video of mother-infant interactions. It emphasizes nurturance, following the child's lead, and reducing frightening caregiver behavior. It specifies that the coach should (preferably) positively comment for each minute of the session. There are various themes in the session that address an infant's defensive behavior, being aware of the parent's own histories that may predispose him or her to negative responses, and parenting responses (Berlin et al., 2016).

The Circle of Security

This program consists of weekly individual or group sessions for parents that focus on *relationship capacities* via teaching attachment theory and research to the parents and assisting them to reflect on their own histories and attachment behavior. A core graphic is used to depict key ideas of attachment theory, children's need for connection and autonomy, and parenting behavior to support those. Another core is a metaphor for children's behavior for the parents called *shark music*. This can be considered a psychoeducational strategy that targets IWMs and misattuned behavior and also educates regarding their children's needs (Berlin et al., 2016).

OCCUPATIONAL THERAPY TREATMENT GUIDED BY PROGRAMS THAT PROMOTE ATTACHMENT

Some useful treatment ideas that emerge in these programs can be incorporated by occupational therapists. In the evaluation process, the infant-parent therapist uses observation skills and introspection (Lieberman & Pawl, 1993). The therapist observes how the infant functions developmentally and emotionally and how the parent experiences or responds to the infant while observing their interaction. Families who are observed usually have a negative idea of the outside bureaucracy that purports to work with them, so the therapist also reflects on the possibility of forming a therapeutic relationship (Kyler, 2008; Schultz-Krohn & Cara, 2000). Occupational therapists can use their own reflective and introspective skills and feelings to get an idea of how their clients might respond to their children, as well as an idea of the cultural family-centered treatment that may be necessary.

Two principles of infant-parent psychotherapy can be incorporated into occupational therapy services and interactions (Lieberman & Pawl, 1993; Seligman, 1994). *Nondidactic developmental guidance* is a method that assumes that the caregiver is the best to use information about his or her child, considering the relationship and emotions between the caregiver and child. The therapist encourages the parent to view the infant's behavior in a way that interrupts viewing the infant from the parent's own negative experiences. This intervention is accomplished not by giving advice, but by questioning or asking the caregiver's observation or experience of what is happening right then. This intervention aims to support a change in behavior as well as the caregiver's perspectives. For example, a toddler may fuss and cry and push away from a parent, but the parent refuses to let the toddler go or to acknowledge the toddler because he or she doesn't want to "spoil the child." A therapist might question the parent by asking, "What do you think will happen if you do acknowledge your child's needs?" Alternatively, the therapist might remark on the active exploration and curiosity of the child. In this way, the therapist does not negate the parent's perspective and may provide a different way of thinking about the child and interaction.

Support and advocacy are activities that support the infant-caregiver relationship (Lieberman & Pawl, 1993). This support provides a role model of a caring relationship that can be emulated by the parent with the infant. These are often concrete interventions that provide relief and also hope for often bedraggled caregivers. For example, a parent may not have enough money to buy diapers, so the therapist may find public health programs that are able to donate diapers. In an incident experienced by the author, a parent was becoming agitated because she did not have a dresser. The author serendipitously found a dresser left on the street that was free for anyone to take and picked it up, drove it to the client's home, and helped the client move the dresser into her home. Occupational therapists provide such advocacy and education.

An occupational therapist recognizes the co-occupations of caregiver and child (American Occupational Therapy Association, 2014), and the *Occupational Therapy Practice Framework* addresses the interacting cultural worlds of the practitioner and family. The occupational therapist uses what he or she learns about the habits, routines, and rituals of the caregiver and child (Kellegrew, 2000; Larson, 2000).

The infant mental health therapist offers support and does whatever is needed to bolster the infant-parent relationship. Likewise, occupational therapy's domain (American Occupational Therapy Association, 2014) specifies advocacy as an outcome and suggests that occupational justice could be a goal of treatment. Whereas the infant mental health therapist offers nondidactic guidance, occupational therapists offer questions that result from the clinical reasoning process. Likewise, the occupational therapist uses clinical reasoning, self-reflection, introspection when working with clients (Taylor, 2008); recognizes his or her use of therapeutic self in the relationship; and models the caregiver role (Schultz-Krohn & Cara, 2000).

Perhaps the concept that comes closest to working with families in infant mental health is the idea of *relationship-centered care* (Kyler, 2008). In relationship-centered care, the client and therapist identify strengths but also include the resources of the caregiver, community, and environment. The therapist understands the influence of social, economic, political, cultural, and environmental contexts. In the work of promoting attachment, the practitioner identifies the strengths of the caregiver-infant dyad and the external forces impinging on the dyad.

The infant mental health therapist pays attention to the ability of an infant to regulate his or her emotions and to organize his or her emotional responses, and the therapist enlists the caregiver to soothe and calm the infant. Likewise, occupational therapists are mandated as part of their practice domain to work with affect regulation (client factor and coping skill) and affect regulation skill (performance skills). Thus, an occupational therapist would work in a family-centered way with parent and child, using strategies of education and therapeutic use of occupations and self to assist the parent in recognizing how his or her infant processes sensory information and to respond in an attuned way to his or her sensory needs. In so doing, the occupational therapist promotes healthy affect regulation and healthy attachments.

CASE ILLUSTRATION 9-4: MARISELA—CONCURRENT INTERVENTION: OCCUPATIONAL THERAPY INTERVENTION AND PROMOTING ATTACHMENT

Marisela, a product of in vitro fertilization, was delivered at 31 weeks' gestation, weighing 3 lb 7 oz, to a 47-year-old mother. Although she did have some respiratory distress, she never received assisted ventilation or supplemental oxygen. She had no neonatal neurological sequelae, but she did have bilateral partial congenital cataracts and underwent a partial bilateral lensectomy around 6 months of age. Afterward, she was referred to a high-risk infant follow-up program. The purpose of this follow-up was to identify neurodevelopmental delays and make referrals to appropriate community-based early intervention programs.

When Marisela was 6 months 15 days old (adjusted age, 4 months 12 days), she attended her first high-risk infant follow-up appointment. At that time, she was noted to have somewhat decreased resting muscle tone, with over-recruitment of her extensor musculature when active. Her muscle strength was moderately decreased proximally with decreased antigravity movement and continuous but consolable motor activity. Her mother, Titi, reported that the pediatrician had characterized her extremity movements as "flailing" and "purposeless." She was irritable and demonstrated limited visual responsivity because she had not yet been fitted with her contact lenses, and she made no attempts to calm herself. These behaviors resulted in moderately delayed abilities in all developmental realms. Luckily, she fed from the bottle easily, enjoyed bath time, and slept all night. Marisela was referred for the local education agency's services for vision impairment and to the local early intervention agency for physical therapy and occupational therapy services.

Occupational therapy addressed sensory processing as it impacted self-regulation, parent-child interaction, and play, in addition to monitoring and promoting Marisela's transition to textured foods. During the evaluation, the occupational therapy practitioner observed Marisela, during which Titi commented that she was worried about Marisela's flailing movements and inability to stop them (a misattunement). The occupational therapy practitioner promoted attachment bonds during the interventions by interpreting Marisela's movements within a sensory modulation perspective and educating Titi about Marisela's signals of distress to her parents. She also asked Titi if it was necessary to "stop" Marisela's flailing movements when sensory treatment might ameliorate them.

Discussion

Although Marisela and her mother, Titi, were referred to occupational therapy for vision impairment and early intervention, the occupational therapist was also able to promote attachment behaviors using observation, education, and questions resulting from clinical reasoning.

Occupational Therapy Application

Infants and their families will be referred to occupational therapy for eating, physical, developmental, and other problems. Within their domain of practice, occupational therapy practitioners can observe and promote the attachment process while conducting occupational therapy interventions. This, then, is the importance of knowing about attachment theory: it is likely that some of the clients that are referred to occupational therapy may have problems with attachment, and occupational therapists can promote attachment bonds in the natural course of their treatment. For example, some programs have been developed by or are used by occupational therapists that are sensory integration–based sensory modulation interventions (Champagne, 2011). Similar to therapeutic use of self, the PACE model, developed by Daniel Hughes (2006), advocates an evidence-based approach (Becker-Weidman & Hughes, 2008) that is playful, accepting, curious, and empathic. The traits advocated for caregivers or others working with foster children, in particular, can be translated into occupational therapy sensory modulation perspectives for the caregiver, such as adjusting breathing patterns to match the infant, using body positioning and language that ensure attunement with each other, matching voice pace and rhythm, and using playful, exploratory, empathic, and accepting attitudes.

Case Illustrations 9-4 and 9-5 are examples of referrals to occupational therapy in which the practitioner was able to observe and provide interventions that promoted attachment. Also, examples illustrate how it is important when working with infants and toddlers and their families to remain broad-minded and open to all perspectives.

Case Illustration 9-6 shows how occupational therapists can observe the attachment system in the course of occupational therapy evaluation and distinguish performance and attachment system difficulties.

CASE ILLUSTRATION 9-5: MARCUS AND JENNIFER—DISTINGUISHING BETWEEN PERFORMANCE OR ATTACHMENT PROBLEMS

When Marcus was referred to occupational therapy, he was 13 months old and newly diagnosed with failure to thrive. He was born at full term to a 36-year-old mother and had no neonatal health problems. He had always been a little small, but over the past 6 months, he had not grown well. His mother, Jennifer, an allied health professional who had quit her job to stay home with Marcus, reported that during the past several pediatric visits, the doctor had told her to "feed him more." The doctor told Jennifer that there was no other reason that Marcus was so small. She and her husband understood the significance of failure to thrive and were frustrated because they felt that they were doing everything they could to get Marcus to eat and that "he just doesn't want to."

Judith, the occupational therapist, visited Marcus and Jennifer in their home, a well-kept condominium, around their usual lunchtime. Marcus's father worked very long hours, typically did not participate in meal times, and was unable to participate in the session. Through interview and a nondirected play session, Judith screened Marcus as being developmentally age appropriate. Marcus was vocal and playful. He spontaneously engaged with toys and Judith's testing materials. He included both his mother and therapist in his play. He easily pulled to stand and cruised along furniture, referencing his mother whenever he moved across the living room from her.

Marcus, Jennifer, and Judith then transitioned from the living room to a dining area that was connected with the kitchen. Marcus showed no resistance to being placed in his high chair at the dining table. Jennifer and Judith sat on either side of him, facing each other. He remained smiling and playful until his mother went into the kitchen to retrieve his lunch. He then cried and tried to get out of his chair, even though his mother kept either vocal or visual contact with him. He calmed when she came back to the table. Food was placed on everyone's plate. He watched with interest as both Jennifer and Judith took a few bites, even reaching out to Jennifer's face. However, he did not make any effort to pick up the same finger food to feed himself. When his mother offered the food, he would close his mouth and turn away. If mother persisted, he fussed. Whenever he wound up with some of the sauce on his face because of turning away at the wrong time, Jennifer immediately wiped his face. Judith suggested that the food be left on Marcus's tray and that the adults continue to eat. After a while, Marcus did begin to play with the food. He soon had it smeared all over his hands. Whenever his hands did become a little messy, Jennifer quickly wiped them off. Periodically, he placed a small bite of soft food in his mouth or he allowed the therapist, not his mother, to give him a small spoon of chunky puree-textured food. With both textures, he demonstrated good oral-facial strength, age appropriate oral-motor skills, and timely transition of the food bolus for swallow. No coughing, choking, gagging, or respiratory changes were seen. He did not show any aversive responses to the textures in his mouth, or on his face or hands, for that matter. When Jennifer left the table to answer her phone or go back into the kitchen, Marcus cried. By the end of the meal, he had accepted more spoons of food from Judith than from his mother and did not fuss with the therapist.

Discussion

Judith had the opportunity to observe Marcus in a broader context, and his feeding difficulties did not appear to have a developmental delay, oral-motor dysfunction, or sensory processing basis as the main issue. Because Judith had some knowledge of attachment theory and treatment, she recognized a disruption in the parent-child relationship; Marcus appeared not to have a secure attachment with his mother. Jennifer clearly showed significant anxiety during the lunchtime observation, and although Judith wondered how much of her anxiety was due to the recent failure to thrive diagnosis, it did seem that Jennifer's anxiety, along with Marcus's unique temperamental response to her anxious behaviors, contributed to difficult feedings and limited intake.

OCCUPATIONAL THERAPY ROLES

Marisela and Marcus (Case Illustrations 9-4 and 9-5) exemplify the range of toddlers who are treated by pediatric occupational therapists. In different ways and at different times, they each demonstrated an attachment relationship with their parents. They have developed varying abilities to discern important social cues; have had feelings elicited during their interactions with their parents and others; and have compared, contrasted, and then encoded their repeated bodily and emotional feelings into their memories.

CASE ILLUSTRATION 9-6: MARISELA AND TITI—COLLABORATIVE TREATMENT: OCCUPATIONAL THERAPY AND INFANT MENTAL HEALTH CONSULTANT

Marisela returned to the high-risk infant follow-up program when she was 10.5 months adjusted age. Since receiving contact lenses, she demonstrated markedly improved visual attention and discrimination in her play and social interactions. Her strength and quality of movement were also improved. Her overall developmental testing scores fell in the low average to mild delay range. She had begun to finger feed and had transitioned to stage 2 pureed foods, but she had no interest in using the cup. She had begun to wake one to two times every night, crying inconsolably. Marisela's parents—Titi and her partner, Gabe—were able to attend the sessions. Her parents reported that she had significant irritable periods during which she "works herself up to a frenzy." Her only self-soothing strategy was to suck on her wrist. They reported that she did not like to be left alone and that they believed that she had significant stranger anxiety. Both Titi and Gabe reported being ineffective in their attempts to help her cope. She was receiving vision therapy services one time per week; physical therapy treatment two times per week; and occupational therapy treatment one time per week for continued interventions for feeding, strengthening, and play. The high-risk infant follow-up program worked closely with the early intervention agency to assist Marisela's parents to access an infant mental health professional for consultation.

Her last high-risk infant follow-up program appointment was when Marisela was 26 months old. Her age was no longer adjusted for prematurity, as is the community standard. Her cognitive skills were age appropriate, as were her fine motor skills. Gross motor skills continued to be moderately delayed due to decreased motor control, decreased dynamic balance, and difficulties with motor planning. Her language abilities scored in the low average to mild delay range. Marisela ate "voraciously" all textures of food, using all the age-appropriate utensils. She enjoyed her bath time. She helped with tooth brushing as well as hand and face washing. Gabe and Titi reported that Marisela "loves to tidy and clean up." Routines were helpful to her. Her favorite play were activities that included her push cars and a trampoline. However, Gabe and Titi reported her to be "extremely willful" and that she would have "complete meltdowns" when her plans were interrupted. She was also described as "clingy and insecure." Marisela continued to receive vision therapy, physical therapy, and occupational therapy in addition to weekly infant mental health consultation.

Marisela's occupational therapist collaborated with her infant mental health consultant. Each discipline had a specific role to play with Marisela and her parents, but both acknowledged the importance of incorporating the other discipline's strategies. The infant mental health consultant understood that, although Marisela's sensory processing difficulties clearly played a large role in her difficulties with being calm and able to look and listen to her parents as an infant, there was now the larger context of how her primary attachment relationships with Titi and Gabe had developed. She continued to have significant self-regulatory difficulties and sought out excessive amounts of proprioceptive input to calm and organize herself. The infant mental health consultant worked with Titi and Gabe on how to read and anticipate Marisela's physical and emotional cues so that they could help her manage her feelings before she had meltdowns. She also worked with them on how they could help her pull herself together when she did fall apart. Strategies incorporated occupational therapy's interpretation of Marisela's fragile sensory modulation abilities and need for more proprioceptive input. Conversely, the occupational therapist continued to include Marisela's parents in treatment sessions rather than asking them to wait in the waiting room.

Discussion

The occupational therapist learned from the infant mental health consultant that Marisela needed her parents to emotionally assist her with her regulatory abilities and that her difficulties were not solely sensory in nature. Therefore, the occupational therapist included her parents in family-centered care and also adapted communication strategies for the parents to include emotional content. Both the occupational therapist and infant mental health consultant worked together to incorporate strategies learned from each other in their respective interventions. Both became consultants and provided education to each other and for the parents in the infant-parent dyad.

Occupational therapy had a different role to play with each child, ranging from more typical developmental therapy using occupational therapy frames of reference such as sensory integration, neurodevelopmental therapy, motor control, and oral-motor/feeding treatment to developmental guidance and parent support. In each instance, occupational therapy also played a role in promoting the attachment process. In the case of Marisela, the occupational therapy role was more typically developmental based on sensory processing, play, and facilitating feeding, but the occupational therapy practitioner was also able to notice a misattunement between mother and daughter. Therefore, she was able to promote attunement and attachment behaviors at the same time that she intervened with sensory modulation, play, and feeding.

OCCUPATIONAL THERAPY INTERVENTION STRATEGIES

Occupational therapy with young children will be most effective in supporting each child's developmental progression if it consistently adapts treatment strategies to support the growing attachment relationship. This perspective suggests that the therapist do the following:

- Plan for each treatment activity to ensure that the child feels safe and secure, both physically and emotionally.
- View the child's behaviors as communication and consistently respond to him or her.
- Assist parents and other people important in the child's life to establish predictable daily rituals and routines.
- Ensure that the parent is involved in treatment sessions as he or she is able because he or she is a primary mediator of the child's emotional life.
- Understand the need for a family-centered approach and to support the parent and provide education through respect and meeting individually with only the parent or family if indicated.
- Consider all possible explanations for a child's behaviors (e.g., clingy behavior due to a sensory processing disorder, poor motor control, or possibly delayed emotional development [attachment processes]).
- Include as a therapy goal that each parent and child will successfully engage in mutually rewarding interactions (Costa, 2006; Holloway, 1998; Holloway & Chandler, 2010; Landy, 2009; Williamson & Anzalone, 2001). In the case of Marcus and Titi, these strategies were demonstrated by further developments in their lives.

Some occupational therapists may not consider themselves to be providing psychosocial occupational therapy services when working with the infant/toddler population. However, successful pediatric occupational therapy services necessarily address attachment because of its foundational role in overall development. The occupational therapist can assist the parent to find those alternate ways of relating that can be more successful and rewarding for both parent and child.

Case Illustration 9-7, with Erik and Junko, is an example of how an occupational therapist facilitated a successful and rewarding relationship.

SUMMARY

This chapter discussed attachment theory, the attachment system, its origins and development, research, and cultural applications. It discussed programs that promote attachment and the relationship of those programs' principles to occupational therapy interventions. It discussed occupational therapy treatment incorporating attachment in early intervention and intensive care and principles of intervention. It advocated for occupational therapists to become knowledgeable about attachment theory, research, and recent advances in neurobiology and to address attachment in early intervention. Furthermore, it advocated that occupational therapists address psychosocial issues in early intervention.

ACKNOWLEDGEMENT

Some material for this chapter, particularly the case material, was provided by Elise Holloway, MPH, OTR/L.

REFERENCES

Adoption and Foster Care Analysis and Reporting System. (2017). *AFCARS report #24*. Retrieved from https://www.acf.hhs.gov/cb/resource/afcars-report-24

Ainsworth, M. D. S. (1967). *Infancy in Uganda: Infant care and the growth of love*. Baltimore, MD: Johns Hopkins University Press.

Ainsworth, M. D. S. (1977). Infant development and mother-infant interactions among Uganda and American families. In P. H. Leiderman, S. R. Tulkin, & A. H. Rosenfeld (Eds.), *Culture and infancy* (pp. 119-150). New York, NY: Academic Press.

American Occupational Therapy Association. (2014). The Occupational Therapy Practice Framework. *American Journal of Occupational Therapy, 68*, S1-S48. doi:10.5014/ajot.2014.682006

American Psychiatric Association. (2013). *Diagnostic and statistical manual of mental disorders* (5th ed.). Washington, DC: Author.

Atkinson, L., Chisolm, V. C., Scott, B., Goldberg, S., Vaughn, B. E., … Tam, F. (1999). Ch. III Maternal sensitivity level and attachment in Down Syndrome. *Monographs of the Society for Research in Child Development, 64*(3), 45-66.

Becker-Weidman, A., & Hughes, D. (2008). Dyadic developmental psychotherapy: An evidence-based treatment for children with complex trauma and disorders of attachment. *Child and Family Social Work, 13*(3), 329-337. doi:10.1111/j.1365-2206.2008.00557.x

Berlin, L. J., Zeanah, C. H., & Lieberman, A. F. (2016). Prevention and intervention programs for supporting early attachment security. In J. Cassidy & P. R. Shaver (Eds.), *Handbook of attachment: Theory, research and clinical applications* (3rd ed., pp. 739-758). New York, NY: Guilford.

CASE ILLUSTRATION 9-7: ERIK AND JUNKO—SUCCESSFUL DEVELOPMENTAL GUIDANCE

Erik was a very small premature infant, born at 24 weeks' gestational age at a weight of 610 grams. He was hospitalized in the neonatal intensive care unit (NICU) for 5 months. He had quite a complicated neonatal history, as demonstrated by his 18-page medical discharge summary. His diagnoses included oxygen-dependent bronchopulmonary dysplasia, retinopathy of prematurity with laser surgery, multiple septic episodes, renal failure, seizures treated with phenobarbital, and significant gastroesophageal reflux.

Erik was discharged home on supplemental oxygen and feeding adequately by bottle. He was never able to transition to breastfeeding. Within 1 week of his NICU discharge, he stopped accepting the bottle. His pediatrician used home health services to place and monitor a nasogastric tube for feedings. He was hypotonic with compensatory arching, exacerbated by his frequent gastroesophageal reflux and vomiting. Although his laser surgery was considered successful, he ultimately was diagnosed with astigmatism and amblyopia, for which he was prescribed glasses at 14 months of age.

Early intervention services have been in place since Erik's NICU discharge. He has received occupational therapy, physical therapy, and infant development services, each two times per week. Erik has been developmentally delayed throughout his life, but recently, as he has neared 2.5 years of age, he has begun to close the gap between his chronologic age and his developmental age in all areas. He began walking independently around 22 months adjusted age. His receptive language has always been around age expectations, whereas his expressive language has been delayed. He has struggled with feeding and was quite slow to transition to pureed and table foods. His overall growth has been slow as well.

Erik's father works internationally, and so his mother, Junko, is a single parent for about 8 months at a time. She has worked part-time and ensured that Erik consistently participated in his early intervention program as allowed by his fluctuating medical status. All of Erik's early interventionists have observed that he and Junko have a loving relationship. He is able to seek her out for comfort when upset but also is able to move away from her to explore in his immediate environment. He is cautious around new people but able to warm up to them after a period of time. From the beginning, Junko was able to read and respond to his cues: his signs of distress and calm, readiness for interaction, and need for rest. She also was able to regulate her own emotional state to help Erik regulate his own. She met him where he was, so to speak, in terms of his physiologic, motor, cognitive, communicative, and emotional needs. As he matured in these different realms, he grew in his emotional independence. Once he was able to sit independently, Erik tolerated being put down on the floor but still close to his mother. When he began using vocal signals to call to his mother, he also stopped fussing when she moved to the other side of the room. She protected him from those people who did not understand that attachment-separation processes come from the development and interaction of all developmental realms and who believed that he should be forced to separate from her to "go to the treatment room" to "learn" to separate from her. Junko did this naturally, with support and guidance from the occupational therapist. Throughout his course of therapy, the occupational therapist acknowledged Erik's emotional response to motor activities, playground play, bathing, and feeding. The occupational therapist guided Junko in observing Erik's messages, supported her in recognizing that Erik proceeded at his own pace emotionally, and planned developmental therapy activities to include and promote Erik's special relationship with his mother. As part of her treatment plan, his occupational therapist assured that Erik would feel safe, calm, and secure by incorporating his mother's presence during playful and safe occupational treatment.

Discussion

Junko used occupational therapy services during self-care and play activities and co-occupations to develop a secure attachment and self-regulation of emotions with him, despite his developmental difficulties and external pressure that urged typical age independence.

Bowlby, J. (1973). *Prototypes of human sorrow. In Separation: Anxiety and anger* (pp. 3-22). New York, NY: Basic Books.

Bowlby, J. (1988a). Developmental psychiatry comes of age. *American Journal of Psychiatry, 145*(1), 1-10.

Bowlby, J. (1988b). *A secure base: Parent-child attachment and healthy human development* (pp. 20-38). New York, NY: Basic Books.

Bowlby, R. (2002). *Attachment from early childhood through the lifespan.* Presentation at the UCLA Lifespan Learning Institute, Los Angeles, CA.

Bretherton, I., & Munholland, K. A. (2016). The internal working model construct in light of contemporary neuroimaging research. In J. Cassidy & P. R. Shaver (Eds.), *Handbook of attachment: Theory, research and clinical applications* (3rd ed., pp. 63-90). New York, NY: Guilford.

Bretherton, I., & Waters, E. (Eds.). (1985). Growing points of attachment theory and research. *Monographs of the Society for Research in Child Development, 50*(1-2; Serial No. 209), 3-35.

Cassidy, J. (2016). The nature of the child's ties. In J. Cassidy & P. R. Shaver (Eds.), *Handbook of attachment: Theory, research and clinical applications* (3rd ed., pp. 3-24). New York, NY: Guilford.

Cassidy, J., Jones, J. D., & Shaver, P. R. (2013). Contributions of attachment theory and research: A framework for future research, translation, and policy. *Development and Psychopathology, 25*(42), 1415-1434. doi:10.1017/S0954579413000692

Cassidy, J., & Shaver, P. R. (Eds.) (2016). *Handbook of attachment: Theory, research, and clinical applications.* New York, NY: Guilford.

Champagne, T. (2011). Attachment, trauma, and occupational therapy practice. *OT Practice, 16*(5), CE-1-CE-7.

Corbin, J. (2007). Reactive attachment disorder: A biopsychosocial disturbance of attachment. *Child and Adolescent Social Work Journal, 24*, 539-552. doi:10.1007/s10560-007-0105-x

Costa, G. (2006). Mental health principles, practices, strategies, and dynamics pertinent to early intervention practitioners. In G. M. Foley & J. D. Hochman (Eds.), *Mental health in early intervention: Achieving unity in principles and practice* (pp. 113-138). Baltimore, MD: Paul H. Brooks Publishing Co.

Cozolino, L. (2006) The social brain [online]. *Psychotherapy in Australia, 12*(2), 12-17.

Creeden, K. (2009). How trauma and attachment can impact neurodevelopment: Informing our understanding and treatment of sexual behavior problems. *Journal of Social Aggression, 15*(3), 261-273.

Delvecchio, E., DiRiso, D., Salcuni, S., Lis, A., & George, C. (2014). Anorexia and attachment: Dysregulated defense and pathological mourning. *Frontiers in Psychology, 5*, 1-7.

Diamond, G. S., Reis, B. F., Diamond, G. M., Siqueland, L., & Isaacs, L. (2002). Attachment-based family therapy for depressed adolescents: A treatment development study. *Journal of the American Academy of Child and Adolescent Psychiatry, 41*(10), 1190-1196.

Dozier, M., & Rutter, M. (2016). Challenges to the development of attachment relationships faced by young children in foster and adoptive care. In J. Cassidy & P. R. Shaver (Eds.), *Handbook of attachment: Theory, research, and clinical applications* (3rd ed., pp. 696-714). New York, NY: Guilford.

Fraiberg, S. (1980). *Clinical studies in infant mental health: The first year of life.* New York, NY: Basic Books.

Fraiberg, S. (1982). Pathological defenses in infancy. *Psychoanalytic Quarterly, 51*, 612-615.

Harder, S. (2014). Attachment in Schizophrenia-Implications for research, prevention and treatment. *Schizophrenia Bulletin, 40*(6), 1189-1193.

Hardy, L. (2007). Attachment theory and reactive attachment disorder: Theoretical perspectives and treatment implications. *Journal of Child and Adolescent Psychiatric Nursing, 20*(1), 27-39.

Holloway, E. (1998). Early emotional development and sensory processing. In J. Case-Smith (Ed.), *Pediatric occupational therapy and early intervention* (pp. 111-126). Boston, MA: Butterworth-Heinemann.

Holloway, E., & Chandler, B. E. (2010). Family-centered practice: It's all about relationships. In B. E. Chandler (Ed.), *Early childhood: Occupational therapy services for children birth to five* (pp. 77-108). Bethesda, MD: ATOA Press.

Hughes, D. (2006). *Building the bonds of attachment: Awakening love in deeply troubled children.* Lanham, MD: Jason Aronson.

Kellegrew, D. H. (2000). Constructing daily routines: A qualitative examination of mothers with young children with disabilities. *American Journal of Occupational Therapy, 54*, 252-259.

Kerns, K. A. (2008). Attachment in middle childhood. In J. Cassidy & P. R. Shaver (Eds.), *Handbook of attachment: Theory, research and clinical applications* (2nd ed., pp. 366-382). New York, NY: Guilford Press.

Kyler, P. (2008). Client-centered and family-centered care: Refinement of the concepts. *Occupational Therapy in Mental Health, 24*(2), 100-120.

Landy, S. (2009). *Pathways to competence: encouraging healthy social and emotional development in young children.* Baltimore, MD: Paul H. Brooks Publishing Co.

Larson, E. A. (2000). The orchestration of occupation: The dance of mothers. *American Journal of Occupational Therapy, 54*, 269-280.

Lieberman, A., & Pawl, J. (1993). Infant parent psychotherapy. In C. Zeanah (Ed.), *Handbook of infant mental health.* New York, NY: Guilford Press.

Mesman, J., van IJzendoorn, M. H., & Sagi-Schwartz, A. (2016). Cross-cultural patterns of attachment: Universal and contextual dimensions. In J. Cassidy & P. R. Shaver (Eds.), *Handbook of attachment: Theory, research, and clinical applications* (3rd ed., pp. 852-877). New York, NY: Guilford.

Narvaez, D., & Gleason, T. (2012). Developmental optimization. In D. Narvaez, D. J. Panksepp, A. Schore, & T. Gleason (Eds.), *Human nature, early experience and the environment of evolutionary adaptness* (pp. 307-325). New York, NY: Oxford University Press.

Papousek, M. (2011). Resilience, strengths, and regulatory capacities: Hidden resources in developmental disorders of infant mental health. *Infant Mental Health Journal, 32*(1), 29-46.

Rutgers, A. H., Bakermans-Kranenburg, M. J., van IJzendoorn, M. H., & van Berckelaer-Onnes, I. A. (2004). Autism and attachment: a meta-analytic review. *Journal of Child Psychology and Psychiatry, 45*(6), 1123-1134.

Rutgers, A. H., van IJzendoorn, M. H., Bakermans-Kranenburg, M. J., Swinkels, S. H., van Daalen, E., Dietz, C., ... van Engeland, H. (2007). Autism, attachment and parenting: A comparison of children with autism spectrum disorder, mental retardation, language disorder, and non-clinical children. *Journal of Abnormal Psychology, 35*, 859-870. doi:10.1007/s10802-007-9139-y

Salter Ainsworth, M. D., & Bell, S. M. (1970). Attachment, exploration and separation: Illustrated by the behavior of one-year-olds in a strange situation. *Child Development, 41*(1), 49-67.

Schore, A. N. (2000). Attachment and the regulation of the right brain. *Attachment & Human Development, 2*(1), 23-47.

Schore, A. N. (2010). A neurobiological perspective on the work of Berry Brazelton. In B. M. Lester & J. D. Sparrow (Eds.), *Nurturing children and families: Building on the legacy of T. Berry Brazelton* (pp. 141-153). Malden, MA: Blackwell Publishing.

Schore, A. N. (2016). *Affect regulation and the origin of the self.* New York, NY: Routledge.

Schultz-Krohn, W., & Cara, E. (2000). Case report: Occupational therapy in early intervention: Applying concepts from infant mental health. *American Journal of Occupational Therapy, 54*(5), 550-554.

Seligman, S. (1994). Applying psychoanalysis in an unconventional context. *Psychoanalytic Study of the Child, 49*, 481-500.

Siegel, D. J. (2012). *The developing mind: How relationships and the brain interact to shape who we are* (2nd ed.). New York, NY: Guilford Press.

Simpson, J. A., & Belsky, J. (2016). Attachment theory within a modern evolutionary framework. In J. Cassidy & P. R. Shaver (Eds.), *Handbook of attachment: Theory, research, and clinical applications* (3rd ed., pp. 91-116). New York, NY: Guilford.

Slade, A., & Aber, J. (1992). Attachments, drives and development: conflicts and convergences in theory. In J. Barron, M. Eagles, D. Wotilsky, & L. David (Eds.), *Interface of psychoanalysis and psychology* (pp. 154-185). Washington, DC: American Psychological Association.

Sroufe, L., & Waters, E. (1977). Attachment as an organizational construct. *Child Development, 48*, 1184-1199.

Taylor, R. (2008). *The intentional relationship: Occupational therapy and the use of self.* Philadelphia, PA: F. A. Davis.

Williamson, G. G., & Anzalone, M. E. (2001). *Sensory integration and self-regulations in infants and toddlers: Helping very young children interact with their environment.* Washington, DC: Zero to Three.

Young-Bruehl, E., & Bethelard, F. (2002). *Cherishment: A psychology of the heart.* New York, NY: Simon & Schuster.

SUGGESTED RESOURCES

James Robertson Films: http://www.robertsonfilms.info/

John Bowlby Attachment and Loss: http://www.youtube.com/watch?v=VAAmSqv2GV8

Secure & Insecure Attachment by Richard Bowlby: http://www.youtube.com/watch?v=MrcNjFyWeWE&feature=related

The Strange Situation: A Study of Attachnment in Infants. https://www.youtube.com/watch?v=m_6rQk7jlrc

The Strange Situation, Mary Ainsworth: http://www.youtube.com/watch?v=QTsewNrHUHU

Mental Health of Children

William L. Lambert, MS, OTR/L

Occupational therapy for children with emotional and behavioral disturbances has been an area of specialization within the profession for many years. Indeed, the practice of occupational therapy with children with mental and behavioral disorders requires knowledge of specific psychiatric and general mental health disorders and conditions; expertise in normal or typical growth and development; and practice skills unique to this population, its issues, and its concerns.

Those providing care to these children often work in collaboration with other health care professionals such as child psychiatrists, psychologists, social workers, and nurses; independently as consultants or contract therapists; or through a private practice. The delivery system for providing occupational therapy for this population has changed dramatically in the past two decades. In the past, the primary sites that employed therapists to provide services for children experiencing psychosocial issues were psychiatric hospitals with children's units or wards, outpatient mental health clinics, and day treatment programs. Currently, therapists who have a particular interest in working with children with emotional or behavioral problems must consider new alternatives and innovative ways to meet the needs of this population due to the move away from medical model/hospital-based treatment. Many programs are being eliminated and clinical services reduced. Secondary to increasingly shorter lengths of stay and limited reimbursement, therapists will necessarily need to be prepared to address the

mental health issues of children in school and community settings not usually thought of as psychiatric/mental health, but rather as pediatric. The reader is encouraged to thoughtfully consider how to apply the concepts and information presented in this chapter in all settings where children are in need of occupational therapy services.

This chapter presents an overview of occupational therapy practice with children who are experiencing mental health problems that are affecting their ability to function in one or more areas of their lives. Basic concepts used in providing occupational therapy to children with mental health issues are described. Occupational therapy programming is discussed based on experience and on successful interventions used in other settings. Treatment, intervention groups with examples of group protocols, and activities appropriate for this population are presented that may be used in a variety of pediatric settings.

DSM-5 Diagnoses

The *Diagnostic and Statistical Manual of Mental Disorders* (DSM-5; American Psychiatric Association, 2013) contains disorders usually first diagnosed in childhood or adolescence under neurodevelopmental disorders. Many of these disorders, such as attention deficit hyperactivity disorder (ADHD), intellectual disabilities, autism spectrum disorder, and Tourette's disorder can continue

MacRae, A. (Ed.). *Cara and MacRae's Psychosocial Occupational Therapy: An Evolving Practice, Fourth Edition* (pp 157-177).
© 2019 Taylor & Francis Group.

to cause problems during adulthood. "Approximately one-half to two-thirds of children who have ADHD continue to have symptoms of the disorder into their teenage years and on into adulthood" (Resnick, 2005). Many disorders that are discussed in other chapters, such as schizophrenia, major depression, bipolar disorder, and posttraumatic stress disorder, may also first be encountered in childhood. However, these disorders may present differently in children. Symptoms of childhood depression include irritability, sadness, social withdrawal, and anhedonia, as well as negative feelings appearing in play. Irritability is especially common in depression and mania in children (Harvard Medical School, 2007). Depression with children sometimes presents with anger, aggression, or acting out. Acting out can be defined as the expression of thoughts and feelings through maladaptive behavior instead of recognizing and verbalizing those ideas. Children may express depressive symptoms in other ways, such as anger, because it is cognitively easier for them to be mad than sad.

A difference in the way that children with bipolar disorder present is that their moods may shift many times within the same day or same therapy session. Additionally, their "symptoms rarely follow a discrete pattern. Children, especially young children, usually do not show the adult cycle of distinct mood swings from mania to depression lasting for several months, with intervals of normal mood in between," but on the other hand, "children may also have more classic and unmistakable manic symptoms" (Harvard Medical School, 2007). Their presentation is further complicated by frequently also meeting the criteria for ADHD and oppositional defiant disorder. "Bipolar disorder in children is especially difficult to distinguish from ADHD, since many of the symptoms—impulsiveness, distractibility, and hyperactivity—are similar" (Harvard Medical School, 2007). A family history that includes relatives who have been diagnosed with bipolar disorder greatly assists in making this diagnosis in children. Knowing which medications were beneficial to blood relatives also makes choosing the appropriate medication for the child easier.

Common diagnoses of children seen or encountered by occupational therapists in various settings include ADHD, oppositional defiant disorder, separation anxiety disorder, and conduct disorder. More recently, attention has been focused on the occurrence and prevalence of reactive attachment disorder (RAD; see Chapter 9 for more information) and autism spectrum disorders.

Children with ADHD often have problematic social interactions with peers, teachers, and authority figures, as well as difficulty in participating appropriately in the classroom and during extracurricular activities. Treatment with medications such as methylphenidate (Ritalin, Metadate) and amphetamine/dextroamphetamine (Adderall) is often at the center of controversy and debate. These and other medications are criticized for being overprescribed and heavily marketed to parents.

The specific causes for RAD are unknown; however, early experiences with caregivers of neglect and/or abuse where the parents did not address the child's basic emotional and physical needs appears to play a role and, more significantly, repeated changes in the primary caregiver or a succession of caregivers early in life appears to prevent the establishment of stable, appropriate attachments. There is a high risk of this disorder in toddlers and children in foster care and orphanages. Children with attachment disorders can be frustrating to work with and to parent. They present with a high need to be in control, frequently lying without reason. Interpersonally, they may be overly affectionate and inappropriately related with others, including strangers, or lack interest in others and not seek attention. They may lack a conscience and deny responsibility or project blame for their actions. Frequently, they hoard or gorge on food in the absence of want. Nondirective play therapy and sensory integrative therapy have been identified as efficacious therapeutic interventions. Treatments under the rubric of attachment therapy have been controversial, lack empirical support, and are thought to be antithetical to attachment theory (Dozier & Rutter, 2008). Close and ongoing collaboration with the child's family and involving parents in treatment is essential for facilitating successful outcomes. At best, therapists can attempt to assist children with RAD to form a more secure sense of self and others and to guide parents and foster parents to help regulate emotions, understand their children's signals, and provide consistent and committed care (Dozier & Rutter, 2008). Case Illustration 10-1 presents the story of a child with RAD and his family in therapy.

Children may have more than one disorder. For example, children with ADHD may also have depression, obsessive-compulsive disorder, or all three. Children with depression may also have an anxiety disorder, and sensorimotor problems may coexist with many disorders.

The presenting problems encountered by occupational therapists treating children with emotional problems are varied. "Typical" psychosocial stressors may include the parents' divorce; emotional, verbal, physical, and/or sexual abuse; other traumatic events, such as the death of a sibling, parent, or grandparent; and socioeconomic conditions. The child may respond to traumatic events by withdrawal, aggressive or atypical behavior, or regression to behavior expected from a younger child. Sometimes the child is confronted by a physical condition such as diabetes, which may limit the child's ability to play and eat what others are eating or require an unusually strict adherence to a medication and blood-monitoring situation. The child may find the illness overwhelming and consequently start acting out at home or become noncompliant with the treatment of the illness in an attempt to exert control.

In other cases, a dysfunctional family situation may have led to treatment. Parents sometimes lack the parenting skills required for rearing a normally developing child. In such circumstances, it may be a lack of parental

CASE ILLUSTRATION 10-1: JOE—FAMILY INTERVENTION FOR A CHILD WITH REACTIVE ATTACHMENT DISORDER

The consulting therapist for the foster care agency arrived at Joe's home and was met at the door by Joe's mother, Debbie, and his father, Clint. Once inside, he was introduced to their adopted foster children, Danny, age 14, and Ellen, age 12, as well as Joe, a preadoptive foster child who is 9 years old. The reason for the referral was family difficulties arising from parenting Joe, as well as the other children. The therapist's interview with Joe's parents yielded that Joe, who has been diagnosed with RAD, has been stealing, hoarding food and other items in his room, and "doesn't clean up his messes," nor does he comply with directions to complete chores around the house. Interpersonally, he is detached and unaffectionate with Debbie and Clint, but they remarked, "He couldn't be nicer to his football coach and teachers, but it's a completely different story when it comes to us."

The therapist asked what chores were assigned to each of the children, and the parents replied, "Whatever we ask them to do—they don't do what they're told anyway, so we just end up yelling and fighting over it." When asked what the children's consequences were for not completing their chores, particularly Joe, whose behavior had generated the referral, the parents said there had not been any.

The therapist suggested that perhaps a consequence for Joe might be not going to football practice or missing a game because it was something that he valued.

Debbie said, "It's too difficult to punish just Joe. All of the kids have activities after school and in the evening, so if he had to stay home, they all would have to stay home because Clint works second shift, and I can't leave Joe home alone while I drive the others to their activities."

Clint said, "Anyway, it wouldn't be fair to Joe's team. It's his responsibility to be there, and it's not the other kids' fault that Joe won't listen to us."

Intervention

The occupational therapist had a family meeting during the initial visit to develop and begin implementation of a family chore list. He established that the parents were in charge of this and asked them to develop a specific list of chores for each child for the next session. Additionally, he asked the parents to develop reasonable consequences for when a child didn't complete his or her chores, and also rewards for their successful completion. The children were asked to consider what their consequences should be as well, all of which would be discussed during the next visit. The therapist then met privately with Debbie and Clint and discussed the causes and symptoms of Joe's RAD. He asked them to not take Joe's behavior personally but to put it into perspective given his diagnosis and to make a list of realistic goals. He also stressed the need to reinforce Joe's positive behaviors by "catching him doing something good" because this is often difficult for parents of children who present with symptoms like Joe. Additionally, he provided them with a pamphlet on the disorder to read and asked them to make a list of any questions they had for the next session.

In the next session, the occupational therapist held another family meeting to implement the family chore list. Each child was informed of his or her assigned chores, and the list was posted on the refrigerator, where it could remain visible and the children could easily refer to it throughout the day. All of the children agreed to give this a try, and also presented possible consequences for not completing their chores such as losing their allowance, having to go to bed early, and not being able to play video games. When meeting with the parents following the meeting, the therapist further discussed with them how Joe's diagnosis affected his behavior and interactions and, consequently, their family and home life, and he discussed how to set more realistic expectations.

Discussion

Many of Joe's presenting problems were the direct result of having RAD. By providing the parents with education regarding the disorder, he guided them to make more realistic goals for a child who is undoubtedly difficult to parent, and the stress on the parents' marriage and home life improved for them and for the family as a whole. The therapist recognized the family's need for structure, consistency, and consequences for behavior, which is illustrated by the family meeting approach that unified the parents and established appropriate roles for them and their children through the various interventions.

(continued)

> **CASE ILLUSTRATION 10-1: JOE—FAMILY INTERVENTION FOR A CHILD WITH REACTIVE ATTACHMENT DISORDER (CONTINUED)**
>
> *Discussion (continued)*
>
> Parenting skills were also addressed in terms of having them consider looking at chores and other household responsibilities as opportunities to reinforce positive behavior and extinguish negative behavior and provide rewards for compliance rather than using inconsistent punishment. RAD is difficult to treat, and many of the presenting problems and symptoms displayed are not necessarily going to be resolved because these children often change very little in terms of their personality, temperament, behavior, and interactions with their adoptive parents. Therefore, as in this example, it is necessary to treat the whole family system to affect change and bring about positive therapeutic outcomes. (For an additional example, see Case Illustration 11-6 in Chapter 11.)

supervision, an inability to set and enforce limits and rules, or the failure to distinguish and differentiate the needs of the parent from the needs of the child. In other situations, parents have placed expectations on children that the latter find overwhelming, such as a parental need to see a child excel in academics or athletics, whether or not the child values these activities. Sociological factors, such as poverty, violence, and crime, may constitute a stressful environment, resulting in depression or anxiety and leading to a need for treatment. Whatever the antecedents that lead to a child receiving professional treatment, the primary reasons are similar to many psychiatric intervention situations. These factors include the following:

- Danger of harming oneself or others
- A breakdown in role functioning, namely appropriate behavior as a sibling, student, playmate, son, or daughter
- A decrease in obedience to, or compliance with, authority figures
- Social withdrawal
- Increase in aggression or other unacceptable or inappropriate acting-out behaviors, such as fighting, truancy, criminal activities such as theft or vandalism, fire setting, and violence directed toward pets or other animals
- Use of drugs or alcohol
- Stopping medications
- Dropping grades

Other conditions that contribute to emotional problems in children include fetal alcohol spectrum disorders (Centers for Disease Control and Prevention, 2018). Fetal alcohol spectrum disorders include fetal alcohol syndrome, alcohol-related neurodevelopmental disorder, and alcohol-related birth defects; the latter two formerly being described by the term *fetal alcohol effects*, which sometimes impair a child's ability to learn from experience or impair the usual responses to medical interventions. The offspring of mothers who used or abused alcohol or drugs during pregnancy may display a wide range of often unpredictable developmental deficits that complicate treatment and may

adversely affect outcomes. These various conditions affect each child differently and can range from mild to severe.

Regardless of the unique circumstances that are part of a child's particular situation, the onset of the illness varies with each child, based on diagnosis, genetic predisposition, level of disability, and equality-of-life factors such as income level, access to health care, and stability of the family situation. Children's emotional and behavioral problems and the consequences of interpersonal and social impairments become more visible once they reach the age where they can be observed by others at day care, preschool, or the school system setting. At this time, difficulties tend to become more evident, and families often seek professional, clinical help.

HELPFUL CONCEPTS FOR TREATING CHILDREN

Because children are developing a self-identity and learning how to behave in their social world, concepts such as structure and consistency, interpretation, time-out, limit setting, avoidance of power struggles, modeling, and a consistent team approach are important to keep in mind when working with them. Although some of these concepts are used when working with adults, who presumably have developed some sense of identity and acceptance of social norms, they are particularly important for the developmental period when individuals are learning who they are and how to function successfully in the world.

Structure and Consistency

Two fundamental principles guiding treatment in pediatric occupational therapy addressing mental health issues are structure and consistency. For individuals with poor impulse control, attention deficits, hyperactivity, or poor response to limits and rules, increasing the amount of structure can improve their response to activity interventions, help them learn how to modulate their own emotions, and assist them in learning appropriate role behavior. The environment itself is used to provide cues to appropriate behavior similar to those used in milieu therapy or therapeutic communities.

Structure can be verbal, such as the tactic of redirection, or physical and tangible, depending on the specific activity or equipment used. Redirection can be defined as a verbal tactic that adds to the structure of therapy by refocusing the child on the assigned or current activity in which the child is participating and providing cues for appropriate involvement or behavior. For example, Holly, a 9-year-old girl, stops painting her suncatcher and, due to her impulsivity, leaves her seat to retrieve another one, even though she has not finished painting the first. Redirection can be provided by the therapist saying, "Holly, you are doing a beautiful job of painting your suncatcher. What color are you going to use next? Why don't you show me?" Such a statement cues Holly about where she should be and what she should be doing in a positive way. Redirection such as in this example proves to be more effective than saying, "What are you doing out of your seat?" which allows for a variety of responses on Holly's part, none of which may be the one desired by the therapist. Activities can begin with the imposition of verbal structure, such as directions and limits or rules regarding the activity. For example, the group leader or therapists may say, "Today in group we are going to share the toys in the playroom. There can be no hitting. If anyone hits someone else, he or she will have to leave the group." This instruction provides an idea or standard that can be referred to throughout the group session that provides structure and consistency that can be established when the therapist removes a child each time he or she hits another child. For children, a poster that lists the rules of the group or activity provides an additional reference point that can be used to remind them of the structure.

Announcements can be used to start a group. The children can be asked to tell something about themselves or their progress toward therapy goals. They can be encouraged to share news such as upcoming family events, plans for the future (following discharge from therapy), changes in their lives, activities in which they have participated, and the like. Announcements provide the therapist with useful information that may explain a child's response to therapy on that particular day. For example, if a child states, "My mom is taking me to family therapy after occupational therapy today," changes in mood or decreases in frustration tolerance might be attributed to anxiety regarding the outcome of the family therapy session later that day. This, in turn, may enable the therapist to make a successful interpretation that can help the child cope more effectively, learn to express feelings more adaptively, and benefit more from occupational therapy that day.

When conducting groups, it is important to ensure that the group begins and ends at the designated times and follows the established routine as much as possible. Naturally, a variety of unpredictable and unavoidable circumstances can interfere with the daily course of programming. For example, a therapist may be sick or on vacation, or special events such as holiday parties may take temporary precedence over scheduled programming. In such cases, it is important to inform clients of changes in the established consistency. This practice can prevent the eruption of acting-out behavior from a client who may otherwise feel unable to trust the adults and the therapeutic environment responsible for his or her care. Box 10-1 provides tips to minimize disruption. A clinical example of acting out can be seen in Case Illustration 10-2, in which a child, Joanie, was not made aware of the impending absence of the therapist who normally ran her group.

A point that may be implicitly understood by occupational therapists is that another way to provide structure is through activities themselves. An example is making a tile mosaic project in a parallel task group. Structure is provided when:

- Each client has his or her own project, which encourages work in a specific spot and focuses attention on a personal project
- An example or sample is provided that may be followed to enhance redirection to task
- The instructions are clear (e.g., "Put tiles in the tray like this"); this encourages following the stated direction
- Steps are graded according to therapy goals (e.g., "Pick up each tile and glue it in place")

Children enjoy the structure of individual activities, which can serve as a means of exploring their abilities and skills and learning about their strengths and limitations. Puppetry, doll play, and drawing provide techniques for dramatizing and externalizing intrapsychic issues. For the older latency-age child, board games may become catalysts for communication and interpersonal relationships.

In general, in planning activities for children, it should be constantly considered whether:

- The activity chosen is age-appropriate
- The activity is broken down into steps that the child can understand
- The steps are age-appropriate for a child to carry out independently
- The therapist wishes the child to carry out the activity independently or by asking for assistance

For example, if an activity should involve a child sustaining attention to a task, perhaps a tile mosaic project involving the selection of a number of small tiles placed in a trivet is the activity of choice. If improving self-esteem is a consideration, an easy-to-do, foolproof activity such as painting a suncatcher or lacing a small coin purse may do. Where individual play skills are lacking, perhaps the creation and assembly of a toy car that the child can use independently or in conjunction with other children is the activity of choice. In any case, the activity should facilitate developmentally appropriate skills and be fun and intrinsically motivating for the child.

Box 10-1. Six Therapy Tips

1. To deal with impulsivity, never put anything on the table where you are having a group activity unless you want the children to touch it.

2. Ease transitions, which are frequently difficult for children with mental illness, with a 5-minute warning before the group ends to prepare them for the change and deal more adaptively with endings.

3. To prevent overstimulation, provide a warm, softly lit environment that is soothing and as free from unwanted noise, disruption, and distractions as possible.

4. Children with emotional disturbances can act out often and produce a considerable amount of maladaptive behavior in therapy. "Catch them being good"—praise positive behavior as often as possible.

5. Maintain an even tone and affect while providing treatment. Your calm demeanor may influence the disruptive child's behavior—at least occasionally!

6. Sometimes, groups just fall apart despite the therapist's best efforts and interventions. Do not insist that the activity occur if the children are not ready to participate. Two effective solutions are to end the group and sit quietly and wait for the children to regain control. Children learn that acting out and disruptive behavior lead to the natural consequence that they lose the opportunity to be involved in the activity. If sitting quietly lasts until the end of group time, they usually realize that their behavior prevented play and say, "Hey, we didn't do anything yet!" Gently remind them that they will need to be in control in the next session if they want the activity to happen.

CASE ILLUSTRATION 10-2: JOANIE—MANAGING CHANGE

When Joanie, age 8, arrived in the therapy room, she learned that the group had been changed from an art group to a play group, which caused her to cry, kick, and scream. When an interpretation was made that the child appeared very upset, she blurted out, "I wanted to have art! I have to paint my project so I can give it to my mother!"

Discussion

Had she been informed of the change beforehand, the incident might have been averted, and Joanie might have been able to present her disappointment and concerns calmly and been provided with options for completing her project, thereby learning how to express her internal feelings and thoughts acceptably.

Although there are common considerations when choosing an activity for any person, for a child, it is particularly important to be mindful of dangerous parts such as sharp edges, toxic chemicals, or toxic paints or parts that can be ingested, such as small wheels found on a toy car for toddlers. Another consideration is whether there are any items that could be used in a suicide attempt or injurious behavior, such as when knives are being used in a cooking group.

Thorough activity analysis, performing sharps counts (i.e., the number of knives, scissors, etc., used in the group), and limiting the length of string or ribbon provided are ways of ensuring safety both during therapy and afterward when projects are taken home. Depending on the participants presenting problems, copper tooling, for example, may be the wrong activity for a group of aggressive children who may not respond to the structure of the activity or may use the materials inappropriately to harm themselves or others.

Interpretation

Interpretation of, or putting words to, behavior is a therapeutic technique that provides a child with an avenue to express feelings with words, which is more often appropriate than other means such as aggression or acting out. This is often an effective way of deescalating a child or adolescent who is displaying behavioral problems that result from an inability to use words for self-expression. In the example of Joanie, interpretation involved the therapist identifying to the child in a clear and supportive manner what she observed. Joanie could then better express the behavior's cause (whether the change in routine, a reminder of a dynamic within her family, or a feeling she could not identify). The identification of these issues by using interpretation clarifies the situation at hand and teaches a more adaptive coping strategy: the use of words to express feelings and reach acceptable solutions to problems. Activities can be used to provide opportunities to externalize intrapsychic issues or facilitate communication. Once issues have been externalized or communicated, interpretation helps children to understand, learn, cope, and adapt emotionally.

Time-Out

Time-out is an intervention technique that results in behavioral changes and increases the child's understanding of his or her role in a situation. If a child is asked to take time-out for kicking a peer while fighting over a toy, he or she will learn that aggression leads to the loss of the chance to play. Time-out also provides an opportunity for the adult to teach the child how to share. Thus, the child becomes better able to perceive the situation and learn from it. Similarly, if a child is removed from therapy for aggression or breaking the rules, he or she will become better able to think about the situation and learn from it. Time-out is the process of removing a young person from a problematic situation to a specific area away from the group and, at the same time, allowing him or her to think about the behavior that led to removal from the group.

The length of time-out should vary with the individual's age and mental capacities. For example, when a child has provoked a fight with a peer, he or she will be removed to a time-out chair, a "think about it" area, or another room, where he or she will be requested to remain for a specified amount of time. Depending on his or her age, he or she may be asked to remain in time-out until he or she can count to 10 or until 1 minute goes by on a timer. An often-stated rule of thumb is 1 minute per year, that is, a 5-year-old would be placed on a 5-minute time-out. However, what may be most effective is for the time-out not to have a specific time in minutes, but to last until the child regains control and can effectively process the situation. Using this approach, one can avoid situations where the child has regained control yet had several more minutes of time-out remaining. To be consistent, the adult would have to maintain the time-out until its predetermined parameter, which may allow the child to begin acting out again and not benefit from the experience. Immediately after the time-out, the child is most amenable to positive interaction and should be engaged in the activity in a constructive way and then praised for constructive behavior. After the activity, it is important to critically analyze the incident. The child and adult should meet briefly to discuss the behavior that led to the time-out, evaluate whether the intervention was useful for the client, and develop a plan of action that will be used in future situations. A plan of action may involve identifying alternative coping strategies with the client (e.g., a self-assigned time-out) or the use of assertive responses (e.g., letting an adult know when he or she is feeling frustrated or agreeing on a code word to indicate the need for a behavior change). This process should be kept as brief as possible so that acting-out behavior is not reinforced. When used properly, a time-out can be efficacious in changing maladaptive behavior to that which is more socially appropriate.

Time-out should not be thought of as a punishment, nor should the individual taking a time-out think of it in this way, but more as a consequence for problematic behavior or actions. It is important to present the time-out as a way to learn new behavior so that a positive learning experience may occur and negative or maladaptive behaviors may decrease.

Limit Setting

Limit setting involves informing others what is permissible and what is unacceptable; it lets individuals know how far they can go. Setting limits is especially important for children because they need, and look for, limits, which eventually become internalized as a set of rules that guide socially accepted behavior. The teaching of behavior, such as learning to respect the property of others and not taking what does not belong to them, begins when children are told, in effect, "Thou shall not steal" (whether this occurs at home, in school, or in a religious setting), and the rule is enforced by the parent. When consistent enforcement of the rule or limit occurs, appropriate behavior will be learned and become a part of that person's internal code of values, morals, or conscience. Children are protected by rules or limits, such as when adults instruct them that they may play in the yard but not in the street or that they must be home before a certain hour. This not only teaches safety and prevents harm, it also shows children that their welfare is the concern of the parent or other adult. Limits that are thus enforced clarify the relationship between the parent (or other adult) and child and teach appropriate role behavior. Limits should be friendly but firm, short, and impersonal. Limits can be put in the context of the group rules, as when the occupational therapist says, "We must share the toys," or when a parent states, "The house rules say that fighting over what program to watch on TV leads to an early bedtime for everyone." Although setting limits may be interpreted as punishment, if stated in a protective, supportive, and friendly but firm way, it will foster more mature behavior. Naturally, the amount of limit setting depends on the needs of the child and the comfort level of the therapist.

An excellent resource for shaping and modifying behavior in children between the ages of 2 and 12 years is Phelan's *1-2-3 Magic: 3-Step Discipline for Calm, Effective, and Happy Parenting* (2016), which develops the child's ability to follow rules and comply with adult authority. Although it is written for parents, any adult working with children who require effective behavior modification could use the concepts.

Therapeutic Use of Self

The therapeutic use of self entails the development of an individual style that works with clients in a specific way to promote change and growth and help to provide

CASE ILLUSTRATION 10-3: KAY—THE THERAPEUTIC USE OF SELF

Kay, a client on a children's unit, could not sustain her interest or complete tasks as assigned. During a cooking group, the occupational therapist assigned her the job of chopping vegetables to be put in a salad. However, Kay did not stay with her task, and, moments later, she was in another part of the room engaging in an activity that had been assigned to another child.

The young occupational therapist, in a raised voice, told Kay, "You are not where you belong," and asked what her task was.

Kay said, "I'm supposed to be chopping vegetables."

The therapist said, "You are driving me crazy," to which she responded, "You sound just like my mother; she always says that."

At that point, the therapist realized he was not being therapeutic and was indeed responding to Kay in the same manner in which adults had always responded to her. Therefore, he acknowledged that fact, apologized for sounding impatient, and redirected Kay to the task at hand (as he should have done previously).

Discussion

As demonstrated by the therapist in this case, the therapeutic use of self involves responding to clients in a way that will guide them onto a new path through developing behaviors that are appropriate and socially acceptable. This involves responding to clients in a different manner than nontherapeutic individuals in past situations.

a corrective emotional experience. This is a difficult concept, or "art," to describe: "The art of occupational therapy involves captivating the child through toys, objects, and games or through the therapist's own actions so that the child becomes involved in the therapeutic process. This art is almost intangible" (Kramer & Hinojosa, 2010, p. 574). An occupational therapist responds to a child in a therapeutic manner, conveying appreciation of the child's uniqueness, kindness, love, and understanding; guiding the child through each step of occupational therapy intervention; and encouraging him or her to accomplish the task that has been chosen to meet the treatment goal. Each therapist will develop a unique and personal style or therapeutic personality for working with patients. The therapeutic use of self requires providing a new response to an old situation, which, in turn, enables the client to respond in a new manner that is both adaptive and appropriate. These concepts are described in Case Illustration 10-3.

Team Approach and Family Involvement

The team concept is particularly essential in providing services, and family involvement in treatment is of utmost importance for children because of their roles as family members. Other family members should be consulted and included on the team whenever possible and be a part of treatment goals and decisions. Developmental life roles also are demonstrated to children and adolescents by other professionals such as teachers and education specialists; other therapists such as psychologists, speech therapists,

psychiatrists, and pediatricians; and activity and sports leaders, such as coaches and community activity leaders. Others who participate in a child's life should be regularly consulted. (Naturally, consultation will be with permission of the client or the responsible parent whenever possible.) Contemporary descriptions of the role of occupational therapy show that more than just sensorimotor or neuromuscular skills are being addressed for the child population. Specifically, programs are suggested that include parent-skills training, parent support and education, and improving families' abilities to function and interact successfully and appropriately.

Medications

Although some medications, such as Ritalin, have received controversial media attention, a variety of other medications are judiciously used in the treatment of children in addition to the psychostimulants. However, there are concerns over the increase in psychotropic polypharmacy (prescribing two or more medications), and rates are on the rise (Zonfrillo, Penn, & Leonard, 2005). Corresponding with the authors' clinical experience, "psychiatric inpatient facilities have higher rates of polypharmacy than outpatient facilities and pediatric offices" and "in all populations, however, a stimulant co-prescribed with other drugs appears to be the most frequent form of polypharmacy. There has been an increase in the rates of prescribing atypical antipsychotics" (Zonfrillo et al., 2005). This increase in prescribing not only includes medications approved by the Food and Drug Administration, but also off-label medications used for children and adolescents (Harrison,

Cluxton-Keller, & Gross, 2013). With regard to using medications to treat bipolar disorder in children (the concerns of which can be universal at this point in time), the concern is that "physicians and mental health professionals turn to pharmacological solutions because of cost-cutting pressure from insurers and HMOs [health maintenance organization]" (Harvard Medical School, 2007). In this author's inpatient experience, insurers considered medications to be "active treatment," whereas patients could access and participate in occupational and other therapies on an outpatient basis. In reality, medications are more readily available in most communities, especially in comparison to rural and underserved parts of the country where consumers live a distance from the urban and suburban centers where therapy services are available and accessible. Medication is often needed to assist the client in gaining control over his or her behavior or stabilizing symptoms so that he or she may more readily participate in therapy. In a clinical setting, medication is often selected after members of the interdisciplinary treatment team, including parents and guardians, have been consulted and, ideally, the client has been observed in a variety of settings. The occupational therapist can contribute valuable observations of the client in various life roles or occupational settings following assessment of the children as they participate in therapy.

Although medication is often needed to assist the client (and a psychiatrist or family physician is ultimately responsible for prescribing medications), it is important for the occupational therapist and other team members to monitor the medicated child's behaviors and physical and mental status carefully. The occupational therapist works closely with the individual and may be the first to observe emerging side effects or changes in behavior. In home, school, and outpatient settings, the same would hold true for family members, educators, and therapists working in the community. It is particularly important to monitor medications closely in young people because psychoactive medication sometimes interacts with the neurochemistry of the synapses and may interfere with development of new neuron networks and neurologically based competencies. Therefore, cognitive and behavioral approaches are usually attempted before a consideration of pharmacology.

CHILD SETTINGS AND PROGRAMS

When considering various program options, the best program will be the most normalized and balanced one, often with the goal of minimizing the need for further intervention. Children's programs may necessarily be based on a habilitative rather than rehabilitative approach. Habilitation involves addressing skills and behaviors that were previously unlearned and undeveloped. This is opposed to the rehabilitative approach often used with adults, which focuses on the retrieval of skills clients already have or had prior to their current illness. (See Chapter 1 for further discussion.)

Inpatient hospitalization, long-term residential treatment, outpatient settings, community-based programs, day programs, and school-based settings may all offer opportunities for the therapist interested in providing therapy to children with mental health concerns; however, opportunities in the more traditional settings are declining. Anywhere there are children, there is a possible treatment setting in which their psychosocial needs may be met. This avenue needs to be pursued if occupational therapists are to continue to use their valuable mental health skills and knowledge with children. Past developments and opportunities within the school system and occupational therapy in partial hospitalization programs are discussed here.

School-Based Programs

Following the Columbine High School shootings in April 1999, the mental health needs of children received a great deal of attention from clinicians as well as the mass media. New roles identified for occupational therapists include conducting screenings for risk factors among students that have been exposed to violence and providing groups to improve appropriate expression of feelings and improving self-esteem.

Anger management is a critical focus. Being part of a critical incident debriefing team in schools that works with students following a traumatic, violent event has also been identified as a role for therapists working in schools.

School districts are required to meet the special needs of their students in cases where performance in the classroom is affected. Depending on the county and the particular office of education, there may be opportunities for the occupational therapist interested in working to meet the school-aged clients' psychosocial needs. Some counties are meeting the psychosocial needs of severely emotionally disturbed students through programs offered on public school campuses. Such programs typically provide services through a special education teacher, psychiatrist, and social worker, as well as teacher's aides and assistants who work with the clinical staff. Occupational therapists are included in some of these programs and may provide services such as assessment, treatment, home programs, school programs, and consultation. In the school-based setting, the goal is to increase the student's function in the special education classroom with the long-term goal of participation in a regular classroom. All treatment goals should indicate progress toward this end. The occupational therapist is able to view students holistically, observe their performance in the classroom, and provide the necessary services for skill development, adaptation, and improved classroom success.

Two pertinent articles (Barnes, Beck, Vogel, Grice, & Murphy, 2003; Case-Smith & Archer, 2008) illuminate the direction occupational therapy in children's mental health must move and present the stumbling blocks that prevent us from addressing their psychosocial, emotional, and behavioral needs. Occupational therapists working in

CASE ILLUSTRATION 10-4: RYAN—MENTAL HEALTH STRATEGIES IN THE SCHOOL SETTING

Ryan is a 10-year-old boy who is home schooled and receives weekly home-based occupational therapy. The therapist is working on Ryan's Individualized Education Plan goals of improving letter formation and spacing, visual-perceptual skills, and attention span. Following participation in a drawing activity and several games of Connect Four (Hasbro) to work on improving prehensile and visual perceptual abilities and increasing his attention to tasks, which he enjoys a great deal, the therapist asks Ryan to write a sentence of his choosing on lined paper designed to improve handwriting skills, a task that has been part of his therapy sessions throughout the school year.

Ryan says, "I can't do that. It's too hard," and begins to lightly hit himself in the head with his hand.

The therapist, who by observation and experience knows that Ryan is not injuring himself, states, "Ryan, I know that this is something that you don't enjoy doing; nonetheless, we are going to work on writing, which is one of the reasons we work together each week."

Ryan lightly taps his forehead on the lined paper on the table and says, "I just can't!"

The therapist says, "Ryan, what is something you did at your grandmother's house last weekend? I know you really enjoy going there. Maybe we could draw a picture of that after you write your sentence. Hey, maybe the sentence and the picture could be about that."

Ryan stops acting out and says, "I played baseball with my cousins and my team won!"

"That sounds like a lot of fun, Ryan. Why don't you make that your sentence?"

Ryan picks up his pencil, writes the sentence, and then draws a picture of the baseball game.

Discussion

This case illustration demonstrates how using mental health interventions such as redirection, interpretation, limit-setting, a client-centered approach, and therapeutic use of self facilitated Ryan's ability to participate in therapy. In addition to the goals in his Individualized Education Plan, the therapist was able to address problems that Ryan faces that impede his ability to complete his assigned school work by addressing his decreased frustration tolerance and his maladaptive coping skills.

---

pediatrics, from early intervention to the school systems, have been slow to provide treatment that, if it were truly holistic, would include addressing all of a child's or student's presenting problems, not just those on the referral.

The school setting remains one of the largest areas of occupational therapy practice, and despite that fact, it has not yet become a noted provider of occupational therapy services that address the mental health needs of students. According to a 2008 study by Case-Smith and Archer, rather than addressing mental health issues, practitioners in school settings stated that disruptive behaviors were barriers to their treatment. They believed that these therapists perhaps did not recognize that the behavior itself could be a target for treatment and perhaps behavioral change was not part their services. Additionally, nearly two-thirds of the participants in their study did not think that they were prepared to work with emotional disturbances. A 2003 study by Barnes et al. found the following obstacles to providing occupational therapy for students with emotional disturbances in the school setting according to practitioners in their study: confusion about the occupational therapy role, limited knowledge or support from the team, and bureaucratic administrative factors, among others. Other professionals believed that the role of occupational therapy was to address handwriting and sensory integration issues and

that addressing the mental health needs of students was out of their purview. At the same time, therapists in this study, as in the study by Case-Smith and Archer (2008), did not believe they possessed the knowledge or preparation to provide mental health interventions. These studies would lead one to believe that either we are not adequately preparing practitioners to address mental health issues or, once in the educational system, they feel confined to a narrowly defined scope of practice. Case Illustration 10-4 provides examples of how a therapist working in an educational system may use mental health practice skills along with those required to provide services to students that address educational issues.

Day Programs

Day programs are sometimes referred to as *day treatment programs*. They are another alternative designed to prevent children from entering or staying in an inpatient hospitalization setting. These programs also provide a useful service of transitioning the client from an inpatient to an outpatient setting or to provide an educational experience when the regular school cannot currently meet the needs of the child with a mental illness. These programs are sometimes affiliated with a mental health unit or residential program in the community. The clients will attend a program during typical school hours and will receive treatment groups or therapy more intensively than if they were only receiving outpatient therapy. The student may attend a program like this to avoid hospitalization or to make necessary adjustments to medication in a supervised setting. As with the school-based program and most treatment programs, the goal is to improve the client's functioning to the degree to which he or she can be placed in a less intensive/restrictive environment.

IMPLEMENTING PROGRAMMING FOR CHILDREN

When developing a program of occupational therapy, it is important to assess the needs of the children, demands of the service delivery system, and structure of the program. For example, if developmental motor lags are an area of concern, sensorimotor groups may be planned. Where play skills are lacking, play groups and opportunities to develop age-appropriate play skills are of prime importance. If children in the treatment setting have difficulty expressing their thoughts and feelings appropriately, programming should address these needs.

The second critical step is to look at the service delivery system itself. In acute care settings, there is relatively little time to provide treatment before discharge looms. Often, it is the role of occupational therapy and the treatment team to begin treatment with the idea that it will be continued outside the hospital setting in the community at school or in an outpatient office. In a longer-term setting, treatment may be carried out entirely in one place, although because of the frequent changes in health care delivery, there may not be an extended period of time to bring about change. In terms of planning occupational therapy for an existing program, it is important to understand how therapy fits into the current program in terms of philosophy and program needs. This makes an understanding of theory important and flexibility imperative. The therapist must assume a systems approach, involving an awareness of the current program, service delivery system, and client's needs.

In addition to occupational therapy assessments based in specific frames of reference, groups and activities are determined by the developmental needs of individual children. For example, a child may be 12 years old chronologically but function at a 3- or 4-year-old level, with a limited ability to express feelings in words and impaired cognitive skills secondary to a diagnosis of pervasive developmental disorder or intellectual disability. Such a child may be placed in a play group that meets the needs of his or her developmental, age-appropriate level. The child's play and social behavior can be observed at the same time he or she is provided with opportunities for developmentally appropriate play activities. When a child is observed to be playing successfully at a developmentally appropriate level, he or she may then be moved up from a play group to a skills group to learn further personal and social skills.

Evaluation and Assessment

General areas of assessment concern the occupational performance areas of self-care and play and also developmental milestone achievement (see Parham & Fazio [2007] for many assessments of play). Play can be evaluated by observing a child at play and obtaining a play history concerning what toys and games the child chooses. The occupational performance mental, sensory, and movement-related functions under client factors to be assessed are primarily sensorimotor, cognitive, psychological, and social. The Child and Adolescent Functional Assessment Scale is widely used (Bates, 2001; Hodges, Wong, & Latessa, 1998). Formal evaluations such as the Test of Visual Motor Skills, the Good-Enough-Harris Draw-A-Person test, or the Erhhardt Developmental Prehension Assessment may further evaluate adaptive motor skills and coordination as well as a basic assessment of achievement on expected developmental milestones (Asher, 2014). A useful tool for a quick assessment of many components is the Kinetic Self-Image Test (Abramson, 1982), developed as part of the Initial Play Interview at Mount Sinai Hospital in New York. In this test, the child is asked to draw a picture of him- or herself doing something. Besides data regarding sensorimotor and cognitive functions and skills, valuable information such as interests, relationships, and self-concept can be determined. Case Illustrations 10-5 and 10-6 show the use of this assessment. The Child Occupational Self-Assessment and Pediatric Volitional Questionnaire (Taylor, 2017) are also some of the tools from Kielhofner's Model of Human Occupation (Model of Human Occupation Clearinghouse, n.d.) that determine interests (Child Occupational Self-Assessment) and motivating environments (Pediatric Volitional Questionnaire).

Intervention

Play is often referred to as the work of the child; it is generally defined as the way children learn basic skills and resolve intrapersonal and interpersonal conflicts.

> From a child's play we can gain understanding of how he sees and construes the world … play refers to a young child's activities characterized by freedom from all but personally imposed rules … by fantasy involvement and by the absence of any goals outside of the activity itself. (Bettelheim, 1987, para. 3)

It is helpful to distinguish play from games because the latter are a predominant occupation of older children and adolescents. Games are usually competitive and have agreed-upon rules that are imposed externally. Games require that the activity be pursued in a prescribed manner,

CASE ILLUSTRATION 10-5: JOSH—KINETIC SELF-IMAGE TEST

Josh, a newly admitted boy, drew a picture of "me, my mom, and my dad going for ice cream." Although the boy was 11 years old, he drew only stick figures and a poorly drawn house. During the evaluation, Josh kept looking at the clock, and he also asked to go to the bathroom several times. When asked if he had an appointment or was waiting or looking for someone, he said, "I have a family session at 3 o'clock." However, when asked if he was leaving group to see if his parents had arrived, he angrily denied it.

Discussion

This simple assessment can be helpful in determining mental age and motor coordination, what the child is thinking about, and the quality of family or personal functioning and relationships.

CASE ILLUSTRATION 10-6: JOHN AND STEPHEN—KINETIC SELF-IMAGE TEST

John, age 10, and Stephen, age 8, were being seen for evaluation during their initial home-based therapy visit. Their parents had recently separated, and the boys lived with their mother, who is a nurse. Their father had been described as having bipolar disorder and alcoholism. Divorce is probable, and their mother was referred to the therapist by an outpatient child psychiatrist after he evaluated the older child. The mother, concerned with the children's reaction to the separation and pending divorce, wished to provide an outlet for the children's feelings and an arena for them to discuss their concerns. Additionally, she has concerns regarding a strong family history of bipolar disorder and alcoholism on both sides of the family and the possibility of these disorders emerging in the children.

In the initial session, the Kinetic Self-Image Test was used to assess the boys. Each was asked to draw a picture of himself doing something. John drew a picture of "playing ball with my dad." Of note was a tall tree drawn in the center of the paper separating the boy from the father. Stephen drew a picture of "John and me playing catch." It included birds, trees, and a yellow sun.

Discussion

Clearly, John's relationship with his father and spending time with him are important, and his concern about the separation is evident in the picture. For Stephen, the focus of the picture was playing with his brother, and its details and pleasant presentation indicates either a more positive approach to family dynamics or denial of the current situation.

without one's personal fantasy, and there is often a goal, such as winning, outside the activity (Bettelheim, 1987). With the basic acceptance of the importance of play (and later, games) as treatment and also with the recognition of play as the predominant occupation of childhood, it is the primary occupation used in pediatrics and the primary activity used in pediatric groups. As stated in a seminal article by Bettelheim (1987, para. 2), "play therapy has become the main avenue for helping young children with their emotional difficulties."

Play is also the primary mode of evaluating children, done through specific assessments and interviews and by ongoing observation. Observation, based on the broad education and the unique and specific knowledge of occupation possessed by therapists, is an excellent evaluation in and of itself. In terms of its use with children, "observation provides the opportunity to document occupation-based assessment without having to depend on youth's willingness and ability to answer questions" (Quake-Rapp, Miller, Gomathy, & En-Chi, 2008). There are various ways to initially evaluate and continue to observe play. Some useful categories to think about while observing play are the following (C. Grandison, personal communication, January 28, 1997):

- Developmental or stage of play, such as solitary, exploratory, parallel, project, or cooperative: A 2-year-old can be expected to engage mostly in parallel play, whereas a 10-year-old can be expected to cooperate with other children in play.
- Entrance to play: For example, does a child hesitate to play or quickly bolt toward the toys?
- Initiation toward play: That is, (1) does a child initiate play independently or wait for someone to start with, and (2) is the same pattern consistent throughout play?
- Energy level: What is the level of energy of the child at play and does it change within or over sessions? Is it the same with or without structure? Is it the same with a parent present?

- Body movement and use of space: That is, does the child know where others are? Does he or she define a small area or fill up every space? Does the child use furniture?

- Emotional tone: That is, what is the emotional tenor to the play (e.g., is it angry or sad?) and does it remain the same over time?

- Materials: What materials does the child gravitate toward and how are they used?

- Symbolic nature of play: For example, does the child use objects and play symbolically? What are the themes of play, and are they consistent throughout?

An ongoing, regularly scheduled play group also provides information about the child's current developmental level of play as reflected in the choice of toys, games, and peers while engaged in play.

Groups

Play group is a nondirective play group that occurs most easily in the context of an occupational therapy playroom. A nondirective play group allows children to gravitate to and engage in the play occupations of their own choosing without the direction or suggestions for participation from the group leader. For purposes of observation and ongoing assessment, this allows for a truer picture of the child's abilities, interests, and play skills and an age-appropriate opportunity for the child to present personal and family dynamics without any leading remarks from the group leader that could bias the child's responses. The group's protocol is illustrated in Box 10-2.

The room includes toys, water and sand play areas, dress-up clothes for fantasy play, and a table and chairs. It serves to encourage the development of play skills, which in turn facilitates the development of social skills. The play group also has the goal of providing an arena whereby children may resolve conflicts and issues that led to their current problems and dysfunction. For example, two children may use dolls to express anger at parents who abused them. They may also recreate arguments or scenes they observed in the home. For example, by using toy sharks, a child may safely and appropriately show anger or jealousy toward a sibling or peer by "eating" him or her during water play or "burying" him or her in the sandbox. A game like Sorry! (Hasbro) helps increase frustration tolerance, and a game like Twister (Hasbro) develops not only laterality, but also the ability to practice being in close proximity to others while appropriately interacting and respecting body space. Beanbag toss games are an appropriate outlet for anger and aggression and also provide the opportunity to engage in turn taking and mild competition. Candyland (Hasbro) and Connect Four are just a few of the many readily available childhood games that can be used or adapted to develop many different skills and prompt conversation and discussion. Inherent in many childhood games such as Duck, Duck, Goose; musical chairs; and dodge ball is a focus on developing a variety of basic abilities. Rolling dodge ball can be played in place of the conventional game. This adaptation involves rolling rather than throwing the ball at peers. This increases safety and prevents the game from becoming overly aggressive.

There are countless ways in which play can help children learn new skills and accomplish treatment goals. For example, it is more efficacious to ask children to try to clean up the entire playroom before you can count to 10 than it is to just command them to clean up the playroom because "it's time to end group." Turning an activity into a game or play, as in this example, is often more effective than other approaches. It is also congruent with the philosophy of occupational therapy and the general approach of using play as a treatment modality. The active experiences of play and the focus on productivity and participation offer intrinsic satisfaction for a child's needs. Aside from conflict resolution, play also offers children the additional ability to work on treatment goals of improving impulse control, developing cognitive skills, mastering the environment, and developing age-appropriate social interactions. Through the mastery of tasks, latency-aged children will be able to benefit from the successful interaction with objects and people in an occupational therapy group and gain mastery over themselves in the process.

Creative task groups also serve as highly effective interventions with latency-aged children. Using tiles to make mosaics, doing wood projects such as creating a bookshelf or making a toy car, painting suncatchers, or participating in seasonal activities such as carving a pumpkin or baking Christmas cookies offer children rewarding experiences. In addition, the experiences teach appropriate interaction and develop cognitive skills, such as the ability to follow directions, complete tasks, and share materials, as well as facilitate increased attention span and concentration. Comments made about the projects often provide a valuable additional perspective on a child's emotions and concerns. Copper tooling is a highly successful creative task project. Children frequently ask, "Can I do more than one?" or, after successful completion of the project, they will ask, "Can we do copper tooling projects again?" Children have remarked, "It's fun to do and easy to make." Indeed, the steps of copper tooling are easy to grade according to the therapeutic purposes of the group, and the completed project reinforces self-efficacy, increases self-esteem, and validates the individual's efforts to affect positive change on the physical environment through the creation of a tangible object that may be personally enjoyed or given as a gift.

Of course, it is important to take safety precautions while completing copper tooling projects such as removing the solution (liver of sulfur) as soon as all group members have used it and conducting the group in a well-ventilated area.

Most often, creative tasks are provided as part of a parallel task group. This structure provides opportunities to

Box 10-2. Play Group Protocol

NAME OF GROUP

Occupational Therapy Play Group

DESCRIPTION

Play is an important part of a child's development. Children learn, express themselves, and develop interpersonal interaction skills through play. Through play, children are able to express inner feelings and conflicts in a nonthreatening way. This group's primary goal is to evaluate skills and provide an adequate environment where the children's dynamics, developmental level of play, and socialization skills can be observed and practiced.

THERAPIST NAME

William Lambert, OTR/L

TITLE

Occupational Therapist

GOALS

1. Provide a stimulating environment where the children will be motivated to play.
2. Encourage peer interaction through play.
3. Provide insightful interpretations related to the play when appropriate.
4. Allow the children to work through dynamic issues through the play.
5. Encourage the highest developmental level of play and interpersonal interaction possible.

ENTRANCE CRITERIA

1. Group members are selected by the occupational therapist according to their developmental levels of play.
2. Five children is an optimal number of group members.
3. Patient has appropriate level of privileges.
4. Patient has been medically cleared by physician.

GROUP RULES

1. Have fun.
2. Share.
3. Listen to staff.
4. Clean up.

FORMAT

Group meets two times per week for 45 minutes with two leaders: the occupational therapist and a member of the nursing staff.

EXIT CRITERIA

1. Change in level of privileges
2. Change in developmental status
3. Discharge from the hospital

develop appropriate interpersonal interactions on a limited basis, share through the use of supplies that are common to the group activity, and develop impulse control by waiting to follow the steps and to see the project through to completion.

Group goals may include learning how to follow simple, step-by-step verbal directions; sharing materials and space; interacting without being intrusive; sustaining and increasing attention span; and developing impulse control. Other information that can be gained through the use of a simple craft project includes dynamic information such as whom the gift or project is to be given and, therefore, who is important in the child's life.

Box 10-3. Skills Development Group Protocol

NAME OF GROUP

Occupational Therapy Skill Development Group

DESCRIPTION

A developmental task group for children who have developed basic play and social skills and need to acquire skills in cognition, interpersonal interactions, and self-expression.

THERAPIST NAME

William Lambert, OTR/L

TITLE

Occupational Therapist

GOALS

1. To improve cognitive skills such as:
   - Problem solving
   - Organization of thoughts
   - Ability to follow directions
2. To improve interpersonal interaction skills and facilitate sharing cooperation
3. To improve ability to express thoughts and feelings appropriately

ENTRANCE CRITERIA

1. Group members are selected by the occupational therapist according to developmental need.
2. Patient should be on appropriate level of privilege to attend groups.
3. Patient is medically cleared by physician.
4. Five to seven children is the optimal number of group members.

GROUP RULES

1. Have fun.
2. Share.
3. Listen to staff.
4. Clean up.

FORMAT

Group meets two times per week for 45 minutes with two leaders: the occupational therapist and a member of the nursing staff. Activities will be planned to develop specific skills through the use of games and creative tasks.

EXIT CRITERIA

1. Change in level of privileges
2. Discharge from hospital

Skill development group assists older children who have adequate play and social skills and need to improve problem-solving, coping, and communication skills. The group's protocol is shown in Box 10-3. Group topics and discussion focus on common problems and situations that children face, as well as the specific problem areas that led to treatment.

Although a variety of activities can be used in the skills development group, including crafts, therapeutic board games are frequently used. The Talking, Feeling, and Doing Game facilitates the expression of thoughts and feelings. This game is highlighted in Case Illustration 10-7. In using a board game format, children are usually willing to participate, and an appropriate amount of structure is provided. Children are often happy to have an outlet for their unexpressed feelings and thoughts and view the game as a safe and nonthreatening means of personal expression. Box 10-4 shows ways to ensure that the environment supports effective group and individual interventions.

CASE ILLUSTRATION 10-7: THE TALKING, FEELING, AND DOING GAME

Seven children aged 8 to 12 years are playing the game with the occupational therapist, a member of the nursing staff, and an occupational therapy student. Sam rolls the dice, lands on a yellow space, and selects a "feeling" card, which reads: "Name three things that could cause a person to be angry." He pauses and then says, "Being told to shut up, being hit, and being lied to."

Dave lands on a white space and selects a "talking" card, which reads, "What kind of work does your father do? What do you think about that kind of job?" Dave answers, "He fixes trucks," although he does not mention that his father is in prison. "I'm going to race motorcycles when I grow up," he says when asked what he thinks of his father's job.

Christine rolls the dice and also lands on a white space. Her card asks, "What is the best thing you can say about your family?" She replies, "They bring me candy and lots of things."

John lands on a red space and picks a "doing" card, which reads, "Skip across the room and then return to your seat." He says, "I'm not doing that," but he agrees to take another card. This one asks him to pretend that he is having an argument with someone and to tell the group what it is about. "I'm arguing with Melissa. She won't share," John replies.

The therapist then rolls and lands on a "feeling" space. His card reads, "When was the last time you cried?" He says, "I cried when my dad died." Then he talks about how crying is helpful in expressing feelings of sadness.

Linda and Rhonda, the other adults in group, reinforce what the therapist has said. This helps the children talk about their feelings and express them appropriately.

Discussion

This game promotes, through talking, the expression of what is on children's minds. The game facilitates the expression of feelings, promotes the discussion of personal problems, and explores family dynamics without threat and in a manner that matches the children's emotional ages. It is important to have a good working knowledge of the children in the group and be familiar with their individual histories and issues to lead a game such as this effectively.

Box 10-4. Tips for Creating an Effective Playroom or Therapy Area

- Soft lighting to provide a calming atmosphere
- Area rugs or carpet to play on
- Colorful but not overstimulating room
- Adequate tables and chairs. These do not need to be child-sized except for younger preschool-age children. Most latchkey-age children can use a conventional-sized table and chairs.
- Materials should be easy to clean.
- An area for water play and larger gross motor groups is ideal, but be adaptive! A bathtub or utility sink can do as needed or on a regular basis, depending on funding, facility, and frequency of use.
- Craft paper in large rolls can be used for many purposes: to cover the table for a craft activity, to do body tracings, to make murals and drawings, and so on. This inexpensive investment goes a long way and lasts a long time!

There are ever-increasing numbers of blended and non-traditional families in the United States. The traditional family may no longer be constituted of a biological mother and father with biological siblings. Children and adolescents may be adopted and raised by extended families, grandparents, relatives, step-parents, or family friends. Whomever the child or adolescent considers to be family may be permitted to join in treatment, as is often the case in the parent-child activity group.

The parent-child activity group involves engaging the parents of the emotionally disturbed child in an activity with the child. It is held weekly in the occupational therapy room, where families work on a project together with the goal of completing it in one session. This group improves the parent-child interaction by engaging them together in a pleasurable, successful activity, something that may not otherwise be possible due to the child's illness. The therapist provides encouragement and support and models appropriate caregiver behavior, such as setting limits on inappropriate actions and giving praise for desirable ones. The occupational therapist assists parents in differentiating between behavior that is maladaptive and behavior that is typical for the child's developmental level. Beyond providing occupational therapy for families and their children, the therapist is able to provide those involved in the child's treatment with information about family interactive patterns, the child's response to therapy with the parents, and how well the parents are implementing what they are being taught about how to interact with their child. The parent-child activity as originally conducted expanded the scope of occupational therapy in the hospital setting to areas traditionally reserved for individual and family therapists. By providing information on the child's behavior and the therapeutic outcomes of the session, occupational therapy has enhanced the interdisciplinary treatment team's ability to see the child and family more globally and respond with more integrated treatment for both. This group can be effectively used in a variety of settings, including the home, school, or outpatient office, both with individual families or several families attending the same session. Depending upon the specific reasons for referral and the expectations of the referral source, clinical information gleaned may be shared with other clinicians involved in the case or used by the group leader with the group participants. At the conclusion of the session, the therapist may choose to process the session with all the participants present, privately with the parents/guardians, or both, which is usually the norm. Regardless, it is generally beneficial to meet with the parents/guardians apart from their children to provide opportunities for questions, discussion, and teaching or reviewing effective and appropriate parenting and intervention skills.

OCCUPATIONAL THERAPY PRIVATE PRACTICE FOR CHILDREN

Therapists have been challenged to follow clients into the community, to consider consulting as an alternative to direct service, and to find new sources of funding, including cash. Clinicians need to present occupational therapy outcomes and market to the needs of clients and community agencies. As the location of care moves out of the hospital and lengths of stay become increasingly shorter, one arena for therapists is private practice and considering private pay for reimbursement of services through community-based practice.

The following are examples of private practices that can be implemented by using the interventions originally used in an inpatient setting described earlier in this chapter in the community. These interventions include consultation and direct service for a foster care agency and home-based therapy. Both involve a family-centered approach and a fee-for-service format for payment (cash or check). Traditional forms of reimbursement, such as private insurance or managed care companies, are not used or accepted. This arrangement also adds an increased measure of confidentiality, and the therapist, family, or agency can determine the number of sessions.

Occupational Therapy Services for a Foster Care Agency

Providing occupational therapy services for a foster care agency brings unique and rewarding challenges and illustrates a new role for occupational therapy in the community in a nontraditional practice setting. "Foster children exhibit diverse psychological, emotional, and behavioral problems, which have been well documented. The literature repeatedly reports that foster children have high rates of mental health, behavioral, and adaptive functioning issues" (Precin, Timque, & Walsh, 2010, p. 152; see also Dozier & Rutter, 2008). The child in foster care can be assisted in adapting to various situations through occupational therapy intervention that increases the child's ability to function in an age-appropriate manner at his or her current level of development. Intervention is aimed at reducing the number of times that a child's life is interrupted so that agency goals of successful pre- and postadoptive placements can be achieved, as well as easing a child's transition from a foster care placement to reunification with the biological parent(s) and birth family. An example of interventions to facilitate family reunification is presented in Case Illustration 10-8.

Foster Care Agency—Expert Witness

In another case of family reunification, the mother failed to attend any of the scheduled parent-child activity sessions. During groups with the occupational therapist, the siblings consistently expressed their desire to remain in the preadoptive foster home and to be adopted by their foster parents. At the custody hearing, the report of the children's desire to be adopted and to have the biological mother's rights terminated to facilitate their adoption was presented to the judge and served as an objective outside opinion as well as an expert witness. In chambers, the children corroborated the therapist's testimony, and the judge ruled for termination based on the children's statements, the occupational therapist's evidence, and the evidence from others involved in the case. This evidence from various sources paved the way for adoption in an appropriate home for these children.

CASE ILLUSTRATION 10-8: REUNIFICATION—THE SMITH FAMILY

Joseph, age 5, lives in a large city with his mother, Rose, age 27. They have just successfully completed family-based therapy sessions with the occupational therapist, which was an essential piece of their reunification plan. Now Rose and Joseph will again have John, Sophia, Carl, and James back in the home. Currently, John, age 10, lives in a foster care home. Sophia, age 8; Carl, age 6; and James, age 3.5 live in another foster care home. Reunification will be facilitated through two separate intervention strategies. First, parent-child activity sessions with the entire family will be conducted by the occupational therapist once per month. Second, the occupational therapist will schedule sibling groups between the family sessions to reacquaint the brothers and sisters with each other. Rose and Joseph arrive for their scheduled parent-child activity on Saturday morning and join the other siblings and the therapist at the occupational therapy office. The initial intervention is for the children and mother to play together using the toys in the room, and later to make pudding to have for dessert, which will follow a lunch provided by the foster care agency.

The occupational therapist begins the activity by asking, "John, why don't you be a big brother and help your little sister and brothers by being in charge of pouring the milk?" This intervention occurs once the therapist notices that Rose appears overwhelmed and makes no attempt to organize the task. The therapist then notices James crawling for the door and retrieves him. "Sophia, will you keep an eye on James so he doesn't get into trouble?" he suggests.

Eventually, Rose opens the pudding package after reading the directions to the children, several of whom are not paying attention, and begins giving her children various tasks to complete. The therapist moves to the periphery of the room to facilitate the mother taking charge of the situation and to assess the parent-child interaction. Once the pudding has been spooned into cups and put in the refrigerator, the therapist cues the family to clean up the dishes. The family is given time to socialize as they wait for pizza to be delivered. The younger children fight over a toy, but the mother redirects them to share. John, as usual, is quiet and isolative. Rose picks up the toddler and attempts to engage James in play with nearby toys. Joseph engages in spontaneous play with his younger brothers and wrestles with them. Sophia, who had been drawing, starts to cry because she feels left out. The occupational therapist suggests ways for her to ask her siblings to play with her, such as asking them to come draw with her or to play a game.

Discussion

Occupational therapy groups were used to facilitate reunification of several siblings living in different foster care homes with their biological mother and an additional sibling residing with her. Sibling groups based on the play group format refamiliarize the siblings with each other during sessions using play, games, and arts and crafts, in addition to developing and building relationships and interactions among the children and provide opportunities for professional observation and assessment. The sibling groups were used in conjunction with a parent-child activity that occurred during the biological mother's scheduled monthly visit with all of her children, a vital part of the reunification process. This group used activities such as making pudding and simple meals, arts and crafts, structured play, and games designed to reinforce roles of mother, older brother, sister, younger brothers, and toddler, with the therapist serving as facilitator. These groups were used to promote appropriate parent-child interactions and establish filial roles. The groups also provided a therapeutic milieu for the mother and children to meet each other in a safe setting, not only for interaction, but also for expression of feelings regarding present and future visitation.

The therapist provided role modeling and suggestions for improving parenting skills. He also solicited the mother's feedback as to how she perceived the reunification process to be progressing. The therapist also provided the foster care agency with ongoing reports, and his assessment of family functioning helped determine when reunification would occur. Following 21 months of occupational therapy intervention, the family was reunited and continues to live together. Although therapy progressed well across time, other factors, such as the mother finding an appropriately sized home, having the home approved, and various bureaucratic requirements, lengthened the reunification process. This case illustrates how the luxury of time and many ongoing sessions can exist when traditional reimbursement sources are not used.

Testifying in court is a unique experience. Some suggestions when testifying are to remember to always address the judge as Your Honor and answer only the questions you are asked succinctly and specifically. The more information volunteered, the more opportunities the opposing side's attorney has to discredit your testimony.

In court hearings to involuntarily terminate parental rights of children in foster care who want to be adopted by their foster parents, the responsibilities of the therapist are specific. They are to assess the children through information from interviews and therapy sessions. Then in court, the therapist presents his or her clinical opinion regarding what outcome the children want, their feelings regarding the termination, and what outcome he or she recommends based on his or her area of expertise and clinical experience.

Being a witness in court includes being a developmental specialist, child advocate, and clinical expert regarding children's behavioral and emotional health through the eye and lens of occupational therapy.

Foster Care Agency—Direct Service

The occupational therapist provides other services for the foster care agency, including family intervention and troubleshooting regarding developmentally appropriate rules and activities for children in foster care. This is especially important in instances where the foster parents require direction and instruction to smooth family difficulties and deal adaptively and appropriately with the children and their diverse issues, presenting problems, and diagnoses.

With the aid of occupational therapy intervention, a foster care or preadoptive home placement can remain consistent and reduce the number of times that a child's life is interrupted. Minimizing interruptions is imperative to the mental health of children in the foster care system (Dozier & Rutter, 2008; Waterman, 2001).

Home-Based Occupational Therapy

Occupational therapists have been encouraged to develop new strategies for serving the mental health needs of children and their families (Dorman & Helfrich, 2001). Therefore, home-based intervention has been cited as a growing area of practice and uses the natural setting of the home to assess and treat areas of behavior, family dynamics, and parent-child interactions (Case-Smith & O'Brien, 2015). Interventions can include anger management, social skills training, and parent-child activities. The parent-child activity discussed previously in this chapter and in the described foster care case interventions is also part of a home-based approach, with the added dimension of using the family home as a treatment setting. This provides an in vivo environment to observe situations and interactions that affect therapy outcomes but are not able to be observed in other settings. For example, the 24-hour television, the dog running through the house barking because of a thunderstorm, the younger sibling who intrudes on the session with his brother and steals game board pieces, dinner late or burning, and so on provide real-life situations and stressors that can be observed and used as intervention points in therapy.

Upon referral from a child psychiatrist, occupational therapists may see children and their families in their own homes to address the variety of psychosocial deficits and problems that led the children and their families to seek professional help. Again, the duration and length of therapy is determined largely by the family and the therapist, with direction provided by the referring psychiatrist. The occupational therapist must possess an extensive background in providing psychosocial interventions to children with emotional disturbances and their families and be able to practice autonomously. An additional benefit to this practice setting is that there is rarely a missed appointment, although a family may forget about the scheduled visit. Receiving payment upon conclusion of the session eliminates the need for billing, and seeing children and their families in their homes eliminates the need for renting office space. However, it does include other incurred expenses that should be taken into account regarding billing and determining the hourly rate, such as mileage, the price of gas, and increased wear and tear on one's car. Also, like many other home health therapists, one's car becomes a clinic where supplies are kept, and for a pediatric therapist, the car often becomes a traveling collection of toys, games, and other therapy supplies.

Infant mental health is a relatively new area of pediatric mental health that offers opportunities to occupational therapists (Bazyk, 2011; Jackson & Arbesman, 2005). Additionally, addressing bullying and other current problems facing young people offers opportunities for therapists wishing to address the psychosocial needs of this population. (See Chapters 10 and 12 for more information on these topics.)

SUMMARY, CURRENT TRENDS, AND RECOMMENDATIONS

The various conditions of children with mental illnesses include depression, bipolar disorder, and posttraumatic stress disorder, in addition to disorders first identified and diagnosed in childhood, such as ADHD, oppositional defiant disorder, and RAD. When connecting behavior and diagnosis, genetic predispositions to mental illness and the symptoms and presenting problems of the disorders should be considered as well as environmental psychosocial stressors such as family dysfunction, abuse, trauma, neglect, violence, and poverty. Developmental level and age-appropriate tasks should also be considered when working with children with emotional disturbances.

Useful concepts to consider when working with this population are structure and consistency, redirection, interpretation of behavior, time-out, a personal therapeutic style, a team approach, and the judicious use of psychotropic medications.

When implementing programming for this population, it is important to consider the needs of the consumers, the demands of the service delivery system, and the structure of the current or planned program. Various assessments, including observation, are useful tools for occupational therapists planning therapeutic interventions. Interventions for children can be based primarily on play and include nondirective play, skill development, creative tasks, and parent-child activity groups.

"Sicker and quicker" has become an often-used phrase when describing the trend toward offering less time for therapy for hospitalized children who may have very severe emotional and behavioral problems. This is currently true in settings outside of the hospital as well. Because managed care often replaces traditional insurance and reimbursement programs, time frames for therapy are becoming shorter and inpatient hospitalizations are being curtailed in favor of community-based care. Unfortunately, cost containment may also limit access to occupational therapy unless therapists make the transition from traditional hospital and medical model practice settings to emerging areas of practice and community-based care. In an attempt to bring their expertise to these other arenas of the continuum of care, therapists need to consider and explore new ways of providing therapy to this population. These new ways include, but are not limited to, foster care, home, public, and private school settings, and exploring the possibilities extant in the unfamiliar territory of the variety of agencies and programs already in place that provide services to children with and without identified disorders who to date have not employed occupational therapists, and those who have, most notably the school systems. Looking to the community for the answers to the question of how we can serve children with mental health issues is the beginning of our journey to provide occupational therapy to what may be considered an underserved population. In addition, our unique ability to address the whole child in every way, including occupationally, needs to become an accepted and well-known fact to enable us to move forward in meeting the largely unmet needs of children with mental health problems and their families.

Children in need of services to remediate mental and behavioral pathology and develop and integrate new skills can be found everywhere—in the hospital, the school, at day care, at home, and in your neighborhood. This is still true. Because children (and often their parents) are not always effective self-advocates, it is incumbent upon therapists to advocate for appropriate services, including occupational therapy, for underserved populations such as children and their families who are struggling with mental health issues. Indeed, the *Occupational Therapy Practice*

Framework (American Occupational Therapy Association, 2014) includes interventions and outcomes that include advocacy and occupational justice for populations and communities.

ACKNOWLEDGEMENT

The author would like to acknowledge Kasey Fitzgerald, MS, OTR/L, who contributed significantly to the editing and research for this chapter.

REFERENCES

Abramson, R. M. (1982). Developmental and diagnostic assessment. In L. Hoffmann (Ed.), *The evaluation and care of severely disturbed children* (pp. 37-44). New York, NY: SP Medical & Scientific Books.

American Occupational Therapy Association. (2014). Occupational therapy practice framework: Domain and process (3rd ed.). *American Journal of Occupational Therapy, 68,* S1-S51

American Psychiatric Association. (2013). *Diagnostic and statistical manual of mental disorders: DSM-5* (5th ed.). Arlington, VA: Author.

Asher, I. E. (Ed.). (2014). *Asher's assessment tools: An annotated index for occupational therapy* (4th ed.). Bethesda, MD: AOTA Press.

Barnes, K., Beck, K., Vogel, K., Grice, K. O., & Murphy, D. (2003). Perceptions regarding school based occupational therapy for children with emotional disturbances. *American Journal of Occupational Therapy, 57,* 337-341.

Bates, M. (2001). Child and Adolescent Functional Assessment Scale (CAFAS): Review and current status. *Clinical Child and Family Psychology Review, 4*(1), 63-84.

Bazyk, S. (Ed.). (2011). *Mental health promotion, prevention, and intervention with children and youth: A guiding framework for occupational therapy.* Bethesda, MD: American Occupational Therapy Association.

Bettelheim, B. (1987, March). The importance of play. *Atlantic Monthly,* 35-46. Retrieved from https://www.theatlantic.com/magazine/archive/1987/03/the-importance-of-play/305129/

Case-Smith, J., & Archer, L. (2008). School-based services for students with emotional disturbance: Findings and recommendations. *OT Practice, 13*(1), 17-20.

Case-Smith, J., & O'Brien, J. C. (2015). *Occupational therapy for children and adolescents* (7th ed.). St. Louis, MO: Elsevier Mosby.

Centers for Disease Control and Prevention. (2018). *Fetal alcohol spectrum disorders (FASDs).* Retrieved from https://www.cdc.gov/ncbddd/fasd/index.html

Dorman, W., & Helfrich, C. (2001). *Psychosocial competence and its impact on function in children and youth.* Paper presented at the meeting of the American Occupational Therapy Association, Philadelphia, PA, April.

Dozier, M., & Rutter, M. (2008). Challenges to the development of attachment relationships faced by young children in foster and adoptive care. In J. Cassidy & P. Shaver (Eds.), *Handbook of attachment: Theory, research and clinical applications* (2nd ed., pp. 698-717). New York, NY: Guilford Press.

Harrison, J. N., Cluxton-Keller, F., & Gross, D. (2013). Antipsychotic medication prescribing trends in children and adolescents. *Journal of Pediatric Health Care, 26*(2), 139-145.

Harvard Medical School. (2007). Bipolar disorder in children. *Harvard Mental Health Letter, 23*(11). Retrieved from https://www.health.harvard.edu/newsletter_article/Bipolar_disorder_in_children

Hodges, K., Wong, M., & Latessa, M. (1998). Use of the Child and Adolescent Functional Scale (CAFAS) as an outcome measure in clinical settings. *Journal of Behavioral Health Services and Research, 25*, 325-336.

Jackson, L., & Arbesman, M. (Eds.). (2005). Children with behavioral and psychosocial needs. *AOTA Practice Guidelines Series.* Bethesda, MD: American Occupational Therapy Association.

Kramer, P., & Hinojosa, J. (2010). *Frames of reference for pediatric occupational therapy* (3rd ed.). Baltimore, MD: Lippincott Williams & Wilkins.

Model of Human Occupation Clearinghouse. (n.d.). Assessment selection tool. *Model of Human Occupation: Theory and Application.* Retrieved from https://www.moho.uic.edu/resources/findTheAssessment/home.aspx

Parham, L. D., & Fazio, L. S. (Eds.). (2007). *Play in occupational therapy for children* (2nd ed.). St. Louis, MO: Mosby.

Phelan, T. W. (2016). *1-2-3 magic: 3-step discipline for calm, effective, and happy parenting* (6th ed.). Naperville, IL: ParentMagic, Inc.

Precin, P., Timque, J., & Walsh, A. (2010). A role for occupational therapy in foster care. *Occupational Therapy in Mental Health, 26*(2), 151-175.

Quake-Rapp, C., Miller, B., Gomathy, A., & En-Chi, C. (2008). Direct observation as a means of assessing frequency of maladaptive behavior in youths with severe emotional and behavioral disorder (2008). *American Journal of Occupational Therapy, 62*(2), 206-211.

Resnick, R. (2005). Attention deficit hyperactivity disorder in teens and adults: They don't all outgrow it. *Journal of Clinical Psychology, 61*(5), 529-533.

Taylor, R. (2017). *Kielhofner's model of human occupation: Theory and application* (5th ed.). Baltimore, MD: Lippincott Williams & Wilkins.

Waterman, B. (2001). Mourning the loss builds the bond: Primal communication between foster, adoptive, or stepmother and child. *Journal of Loss and Trauma, 6*(4), 277-300.

Zonfrillo, M., Penn, J., & Leonard, H. (2005). Pediatric psychotropic polypharmacy. *Psychiatry, 2*(8), 14-19.

SUGGESTED RESOURCES

American Psychiatric Association: https://www.psychiatry.org

American Psychological Association: http://www.apa.org/pi/families/children-mental-health.aspx

American Academy of Child & Adolescent Psychiatry's substance use resource center: http://www.aacap.org/AACAP/Families_and_Youth/Resource_Centers/Substance_Use_Resource_Center/Home.aspx

Images of children's mental health: http://www.google.com/search?q=children's+mental+health&start=30&hl=en&sa=N&biw=1264&bih=620&prmd=ivnscm&tbm=isch&tbo=u&source=univ&ei=911BTtmYD9KvoAGM7Z3LCQ&ved=0CGQQsAQ4Hg

Mental Health America: Resources for children's mental health: http://www.nmha.org/go/children

National Alliance on Mental Illness: Teens & young adults: https://www.nami.org/Find-Support/Teens-Young-Adults

National Center for Children in Poverty: Children's mental health: http://nccp.org/publications/pub_687.html

National Federation of Families for Children's Mental Health: http://ffcmh.org

National Library of Medicine Medline Plus: Child mental health: https://medlineplus.gov/childmentalhealth.html

National Institute of Mental Health: Child and adolescent mental health: http://nimh.nih.gov/health/topics/child-and-adolescent-mental-health/index.shtml

Substance Abuse and Mental Health Services Administration: http://www.samhsa.gov

Mental Health of Adolescents

*William L. Lambert, MS, OTR/L
and Elizabeth Carley, OTD, OTR/L*

What comes to mind when you think about adolescence or being a teenager? The responses could be as varied as the lived experiences of individuals in this developmental stage. As with other stages of development across the lifespan, there may be common characteristics, but just as many differences that depend on a number of factors. We tend to think of adolescence as a period of fluctuating hormones, moodiness, and an angst-filled search for identity, all of which are true. Oftentimes, adolescence is conceived of as a necessarily difficult passage, and it frequently is for those individuals having mental health issues, but most likely not more so than people of any age. Are all childhoods happy? Is midlife always met with a crisis? Do the elderly consider themselves to be living in their "golden years"? How many times has an adolescent been told that they should be enjoying themselves because "these are the best years of your life"? This romantic notion is described by Bruce Springsteen in his song "Glory Days," where he tells of tales of reflections of adolescent experience:

> I had a friend who was a big baseball player back in high school. ... There's a girl that lives up the block; back in school she could turn all the boys' heads. ... Glory days, well, they'll pass you by.

Stereotypes and misconceptions may cloud our ability to see adolescents as unique individuals whose mental health problems reflect external as well as internal factors. Client-centered care would inform us to consider the individual adolescent and his or her mental health issues in context. Personal factors such as heredity, the family's structure and place on the function–dysfunction continuum, level of ability to cope, self-efficacy, resilience, available support systems, and access to mental health services and health care in general all play a part in whether an adolescent will develop a mental illness. Equality-of-life issues such as socioeconomic status, neighborhood composition, education, access to care, and availability of social participation present external factors that can play an important role not only in developing mental health problems, but also in how easily they can be resolved.

This chapter will combine the knowledge gained by the authors through decades of working in the field with adolescents with emotional, behavioral, and mental health issues with currently available data and evidence-based information to guide effective and rewarding occupational therapy intervention with this population. Thus, in keeping with the principles that run through each edition, this chapter will rely on theoretical and clinical evidence.

MacRae, A. (Ed.). *Cara and MacRae's Psychosocial Occupational Therapy:
An Evolving Practice, Fourth Edition* (pp 179-200).
© 2019 Taylor & Francis Group.

ETIOLOGY OF ADOLESCENT
MENTAL HEALTH OR ILLNESS

Many current views of mental illness focus on heredity and genetic predisposition as probable causes, just as these factors are often taken into consideration in the development/acquisition and diagnosis of other physical conditions such as cardiac disease, certain types of cancer, diabetes, arthritis, and so on. The nature versus nurture argument is an old one, but looking at both factors together may be useful. For example, an adolescent possessing a strong family history of depression suffers the loss of a parent, which in turn leads to financial problems that necessitate moving to a smaller home in a different neighborhood. The move facilitates leaving friends behind and going to a new school. The multiple losses and the consequences (e.g., loss of support system and social life) of moving experienced by this individual may lead to a major depressive episode that includes suicidal ideation, plan, and intent. However, a different teen without a family history of depression may possess enough internal resources that allow for recovery through the possession of sufficient adaptive coping skills and the ability to use family and others for support. In addition, possibly the use of an antidepressant medication and/or outpatient therapy might help resolve this person's grief and loss issues.

A variety or combination of psychosocial stressors may impact an adolescent's mental health, such as physical, sexual, or emotional abuse; experiencing a traumatic event; social isolation; and a dysfunctional family system. Just as these risk factors may increase the likelihood of an adolescent developing mental illness, certain individual strengths can act as protective barriers against the onset of mental health problems. Among these strengths are courage, hope, optimism, interpersonal skills, and perseverance. Being a part of a strong, healthy family system can also support an adolescent in his or her resiliency against mental illness. Although the two complement each other, a distinction has been made between the practices of mental illness prevention and mental health promotion. Prevention focuses on the avoidance of risk factors, whereas mental health promotion seeks to improve an individual's protective mechanisms, including increasing self-esteem, mastery, well-being, and social inclusion (National Research Council, Institute of Medicine, 2009). Depending on the practice setting and the needs of the individual, occupational therapists can be effective in both prevention and mental health promotion with adolescents. Effective treatment often consists of concurrently reducing risk factors and promoting protective barriers to help our clients achieve and maintain their highest possible level of mental health.

Social and Cultural Considerations

The developmental tasks of adolescence are determined not only by biological and physical development, but also by cultural and environmental influences. Adolescents from different ethnic and cultural backgrounds can face different expectations in their roles as teenagers. As the United States becomes increasingly diverse, children of diverse cultural backgrounds and children of immigrants enter adolescence with cultural beliefs and values that influence their identify formation and development. Children of immigrants live in families with median incomes 20% lower than the family incomes of children whose parents were born in the United States (Chaudry & Fortuny, 2010). Due to economic hardship, the children of lower-income families sometimes face pressures to assist their families, which can lead to a decrease in the youth's motivation or ability to achieve academically. These pressures include parents encouraging their teenage children to work part-time or full-time to help the family financially or for the teenage girls to stay home and care for their younger siblings while their parents work.

In addition to economic and educational outcomes, youth who have immigrated to the United States face multiple barriers in their developmental trajectory. With immigration comes uncertainty, as families leave support systems and familiar language and culture behind as they move. Immigrant children must often learn a new language in order to succeed in school, and to develop a support system in their new country. For those who are undocumented, the threat of deportation looms, and if deported, families can become separated. Many factors contribute to higher rates of emotional and behavioral concerns among this population of youth, as they face poverty, discrimination, difficulty with acculturation, and traumatic experiences including family separations (Henderson & Baily, 2013). Immigrants who are undocumented can feel like they are "living in the shadows" and, because of this, may be less likely to seek out necessary mental health services for themselves or for their children (Derr, 2016). Case Illustration 11-1 highlights the mental health struggles of an adolescent immigrant in the United States.

Cultural and ethnic differences also affect the ways in which adolescents experience role identity through the transition from childhood to adulthood. Cultural experiences act as rites of passage for adolescents. Many teenagers attend school dances and begin to date and, through experiences like these, begin to develop an identity separate from that of their parents and family. For example, in many Latin American cultures, the Quinceañera, or the celebration of the 15th birthday, represents a girl's entrance into womanhood, and this practice has been adopted by many of Latin American descent who are living in the United States. This idea of a rite of passage can help adolescents identify a concrete point that symbolizes their becoming an adult, although in reality, this is a long process, lasting through the years of adolescence. Similar rites of passage include bar and bas mitzvahs and confirmation, although how much this is experienced as entering adulthood in modern culture is questionable with the current consideration of the period of adolescence extending beyond the teen years and into the early and mid-20s.

CASE ILLUSTRATION 11-1: THE IMPACT OF IMMIGRATION—ADJUSTMENT AND TRANSITION

Daniel, who is 14 years old, immigrated to the United States with his family when he was 10 years old. Two years after their arrival, Daniel's father was deported to Mexico, and Daniel began exhibiting aggressive behaviors. He was recently referred to a community-based mental health agency by a counselor at his school, as he frequently gets in fights with peers and has difficulty getting along with teachers. He has received a diagnosis of adjustment disorder and has also reported conflict at home with his mother and sister. An occupational therapist and social worker are currently working with Daniel in a group setting to help him identify triggers, coping strategies, and ultimately decrease conflict with peers and family members. The group sessions include cooperative games and activities that promote social skills, anger management, and cooperation, as well as group discussions surrounding Daniel's experiences immigrating and then his father's deportation. In this space, Daniel has been able to share his sadness surrounding the loss of his father and the difficulty he experienced during their transition to the United States. Daniel shared his experience learning English and how he struggled academically at school. He also spoke about the loss of his friends and extended family he had as a support system in Mexico. Because Daniel has recently been expressing his anger and frustration toward his mother and sister at home, the therapists have also determined that family therapy sessions could be beneficial for Daniel to be able to process his experiences and his feelings within the family.

Discussion

Daniel's case illustrates an experience common in the United States. With immigration and the transition to a foreign country often comes the loss of one's culture and support system. Children are often separated from their caregiver (either temporarily or permanently) and can experience loneliness and social isolation, especially if they do not speak English. Often, there is uncertainty surrounding the future for families who migrate, and children and youth can experience this journey as traumatic. Using a trauma-informed perspective when working with youth who have immigrated or whose family members have been deported is essential to assist these youth through this period of so many transitions.

DISORDERS, DIAGNOSES, AND PRESENTING PROBLEMS

Mental health diagnoses are currently defined in the *Diagnostic and Statistical Manual of Mental Disorders* (DSM-5; American Psychiatric Association, 2013) and typical diagnoses for adolescents vary to some degree according to the treatment setting. Two diagnoses frequently encountered in an inpatient program, where admissions are limited to those in an acute or crisis phase of their disorder, are major depression/major depressive disorders and bipolar disorder, with hospitalization facilitated by being assessed as a serious danger to self or others. Additionally, individuals whose decompensation includes self-mutilation or cutting; threatening physical violence; suicidal ideation, intent, or plan; or a psychotic episode that may be a precursor to a formal thought disorder such as schizophrenia may also present for treatment in this setting. Other common diagnoses are conduct disorder, attention deficit hyperactivity disorder, personality disorder, attachment disorders, or any of the diagnoses found in the DSM-5 that may be assigned to an adult, such as obsessive-compulsive disorder or posttraumatic stress disorder (PTSD).

The diagnoses encountered in outpatient or community-based settings tend to be less acute or serious than among those who have been admitted to an inpatient hospital program. Among the most common are adjustment disorders, depressive disorder, attention deficit hyperactivity disorder, oppositional defiant disorder, and PTSD. Disorders can be co-occurring, and individuals may also present with substance abuse issues or eating disorders.

Regardless of the setting, the current physical health status and the presence of any acute or chronic medical issues should also be taken into consideration. This provides for a more holistic approach, and the presence of these types of issues may contribute to the overall mental health status of the adolescent and how he or she is able to perform and partake in his or her preferred, valued, and necessary interests and occupations.

Presenting Problems

Changes in occupational functioning, role performance, affect, and mood often signal the development of a mental health problem. The inability to adequately perform occupations in areas of activities of daily living, instrumental activities of daily living, education, work, sleep/rest, play and leisure, and social participation that had previously been successful may indicate an evolving mental health issue. Often, schizophrenia emerges during late adolescence, and a scenario such as changes in grooming, taking care of one's pet, ability to concentrate on school work,

TABLE 11-1. PRESENTING SIGNALS FOR MENTAL HEALTH SERVICES

CHANGES IN BEHAVIOR	CHANGES IN AFFECT OR MOOD	CHANGES IN RELATIONSHIPS	PRESENTING A DANGER TO SELF OR OTHERS
• Social withdrawal • Opposition, defiance, and lack of respect for authority figures • School avoidance/truancy • Decreased impulse control • Decreased frustration tolerance • Aggression	• Anger • Hostility • Sadness • Lability • Grandiosity	• Parent-child • Siblings/extended family • Peers/friends • Teachers/religious leaders	• Suicidal ideation, intent, or plan • Threatening harm or death to others • Risk-taking behaviors • Use of drugs and alcohol (beyond teenage experimentation)

restlessness and an inability to relax, and participation in formerly rewarding free time activities such as computer games or playing golf with friends, along with emerging positive and negative symptoms, could be representative of someone developing a thought disorder. Performance for this adolescent would likely decrease in the roles of family member, student, or friend/peer, as in carrying out the role of emerging young adult who is capable of being well-groomed, appropriately dressed, and able to carry out expected responsibilities in his or her home, school, and community. Other clinical manifestations represented here would be possible positive symptoms of schizophrenia, such as auditory hallucinations and negative symptoms such as a flattened affect and avolition (American Psychiatric Association, 2013). The regression in this scenario, or decompensation, illustrates how treatment for adolescents would tend toward being rehabilitative, rather than habilitative, as is often the case with children because the adolescent would need to recover lost skills and abilities at which he or she had previously been proficient. Often, it depends on the symptoms and characteristics of the diagnosis and the client factors, as well as the context of the adolescent. It can be useful to view mental health and/or illness as a continuum, where one can move back and forth; it is unique to the individual. Presenting problems may be seen in overt behavior, sometimes referred to as *externalizing*, whereas other, internalizing symptoms are dependent on the report of the adolescent.

The presence of internalizing and externalizing behaviors and symptoms depends on the diagnosis and the presentation of the individual. Diagnoses like depression often include feelings of sadness, social isolation or withdrawal, or symptoms that are not necessarily displayed outwardly. Oppositional defiant disorder, on the other hand, is marked by defiance toward authority figures such as teachers or parents and is often displayed by verbal outbursts, fighting, or otherwise disruptive behaviors. The type of symptoms and behaviors being exhibited can affect the identification

of mental illness. For example, those with depressive symptoms that are internalized can be viewed as the quiet or "good" kids in the classroom and are not identified as having any issues for which they need to receive treatment or support. Those adolescents with disorders that include externalizing behaviors are more frequently identified as "problem" kids with more referrals to the dean or principal for disrupting their class and peers. Therefore, those with externalizing behaviors related to their mental illness can be much easier to identify and diagnose. Because of this, it is important that teachers and other adults who work with adolescents not ignore those individuals who are quiet and may not act out or display disruptive behaviors, so that all youth with mental illness receive the treatment and support they need. Table 11-1 lists potential presenting problems for adolescents with mental health issues that may signal the need for mental health services.

SUICIDE

Suicide was the third leading cause of death for young people aged 10 to 14 years and the second leading cause of death for people aged 15 to 34 years in 2015. Statistically, the suicide rate was four times higher for males as compared with females. In 2016, adults aged 18 to 25 years were among those who had the highest percentage of attempted suicide. According to statistics from 2015, the most common method used for people who have died by suicide was firearms (National Institute of Mental Health [NIMH], 2017). According to the Centers for Disease Control and Prevention (2015), 13.6% of students in grades 9 through 12 have written a plan for suicide, whereas 8% have completed an attempt.

A variety of factors may cause an adolescent to consider ending his or her life; for example, the antecedent for an adolescent suicide is in response to an event in the past 24 hours, such as rejection-related events by a peer group or a relationship or being in trouble and facing legal or disciplinary action (Gutman, 2005). Box 11-1 lists common risk factors for suicide.

Frequently, it is difficult for professionals, as well as family members, peers, and others, to believe that an adolescent or any individual is seriously considering suicide. However, *all* suicidal verbalizations or gestures need to be taken seriously. Case Illustration 11-2 shows measures taken in a hospital with a young woman who demonstrated self-harm and suicidality.

The NIMH (2018) advises that the mere mention of suicide should not be considered an attention-seeking behavior but rather a sign of serious emotional distress. Suicide is often looked at in terms of ideation, plan, and intent. *Ideation* refers to thoughts of committing suicide. *Plan* refers to the means one would use to carry out suicide; how one would do it, such as using a gun, by hanging, or by ingesting poison; and when one would do it, such as upon discharge, after Christmas, or if forced to end a relationship. An individual who has suicidal ideation is unable to reflect back on positive aspects of the past but rather is focused on the current unpleasant, negative experience or thoughts. This obsessive thinking of unpleasant, negative experience or thoughts overrides one's memories and is thought by neuropsychologists to facilitate in the brain a network of memories that can lead to suicidal ideation (Gutman, 2005). *Intent* refers to whether the person is intending to carry out the plan. It is essential that an individual who has intent and is suicidal should immediately seek mental health treatment; this should not be postponed nor should the suicidal person be left unattended (NIMH, 2018). Additional interventions include the following:

- Attempt to get the person to seek help from a doctor or the nearest emergency room
- Dial 911
- Eliminate access to firearms and other potential items for self-harm, including unsupervised access to medications
- Consider ideation, plan, and intent
- Take personal responsibility as a professional to keep the individual safe

Prevention Programs

One prevention program identified adolescents in high schools to be peer leaders who modeled and trained their peers to identify adults they could trust in an effort to enhance protective factors associated with reducing suicide. The intervention program increased perceptions of adult support for suicidal adolescents and increased the acceptability of asking for help (Wyman et al., 2010). Adolescents who are having suicidal ideation often do not know where to turn, and increasing their comfort in asking for help or identifying those adults they feel they can trust could potentially save lives. Occupational therapists working with youth who are depressed and considering suicide can play

> ## Box 11-1. Risk Factors for Suicide
>
> - Depression and other mental health disorders
> - Prior suicide attempt
> - Family history of mental illness/substance abuse
> - Family history of suicide
> - Family violence; physical or sexual abuse
> - Firearms in the home (used in half of all suicides)
> - Incarceration
> - Exposure to the suicidal behavior of others
>
> Adapted from National Institute for Mental Health. (2017). *Suicide prevention.* Retrieved from https://www.nimh.nih.gov/health/topics/suicide-prevention/index.shtml

this important role. Developing the rapport and the trust necessary to build an effective therapeutic relationship could also be vital in gaining the trust of a hopeless teenager who may feel he or she has nowhere else to turn. It is also important that, as occupational therapists, we know how to access the appropriate resources in terms of therapists and crisis intervention to which to refer suicidal youth because these individuals may be in need of hospitalization or less restrictive environments in which to receive psychotherapy and other supportive services and possibly medication to treat their symptoms.

Other preventive measures include increasing suicide awareness among this population, their families, and the communities in which they live; developing emergency or safety plans; and focusing on medication compliance, particularly where the medication may have unpleasant side effects. Patient education is also needed to help individuals recognize emerging symptoms and to seek immediate help (Gutman, 2005). Emergency plans, contingency plans and contracts, and specifying what to do if suicidal ideation occurs are essential (Gutman, 2005). A contract is sometimes called a *contract for safety*. The contract for safety asks the patient to contract, or commit, to telling an appropriate person or persons if he or she is having thoughts of suicide. In a hospital or other clinical settings, this may be any member in the therapeutic environment. In the community, this may be a parent, guardian, or other involved appropriate party whom the client has agreed to contact in the event of relapse or decompensation.

Occupational Therapy

Occupational therapy intervention for at-risk youth focuses on fostering self-understanding through reality-based treatment where participants can develop social and communication skills and identify adaptive coping strategies through meaningful occupations. Occupational

CASE ILLUSTRATION 11-2: NECESSARY PRECAUTIONS—SELF-HARM AND SUICIDALITY

Mary was an 18-year-old hospitalized on an inpatient adolescent unit with presenting problems of self-mutilation and suicidal thoughts, ideation, and plans. She attempted suicide prior to her admission as well as during her hospitalization. She presented with a high degree of lethality and potential for self-harm. For example, her arms and legs were covered with scars and recently inflicted cuts serious enough to put her at risk for infection. On one occasion, program staff discovered razor blades in a letter sent to her in response to the request she had made for them in a recent contact. While Mary was a patient on an acute inpatient unit, her length of stay was weeks rather than days due to her frequent attempts to kill herself, even while on suicide precautions that required a member of the nursing staff to be within an arm's length from her at all times around the clock. Once, she attempted to use a washcloth to commit suicide while a female staff member was present.

Her hospitalization was an ongoing cycle of being on and off suicide precautions and earning privileges to go to meals in the cafeteria and occupational therapy groups held off the unit. Mary was a bright young woman who, despite her current problems, planned to finish high school and attend college. She responded especially well to occupational therapy and was an active participant in groups with treatment goals for increasing Mary's self-esteem, self-concept, and self-worth, as well as developing adaptive coping skill and strategies to deal more effectively and appropriately with expressing feelings in a nonharmful manner. The therapist had established a strong rapport with her in occupational therapy, providing her with interventions that she could use currently to address her problems in a group setting and providing her with encouragement and support regarding getting well and with a future-oriented outlook for continuing her education and transition to adulthood.

After 1 to 2 months of this ongoing cycle, the treatment team was considering transfer to a state long-term care facility because her response to the program, therapies, and medication did not appear to be producing any lasting results and improvement. Additionally, discussion focused on restricting her to the unit and not allowing her to attend occupational therapy because the nursing staff felt she was unable to be kept safe in that environment. This presented a dilemma: Was Mary's safety a greater cause for concern than her involvement in therapy, and if so, how could her attendance in occupational therapy continue until she was transferred to a long-term care facility, where an opening could be months away? Necessarily, Mary needed to be kept safe from self-harm, but she also benefited from the active treatment provided by occupational therapy.

A compromise was reached that involved Mary in the decision-making process. Mary would remain on suicide precautions and be accompanied by a member of the nursing staff at all times, including while she was in occupational therapy. The therapist and nursing staff presented Mary with the choice of submitting to a body search following her return from occupational therapy to ensure her safety or remaining on the unit until discharge. Mary chose to continue to attend occupational therapy and to comply with the body search after group. Mary remained on suicide precautions for the remainder of her hospitalization and was an active participant in occupational therapy, which she attended without incident. Once regularly attending occupational therapy, Mary and the therapist, along with a Level II occupational therapy student, planned an adolescent program event involving all the other patients and staff based on a reality television show that Mary especially liked and watched with her peers; the program proved highly successful and enjoyable for the entire program one afternoon.

Discussion

Mary's case illustrates many of the concepts involved in planning and implementing appropriate care and treatment for a severely mentally ill adolescent. For the nursing staff, the primary goal is to keep Mary safe, which they accomplished through their thorough room searches for contraband and being present when Mary opened her mail or received gifts to inspect for items that could provide Mary with the means of self-harm or suicide. They carried out the protocol for suicide precautions, a written doctor's order, which prevented her from committing suicide on the unit. The psychiatrist provided ongoing assessment, prescribed antidepressant medication, and directed the interdisciplinary treatment team. The occupational therapist used therapeutic use of self in relationship and a positive, client-centered approach in providing intervention. The adolescent program offered structure and consistency to provide a framework for treatment in general, and the program staff enforced limits. The interdisciplinary treatment team planned Mary's ongoing treatment with input from all of the disciplines mentioned, including social work, which provided Mary with individual, group, and family therapy. This case also illustrates the need to adjust the structure and the established program and to remain flexible and creative in order to provide treatment interventions that best meet the needs of the patient when unusual circumstances arise.

therapists can assist adolescents to develop self-management skills and ways to organize the environment to decrease excess stress and pressure. With the client-centered focus that occupational therapy provides, therapists can engage clients in activities that they personally find meaningful and purposeful and that can improve resiliency and self-esteem. These activities can also aide in decreasing feelings of hopelessness characteristic of depression because many individuals who attempt suicide meet the criteria for a mental health diagnosis (Gutman, 2005; NIMH, 2017). Occupations that are selected should teach strategies to manage suicidal thoughts and alternative activities that the adolescent can use to stop or divert him or her from negative thoughts or suicidal ideation. Therapeutic activities should be chosen that can provide the adolescent with hope and a future-oriented focus while also being developmentally appropriate and satisfying. Helpful occupational therapy interventions, according to Gutman (2005), include:

- Educating patients and families about suicide and mental health disorders
- Facilitating the ability to manage relapse and disappointment with progress with an effective plan in place
- Assisting patients in making realistic choices despite feelings of hopelessness
- Reinforcing the need to remain actively involved in treatment
- Encouraging ongoing medication compliance
- Involving family members
- Identifying support groups and other resources
- Fostering understanding of and strategies to handle setbacks in the recovery process

As people stabilize, they can experience a period where they do not appear suicidal; however, their positive mood often belies the fact that they have made the decision to kill themselves. This is commonly believed by many clinicians in the field. Patients are also often disappointed with the course of recovery because setbacks and relapses can and do occur as recovery is not always complete (Gutman, 2005).

It is difficult to listen and deal with the circumstances that lead adolescents to consider and attempt suicide. It is even more difficult to have a patient commit suicide while under your care or the care of your facility, or after he or she leaves your treatment program. In consideration of working with at-risk youth, this must be clearly understood. The therapist needs to reach a comfort level with addressing what are literally life-and-death issues. Using therapeutic use of self, a self must be developed that can comfortably, empathically, and effectively deal with adolescents who are, have been, and may again be suicidal, as well as those whom treatment did not prevent from taking their own lives. This is perhaps the most difficult treatment issue to leave at the workplace and not take home with you at the end of the day.

SELF-MUTILATION

Self mutilation or self-injury is "typically not meant as a suicide attempt. Rather, this type of self-injury is an unhealthy way to cope with emotional pain, intense anger and frustration" (Mayo Clinic, 2017). Common forms of self-mutilation include cutting, burning, scratching, and skin picking. Those engaging in cutting behaviors are often referred to as *cutters*, a rather inappropriate reference as opposed to the more client-centered and respectful *a person who cuts or self-mutilates*. Considering that therapeutic use of self in relationship is essential in providing occupational therapy and in our responsibility to treat our clients with dignity and respect, it behooves us to not refer to individuals as their illness or condition, particularly when addressing a behavior that can leave lasting scars, both on the physical body itself and on the psyche of the individual.

Why Does It Occur?

Individuals who self-mutilate often have difficulty expressing their feelings, and the reason for its occurrence may be that it serves as a coping strategy, relieving anxiety and tension (Moro, 2007; Williams & Bydalek, 2007).

The following informal interview of a patient who engaged in self-mutilation supports Williams and Bydalek's (2007) finding. It is worth noting that she clearly seemed to present that it was a coping skill that worked for her, and it illustrates how effective she believed her coping strategies to be and how difficult the former one may be to replace with something more appropriate.

Therapist: Why do you participate in self-mutilation?

Client: I do it to let out my feelings. They build up, and when I cut I watch the blood flow and I feel better.

Therapist: Does it hurt?

Client: I don't really feel it.

Occupational Therapy Interventions

As in most occupational therapy treatment, the focus is on everyday functioning and the occupations that the client engages in on a daily basis. Occupations and activities related to school, relationships with friends and family, work, and socializing activities (e.g., sports, clubs, driving, and going out) are their primary focus. Therapeutic frameworks such as cognitive and sensory therapies (Kaiser, Gillette, & Spinazzola, 2010) have been found to be efficacious for those with this condition. Interventions using these frameworks include self-management as it relates to stress, anger and emotional management and regulation, problem solving, and time management (Moro, 2007). Using cognitive-behavioral therapy approaches, therapists can focus on maladaptive thinking, which prevents occupational performance in daily life (Moro, 2007):

Additionally, the occupational therapy sessions address "problem solving, skills training, relationship strategies and contingency management" (Moro, 2007, p. 62). Also, some settings use sensory interventions, such as tactile stimulation and massage, to decrease incidents of self-mutilation. In addition, Williams and Bydalek (2007) suggested interventions such as exploring with clients what measures might be self-soothing and training in communication skills so that clients could express their feelings instead of acting them out on their bodies. In this author's clinical experience, teaching strategies that mimic the actual destruction of body tissues but cause no lasting effect, such as holding an ice cube to the skin or snapping a rubber band around the wrist, can be effective to replace self-harm behaviors when the individual is transitioning between maladaptive and adaptive coping skills.

EATING DISORDERS

There are few articles on the topic of eating disorders in occupational therapy literature that focus on adolescents and eating disorders. This would seem to indicate a strong need for occupational therapists to publish their work with this population to establish an evidence base and increase referrals for clients with eating disorders to occupational therapists who seem well-positioned to treat them. This would also appear to be an emerging practice area for occupational therapists desiring to work in mental health in a very vital role. In fact, some occupational therapists believe that occupational therapy can provide successful interventions that focus on self-efficacy or self-concept for teens with eating disorders (Gardiner & Brown, 2010).

Eating disorders are known by their DSM-5 diagnosis of Anorexia Nervosa, Bulimia Nervosa, and Other Specified Feeding or Eating Disorder. Binge-eating disorder may be encountered by occupational therapists secondary to concomitant health problems being treated by occupational therapy (Costa, 2009). Occupational therapists working with clients with eating disorders use a variety of approaches, including psychodynamic, cognitive, developmental, behavioral, family oriented, and medical (Gardiner & Brown, 2010). Gardiner and Brown further suggest that occupational therapy practitioners are well-prepared to address the needs of the eating disorder population. Occupational therapy practitioners understand occupations, behaviors associated with those occupations, and cognitive processing; through cognitive-behavioral therapy, occupational therapists address individuals' issues. These skills complemented by psychosocial training enable the practitioner to customize interventions specific to the client using a structured, symptom-focused treatment approach. Furthermore, the occupational therapist's training to use groups in all practice settings and keen sense of the importance of psychosocial relationships assist the practitioner to effectively facilitate family intervention–related groups as well as peer self-help groups. It has been shown that mental health treatment that involves the family is more effective in the long-term outcomes for individuals with anorexia nervosa than is individual treatment (Lock et al., 2010). Occupational therapists often work with adolescents with eating disorders in inpatient and outpatient settings; however, treatment of eating disorders and concomitant altered body image concerns (Shearsmith-Farthing, 2001) is an area of specialization within adolescent mental health and mental health practice in general.

Intervention Specific to Adolescents With Eating Disorders

Treatment can include working with the individual to establish eating routines and working with the family to assist the client to understand the disorder and how the family can affect the course of the disorder. Occupational therapy practitioners commonly use groups when treating adolescents with eating disorders. Some of the groups are self-expressive, which includes body image, or psycho-educational, which may include stress, anxiety, or time management (Kloczko & Ikiugu, 2006). As mentioned previously, meaningful occupation-based groups that are very structured and objective-focused are highly effective; these may include meal planning, shopping, cooking, and dining together.

Individual therapy with adolescents with anorexia nervosa can be based on psychodynamic therapy (Lock et al., 2010). Interventions based on this approach help teens to build autonomy, self-reliance, and assertiveness, presumably based on self-awareness and the ability to self-reflect. Therapists working with adolescents in family-based therapy focus on a safe and reassuring environment. The ultimate goal is for the adolescent to have a healthy autonomy at meal time and to feel supported and not blamed (by the family members) and to assist the parents to support and encourage healthy eating (Lock et al., 2010).

The use of activity analysis and therapists' ability to grade activities are among the unique contributions occupational therapy can make in providing treatment for this population (Gardiner & Brown, 2010). In family therapy approaches based on a highly researched and commonly used approach in recovery for those with anorexia nervosa, initial treatment necessitates that the individual or caregivers select and prepare the food; however, over time, the responsibility is shared, and then the responsibility given to the adolescent (Gardiner & Brown, 2010). It is in this treatment that food-related fears and rituals need to be addressed, and the graded reintroduction of food selection, food preparation, and eating in social settings, facilitated by the occupational therapist, could be vital in achieving full recovery.

The occupational therapist has the unique ability to use these occupations as a therapeutic tool by analyzing, synthesizing, adapting, grading, and using the activities in intervention as suggested by the *Occupational Therapy Practice Framework* (American Occupational Therapy Association, 2014). Some examples of treatment are to facilitate engagement in appropriate levels of leisure and exercise activities, acquire social skills, and select or reintegrate into vocational experiences that will support and promote mental health and recovery.

Essentially, an eating disorder is a maladaptive coping mechanism that has to be addressed and changed before adaptive behaviors emerge. The unique benefit of occupational therapy with this population is that the approach is holistic and incorporates tasks and occupation-based activities where the adolescent can practice and learn to apply healthy adaptive ways of coping in a safe and supportive environment.

It should be noted that a major lifestyle change is necessary for treatment to be successful (Costa, 2009) and that while emphasizing more appropriate behavior in terms of the health of one with an eating disorder in treatment is important, alternative ways of coping can only be adopted when the therapist understands the needs that are addressed by the disordered eating. A practitioner cannot just point out healthier eating behavior but must acknowledge the feelings behind the eating disorder in addition to recognizing the attention the behavior promotes.

BULLYING, CYBERBULLYING, AND SCHOOL VIOLENCE

Bullying and school violence is a growing epidemic in the United States. Since the time of the 1999 Columbine High School shootings, and through countless incidents of school violence since, bullying has received increasing attention (Centers for Disease Control and Prevention, 2015; Goertz et al., 2008; Mental Health America, n.d.) and continues to receive frequent media coverage. The increased awareness makes bullying a significant issue that must continue to be addressed in school settings. With the advent of social media and its prevalence within adolescent culture, cyberbullying has presented new and often more covert effects for youth than traditional bullying in schools. Although social media may provide benefits to children and adolescents, including socialization, communication, learning opportunities, and access to health information, there are also many risks (Ito et al., 2008). These include cyberbullying or online harassment, which can emerge from relationship problems between people who know each other and access to individuals the youth may not know in real life. Hoff and Mitchell (2009) found that cyberbullying disproportionately affects females, with 72.1% of those

surveyed reporting that they had experienced cyberbullying, compared with 27% of males. Effects of cyberbullying include negative psychological effects such as fear, powerlessness, and sadness that often lead to individuals becoming withdrawn and disassociating from friends and peers. Some adolescents report feelings of anger, which can lead to aggressive behaviors through social media and in school. Researchers have identified a phenomenon called *Facebook depression*, which occurs when adolescents who spend much of their time on social media begin to experience classic symptoms of depression (Schurgin O'Keeffe & Clarke-Pearson, 2011). Individuals experiencing these symptoms may be more likely to turn to websites with inappropriate content or to interact digitally with individuals who may prove to have a negative influence on them. Bullying and school violence can have the negative effect of causing depression, moodiness, and an increase in the number of days adolescents miss from school (Centers for Disease Control and Prevention, 2015; Mental Health America, n.d.).

Community and school violence affect some adolescents' access to participation in healthy or productive occupations. Frequent internet and social media access have been correlated with an increase in depression, impulsivity, anxiety, and internet addiction and concurrent sleep deprivation (Weinstein & Lejoyeux, 2010). (Further discussion can be found in Chapter 6.) An occupational therapist working with adolescents can assist youth in identifying other productive occupations and to create a balance in their time use in order to decrease the negative effects of frequent internet and social media use.

In addition to cyberbullying, bullying, and violence on school campuses, for many youth, gang violence poses a serious threat. Youth growing up in inner cities are often born into a world in which they are forced to pledge allegiance to a certain neighborhood or gang for their own safety. Even if youth try to avoid the gang world, they are often caught up in the violence by simply being born on a certain block or by being mistaken for someone who is gang affiliated. The violence and danger in these neighborhoods seriously impede participation in those activities typical of high school. If a teen's neighborhood is not safe enough to walk home after dark, they will miss out on after-school sports or dance teams or other occupations that can be pivotal in character building or feeling occupationally fulfilled. These youth suffer not only from occupational deprivation, but often from symptoms of PTSD. Gang conflict often leads to violence and shootings, and many youth have experienced the loss or injury of a family member or friend. This loss or the witnessing of such traumatic events contributes to mental health issues, including PTSD and depression, among this subsection of adolescents. Occupational therapists who encounter these youth through community agencies, schools, or hospitals have the responsibility of increasing their actual and perceived levels of safety. This can be done by encouraging youth to share their experiences and to deal with their effects. Because violence is commonplace in many of these communities, without the services provided by occupational therapists and other mental health professionals, youth often do not realize that these traumas have a lasting effect on their emotional well-being and overall functioning.

HELPFUL CONCEPTS FOR TREATING ADOLESCENTS

Structure and Consistency

The teenage years are marked by transition and instability because teens must navigate the often-chaotic path from childhood to adulthood. This is not to say that the transition is necessarily difficult. Many adolescents enjoy their teenage years and transition to adulthood with minimal difficulty. In addition to the typical transitions all adolescents experience, those who are identified as having a mental health issue have often experienced trauma, loss, or other environmental stressors that have contributed to the development of their mental illness or presenting problems. These stressors could include a family changing residences (and, therefore, schools) frequently, the death or loss of a loved one, violence in their neighborhood, abuse, or other problems within the family system. Because many teens who are receiving mental health treatment lack consistency or support within their home environments, providing this structure and consistency in the treatment setting is crucial. Consistency can be achieved in many ways, including ensuring that the mental health staff working with the youth remains constant, the time and place of the sessions are the same every week, and the structure of the session or group remains the same so that the adolescent knows what to expect. This structure will facilitate the establishment of trust in their therapist and their peers and will allow the adolescents to disclose more and work more honestly and openly toward their treatment goals and objectives.

Limit Setting

Pushing the limits is something that comes naturally to most adolescents. Part of navigating through this period of transition is pushing and testing the limits set by authority figures to see what happens and for adolescents to test their own autonomy and maturity. Setting limits in a mental health setting ensures consistency and makes it clear to the adolescent what to expect. Because teenagers are in the process of gaining more independence and control over their own lives, it is important to allow adolescents to take some responsibility in helping to develop the expectations and rules for the group. Most teens are more likely to

follow the rules and adhere to the expectations of treatment if they were involved in their creation, instead of having rules imposed on them. Providing positive reinforcement instead of just negative consequences can be very helpful in setting limits for the participants. Adolescents, especially those with disruptive behaviors, are very accustomed to suffering negative consequences (e.g., referrals to the dean or suspension from school) and are not used to being positively affirmed for their behavior. Thus, the use of praise and positive reinforcements, including incentives, can be extremely effective in improving behavior and adherence to rules in mental health treatment settings. Incentive program are used to encourage positive behaviors and teach consequences in mental health groups. In one model of an incentive program, youth receive points for positive behaviors and participation, including volunteering to share first or assisting their peers or staff with activities. At the end of the group session or an allotted number of group sessions, the participant with the most points receives an incentive that was decided upon by the group initially, such as an award, a gift card, or whatever the youth had decided was a motivator in the beginning of the group. When the incentives are chosen by the client, the youth are more motivated to work toward receiving these points so that they will be rewarded.

Avoiding Power Struggles

Adolescents have more life experience than children and are usually more mature. Because of this, they are more capable of negotiating with adults, as well as manipulating staff, rules, and systems. By allowing adolescent clients opportunities to make decisions and have control in the group setting, a therapist can fulfill adolescents' need to express autonomy and act independently. Engaging with youth in struggles for power within the treatment setting can be detrimental to the therapeutic process because it can cause role confusion for the therapist and the youth and encourage youth to perpetuate negative, challenging behaviors. The occupational therapist must take care in allowing the adolescent client enough autonomy to not feel as though he or she is being treated like a child, but provide enough structure to maintain a therapeutic environment for the client. One effective method of avoiding power struggles is by providing choices. Providing choices gives the adolescent the opportunity to have a sense of control and the ability to express autonomy in an acceptable, positive manner. One study showed that "[o]ffering choices to adolescents living in a psychiatric setting elicited a statistically significant difference in performance" and "provided evidence that choice making within parameters set by the occupational therapist can enhance performance among adolescents living in behavioral treatment facilities" (Schroeder Oxer & Kopp Miller, 2001). The following are examples of providing choices:

- Allowing the adolescent to choose between two or three different types of activities that will all be effective in meeting a treatment goal. For example, if the therapist is working on the objective of increasing social interaction through a parallel task group, giving the client the choice between painting suncatchers and making a tile mosaic provides an opportunity for decision making and a sense of control over his or her own treatment. It is also an example of client-centered care.

- Asking a group to plan the menu for a cooking group. Ways of providing parameters that will guide them in making reasonable and appropriate selections include a budget they must stay within, sample menus; a theme such as a picnic, spaghetti dinner, or Italian night; and a time frame for preparing, eating, and cleaning up after the meal.

- Avoiding a potentially dangerous or assaultive situation by offering an adolescent who is becoming angry and verbally threatening choices that teach adaptive coping and anger management skills through a therapeutic interpretation: "Brittany, I can see that this group is becoming frustrating and upsetting for you. Would you like to leave and take a few minutes by yourself, or would you rather step out into the hall with me and we can talk about what's bothering you?"

Therapeutic Use of Self in Relationship

Given this phase of development, where teenagers may gravitate away from relationships with adults, and the peer group becomes all-important, it is vital for the therapist to master the therapeutic use of one's self in the relationship to foster successful outcomes (American Occupational Therapy Association, 2014). Oftentimes, adolescents with mental health problems have had actual or perceived negative relationships with adults. Instances of this may include past abuse, rejection, and broken promises by adult authority figures; abandonment, real or imagined, by their family members; and interaction with law enforcement officers, school officials, and members of the community brought on by the symptoms of their particular disorders or conditions. (See Chapter 9 for more information on attachment through the lifespan.) The following are some key points to consider:

- Create a feeling of acceptance and worth, especially important for those with low self-esteem and poor self-concept.
- Establish and maintain trust and rapport.
- Provide a safe environment for self-disclosure.
- Provide active listening and take responses seriously. Many times, adolescents have been waiting for the opportunity to talk to adults who want to hear about their problems, symptoms, and personal issues.
- A sense of humor is essential.

- Be a reliable and available resource and confidant; however, maintain an appropriate therapeutic role by keeping in mind that you are not trying to be their friend or peer, but an adult who can be trusted.

- Do not pretend to be something you're not. Adolescents can see through any phony and insincere behavior on the part of the therapist, which will prevent trust and appropriate rapport from developing.

Team Approach

There are many advantages to having the opportunity to practice in a setting that uses an interdisciplinary treatment team approach. In an interdisciplinary treatment team approach, clinicians from a variety of professions gather to share their observations and assessment of the client's behavior, the client's response to treatment, and their suggestions for the direction and outcome of treatment. This provides valuable insights to each member of the team, including the occupational therapy practitioner, for planning intervention and working in concert with other professionals to help clients achieve their treatment goals. In the absence of working in a setting that uses this approach, it would be beneficial for the clinician to have mentors and colleagues with whom to confer to lend direction and clarity to a case and assist with troubleshooting when questions or difficulties arise. If a psychiatrist has been the referral source, contact and discussion regarding the course of treatment can be of great benefit, especially for the therapist who is practicing autonomously, such as in private practice.

Trauma-Informed Care and Promoting Resilience

Throughout this text, there are multiple discussions regarding trauma-informed care, but as shown in the previous sections, adolescents have some unique exposure to trauma and the resulting sequelae. Many of the adolescent clients that an occupational therapist will work with have been exposed to traumatic experiences in their early development or may currently be exposed to toxic or traumatic events and environments. These adverse childhood experiences disrupt development, causing social, emotional, and cognitive impairment. Individuals may adopt health risk behaviors in response, leading to greater disease, disability, or social problems and/or death. These experiences also lead to impacts on occupational performance, including social participation, activities of daily living, education, work, play, leisure, and sleep and rest (Petrenchik & Weiss, 2015). Many (if not most) adolescents are "able to succeed and thrive in toxic and/or traumatic environments by inheriting/acquiring certain individual strengths and benefiting from various environmental protective factors" (Richards, Lewis, Sanderson, & Deane, 2016, p. 1). Occupational therapy can assist an adolescent client by providing trauma-informed

CASE ILLUSTRATION 11-3: OCCUPATIONAL THERAPY IN GROUP SETTINGS—THE ISSUE OF PEER CONFIDENTIALITY

Liz, the occupational therapist, co-led a group with a clinical social worker at a public high school with ninth graders who all have substance abuse issues. Ninth graders tend to be very self-conscious and respond greatly to the influence of their peers. Week after week, various group members came to group after smoking marijuana and were asked to return to class because they could not be present in the group while under the influence of substances. Aside from the substance use, all members were reluctant, and some refused to participate in activities because they were self-conscious around their school peers and were concerned with what they would think of them if they participated and shared private information.

Over their winter break from school, the therapists decided to take them on a field trip out of the school setting to see if a change of scenery could help build rapport and establish trust within the group. Sure enough, bringing the group to the youth center and baking cookies helped to build rapport in an alternative setting, made them more comfortable, and helped them open up and share personal experiences with the group.

Discussion

The group leaders figured out how to address an issue that is prominent with teenagers in school: confidentiality with peers they see outside of the group every day in other settings. Essentially, the therapists' changing the environment and offering therapeutic occupational therapy groups in which the teenagers were more relaxed and able to develop trust and rapport with each other ultimately led to the achievement of their treatment goals.

---

care to enhance his or her own protective factors and to promote resilience (Guarino, Soares, Konnath, Clervil, & Bassuk, 2009). Trauma-informed practice realizes the prevalence of the impact of trauma, understanding potential paths for recovery as well as recognizing the signs and symptoms of trauma and responses to a client's experiences accordingly. *Resilience* is a dynamic and interactive process between an individual and his or her environment (Masten, 2001); therefore, protective factors can be identified within an individual as well as in his or her environment. Internal factors that occupational therapists address include social competence, problem-solving skills, autonomy, and sense of purpose. External factors that should be identified and developed include caring relationships, opportunities to participate and contribute, and high expectations in the home, school, and community environments (Richards et al., 2016). If a client is able to improve in these areas, his or her self-efficacy and ability to cope with triggering situations may improve. Assisting adolescent clients with these areas can help develop resiliency and thus improve future functional outcomes. A longitudinal study, the Kauai Study (Werner, 2005), showed the positive effects of developing these internal and external factors in individuals who experienced adverse childhood events and the positive outcomes in terms of relationships, employment, and coping skills later in life. Developing supportive factors and coping skills and identifying opportunities to participate and contribute in meaningful occupations should be central to an occupational therapist's interventions with adolescent clients.

Group Versus Individual Services

Adolescents can be seen by occupational therapists individually or in groups in their schools or clinics. Individual sessions allow occupational therapists to focus on individual areas of need more directly to build the skills necessary for the youth to meet their mental health goals. Groups allow a space for youth to connect with each other, building social skills and allowing them to accept their own issues because they see similar issues in others. Groups also help adolescents build trust by opening up to peers and adults with whom they would otherwise not interact. Group dynamics are an important concept to address because one new adolescent in the group can affect trust and disclosure. Case Illustration 11-3 shows the issues of confidentiality among peers and the effects that a change in environment can have on group dynamics.

EVIDENCE-BASED PROGRAMS

One of the foundational concepts of the New Freedom Commission on Mental Health (2003) is that evidence-based practice is germane to transforming the nation's mental health services system. Certainly, there is a range of what is considered efficacious evidence-based research and practice; however, practitioners, researchers, the mental health community, policy makers, and key stakeholders are closer to an agreement on those essential items that are broadly accepted.

For example, the National Registry of Evidence-based Programs and Practices has established a peer-review database of programs and approaches that have been found to be effective. This site is under the jurisdiction of the Substance Abuse and Mental Health Services Administration (2018) and has an exhaustive list of programs that describe efficacious programs and program design to consumers and practitioners. There are also training materials and tools to assist practitioners in the field who would like to submit their program for peer-review. Following are examples of some evidence-based programs that are used with the adolescent population, the first of which was developed by occupational therapists. The other programs were developed by psychologists, social workers, and other disciplines but have been adapted and implemented by occupational therapists for the adolescent population.

An evidence-based program developed at the Occupational Therapy Training Program (OTTP, 2018) in Los Angeles is a 20-week family therapy program called *Loving Intervention for Family Enrichment*. The entire family attends weekly sessions in which the parents or guardians go through the Parent Project's A Parent's Guide to Changing Destructive Adolescent Behavior program (2018), which focuses on the challenges of parenting adolescents. This curriculum includes methods of discipline, including how to implement consequences, and psychoeducation on drugs and alcohol and mental health. The youth are divided by age group and participate in mental health groups cofacilitated by an occupational therapist and a clinical social worker or marriage and family therapist. All groups follow a curriculum of topics and engage in arts and crafts activities, cooperative games, and psychoeducation. At the start and at the end of the 20 weeks, the families come together for multifamily activities facilitated by therapists, in which the families learns to work together, bond with each other, and treat each other with love and respect.

Aggression Replacement Training (Glick & Gibbs, 2010) is a multimodal curriculum that includes the components of Anger Control, Skill Streaming, and Moral Reasoning. This model was developed by mental health professionals but is a good fit for occupational therapists because it uses a skill-building curriculum to improve daily life functioning and allows for creativity and individualization (e.g., using artwork for clients to express themselves). The model is very interactive, and youth role play experiences from their own lives and learn to change negative behavior.

Family Connections is a multidisciplinary program in which occupational therapists can work with clinical social workers or marriage and family therapists to provide holistic services for the entire family, in the home and community (DePanfilis & Dubowitz, 2005). This program includes case management, identifying appropriate resources for the family, working with parents to improve parenting skills, and developing skills for all of the family members involved. Occupational therapists are uniquely positioned to provide services under this model because we are trained to view individuals holistically, including social and environmental influences and viewing the family as a unit that is part of a community, which is a concept central to this program.

The Seeking Safety program (Najavits, 2002) is designed for youth who have experienced trauma and/or substance abuse. The program is present-focused, which makes it a good fit for occupational therapy practitioners because it does not involve processing the trauma but instead focuses on coping with the symptoms and effects. Occupational therapists assist youth in building the skills to decrease negative symptoms and behaviors and increase positive coping.

ASSESSMENT

Assessment methods may vary greatly from setting to setting. Oftentimes, standardized tools are not the norm, and each facility may either have their own or present the need for you to develop an appropriate assessment, which may include creating a screening tool as well. Observation often proves to be a very viable form of assessment. Astute observation that clinically analyzes body language, verbal and nonverbal communication, and situational behavior is an invaluable tool for the occupational therapist working in mental health. (See Chapter 4 for further discussion.) Observation and completion of a particular assessment activity, such as a magazine picture collage where adolescents are asked to represent themselves through words and pictures of their own choosing, or the Kinetic Self-Image Assessment discussed in Chapter 10, may serve as an initial assessment that provides information about task skills and dynamic information that may cast light on the internal and external issues that led to mental health or mental illness issues, thus providing the therapist with information that will be helpful in planning client-centered intervention. Observation allows for an occupational therapy practitioner to assess the adolescent in a nonconfrontational manner versus a question-and-answer session or direct interview of the adolescent.

Some standardized assessments that are discussed in the current literature as having been used with adolescents include the Child and Adolescent Functional Assessment Scale (Bates, 2001), the Adolescent and Adult Sensory Profile (Brown & Dunn, 2002), the Canadian Occupational Performance Measure (Law et al., 2015), and the PTSD Reaction Index (Steinberg, Brymer, Decker, & Pynoos, 2004).

Achenbach's Child Behavior Checklist and Youth Self-Report (2001) have been used in outpatient settings because these assessments provide comprehensive information about clients' behaviors as well as their occupational performance and functioning. When used together, a therapist can obtain both a youth's self-report and input from his or her parent or guardian about these areas. When administered as pre- and posttests, these assessments can help in developing treatment plans as well as measuring a client's progress.

CASE ILLUSTRATION 11-4: CLIENT-CENTERED AND MEANINGFUL INTERVENTION

It is a cold January day in the northeastern part of the United States. A foot of snow covers the grounds of the adolescent treatment facility, which includes a basketball court. The occupational therapist asks during group what the members would like to do for occupational therapy that week. They reply that they would like to play basketball. When the therapist states the obvious, that the court is buried in snow, they ask if they could shovel the snow and then play basketball. The adolescent classroom teacher and the occupational therapist on the program offer to bring in snow shovels, and when they do, the adolescents quickly shovel the snow off the basketball court and then engage in several games, looking and behaving like typical adolescents and not individuals with severe mental health problems, several of whom had made suicide attempts in the week prior to their admission into the program.

Discussion

It is easy to dismiss the requests of clients, who in this case want to play basketball during the winter, and offer seemingly more sensible choices such as indoor activities. However, by involving the clients in the decision-making and problem-solving process and giving them a sense of control over their environment and their treatment, the therapist in this example allowed the group to choose and execute their own activity, which provided them the opportunity to behave and interact in an age-appropriate and pleasurable manner, despite (possibly temporarily) overcoming their considerable mental health issues through social participation in meaningful occupation that they themselves determined.

INTERVENTION

Adolescents love doing. Although some may balk at a given activity as childish, most readily participate in arts and crafts activities and group activities in general, which may include group games such as Pictionary (Mattel), which serves to increase the level of arousal and social participation, among other skills, or basketball, a familiar sport that provides a real-life context.

Occupational therapists working with adolescents in an outpatient setting have many possible intervention activities to choose from. Craft activities are often used, and adolescents tend to enjoy these tasks. Because school systems are experiencing budget crises and art programs are being cut from many educational curricula, especially in high schools, occupational therapy sessions can be an adolescent's only access to artistic activities. In addition to the relaxing or soothing effects arts and crafts have for many, these craft activities serve countless purposes in outpatient mental health treatment. Completing a simple craft activity can provide an opportunity for the therapist to work with his or her clients on life skills, including problem solving, social interaction, time management, decision making, and frustration tolerance, and can be an effective intervention in increasing self-esteem and self-efficacy. One benefit of outpatient treatment for adolescents with mental health issues is the access a therapist can have to the youth's real life and environments. Engaging in these interventions in the youth's home or school can make the transfer of learned skills to their real life smoother. In outpatient settings, mental health interventions with adolescents can include actual daily occupations, for instance searching for employment or seeking out other community resources. A community-based occupational therapist may take a teenage client out job searching, using the tasks involved in this process as actual interventions. This intervention can be very effective because most teenagers are motivated to gain part-time employment because they desire their own source of income and the autonomy that comes with this. Activities such as encouraging the client to ask potential employers for job applications him- or herself versus having assistance or supervision can be used as intervention in the community. Employment readiness interventions and assessments will be discussed in a subsequent section. Occupational therapists have experience grading occupational tasks up or down depending on the needs of a client, and they can grade these real-life tasks in the community as well, to appropriately challenge adolescent clients and provide opportunities to learn and grow. As in all occupational therapy settings, the most effective outpatient interventions are meaningful and culturally relevant to the adolescent client. Case Illustration 11-4 shares an example of such an intervention.

In both inpatient and outpatient settings, occupational therapists must consider safety issues and use thorough activity analysis to ensure that participation and the activities themselves can only provide positive outcomes. Successful interventions used in occupational therapy settings with adolescents are discussed in the following sections.

Arts and Crafts

Arts and crafts activities such as suncatchers, velvet art, coloring sheets, tile mosaic trivets, murals, and seasonal

CASE ILLUSTRATION 11-5: CREATIVE EXPRESSIVE OCCUPATIONAL THERAPY

At a community-based mental health agency, youth have the opportunity to participate in a music program as part of their treatment. For this program, an occupational therapist works with another staff member who used to be a professional music producer, and the group leaders engage the youth participants in activities designed to build self-esteem, increase self-expression, and learn life skills through music. Through writing music and poetry and creating their own music and beats using state-of-the-art computer editing software, the youth create their own album. The curriculum takes clients through the full process of the music industry, including creating the music, learning about the business side (e.g., contracts, labels, negotiating), writing their own biography, and participating in a photo shoot for the cover of their album. Through this process, the occupational therapist incorporates training in life skills that are required for each step as the youth create their music. For example, communication and social skills are learned through collaborating and negotiating, and frustration tolerance is improved through what is often a challenging process for the youth.

Discussion

Through this creative, expressive process, the youth learn to overcome any insecurities they may have about expressing themselves, and they are able to tell their own story using music, a culturally relevant occupation.

decorations and activities have been successful in the inpatient setting. Creating a group banner or mural with a theme decided upon by the group can create camaraderie among adolescents who have just met and may only be in group together for a few sessions. One year in an inpatient setting, this concept was expanded to a door decorating contest near Christmas where roommates worked together using a variety of media. The adolescents became very invested in the activity and asked to work on the project outside of the designated occupational therapy time, which extended therapy into the milieu. Following completion, the therapist organized a panel of judges from the administration of the facility, and all participants won an award of some type—most colorful, best use of materials, most creative—to be posted beside their door, along with Christmas candy. There are a great many activities that can be created from a roll of white craft paper, from this contest to drawing and designing a city. Having adolescents draw a city as a group project successfully increases social interaction, facilitates teamwork, improves affect, and increases the level of arousal. Both the process and the end product provide interesting opportunities for conversation and discussion regarding the content of the drawing, as well as projective information about the participants through their individual contributions to the group project. (Further discussion on both arts and crafts and creative expression can be found in Chapter 4.)

Creative Expression

Creative activities generally work well with adolescents because they give the youth a chance to express themselves in a less threatening way than just talking and sharing personal information. Writing activities in which youth write about their experiences in the form of stories or poems can be a safe and powerful way to let youth express themselves in a way that feels safe and nonthreatening. Artwork, music, drama, or any other creative expression can also be useful modalities in working with adolescents. As in any occupational therapy treatment, the intervention should be client centered and client driven; therefore, whatever modality the youth is motivated by should be used. Case Illustration 11-5 is an example of the use of creative expression as an intervention.

Board Games

The Game of Life (Hasbro) provides an opportunity for discussion of future plans and facilitates sharing and self-disclosure, as well as providing socialization around a fun game. Pictionary is a game that a large group can play in teams using white craft paper or a chalk or dry erase board that provides some competition and also a lot of humor and laughing with peers. The game Taboo (Hasbro) offers a therapist an opportunity to work with adolescents on communication skills and social skills while giving quieter or more shy youth an opportunity to overcome their insecurities and boost their self-efficacy. Games such as these can seem almost too simple to be therapy, especially to other clinical staff who do not understand the therapeutic value that common occupations such as games possess. How valuable is a group that can make depressed adolescents smile, socialize, and laugh? Many effective resources have been developed specifically for therapy with adolescents. One such game is Talk It Out by Gordon Greenhalgh, PhD (available through Western Psychological Services; see Suggested Resources), which uses a board game format to help teenagers discuss age-related issues and values and facilitates problem solving, self-disclosure, and discussion of adolescents' personal problems and feelings.

Box 11-2. Rewards of Working With Adolescents in Mental Health

- Their gratitude for a listening ear
- Their eagerness to discuss problems
- Their candor about their circumstances
- Their acceptance of others/peers (e.g., sexual orientation, race, interests)
- Their desire to be or return to normal
- Their ability to see that things may not work out as planned

Job Training/Job Readiness Programs

Employment is often a meaningful occupation for adolescents because they begin to understand the importance of becoming self-sufficient; many need to work out of necessity. For adolescents with mental health concerns or other barriers, employment can provide additional challenges to their occupational functioning. Many life skills occupational therapists work on with adolescent clients apply directly to job readiness, including time management, social skills, problem solving, and impulse control. The OTTP in San Francisco (OTTP-SF) developed an occupation-based work skills assessment that is used to identify job-related skills and areas of needed improvement. The assessment, Double OT, is a mystery-solving game through which various skills are assessed through an engaging and occupation-based, client-centered approach. (A case illustration showing the administration of this assessment and a sample of a completed reporting form can be found in Chapter 4.)

Occupational therapy practitioners working at OTTP-SF provide services for adolescent clients involved in the justice system though a program called *Youth Workforce Development*, with a goal of assisting the youth with finding meaningful employment aligned with their interests and skills (Haworth & Cyrs, 2017). Occupational therapists working with adolescents who are interested in obtaining employment can assist their clients with identifying career goals and interests and in finding work opportunities that are aligned with these. Supporting clients with their employment and assisting with time management, impulse control, and any other areas of needed improvement can be an ongoing focus of occupational therapy intervention.

ADOLESCENT TREATMENT SETTINGS AND EMERGING PRACTICE

Opportunities for providing mental health interventions for adolescents exist in a variety of traditional and nontraditional settings, which are described throughout this text. Several innovative programs have also been described in this chapter. As discussed in Chapter 2 on psychiatric hospitals and institutions, many facilities have been closed or downsized, resulting in a lack of access to services and a shortage of providers. This necessitates broadening our scope of treatment in settings not usually thought of as being mental health and creating new models and programs to meet the burgeoning psychosocial needs of adolescents. One avenue for providing adolescent intervention is private practice. (Also see Chapter 3 on community behavioral health services.) Case Illustrations 11-6 and 11-7 are examples of interventions based on the private practice of the first author, which illustrates how the concepts discussed in this chapter can meet mental health needs of adolescents in nontraditional and flexible ways.

SUMMARY

As seen in this chapter, the needs and issues surrounding adolescents are vast and depend greatly on the demands and supports of their environment, as well as their predisposition to mental health or illness. Occupational therapists can effectively provide the skills and support needed for adolescents to make it through these years of transition through the varied array of interventions appropriate to this population described in this chapter. Indeed, there are many rewards of working with adolescents, as described in Box 11-2.

However, those who wish to work in this very gratifying area of practice will need to conceptualize and develop new ways of meeting their mental health needs in new contexts. Occupational therapists will need to address the mental health needs of adolescents in schools and other nontraditional settings. OTTP, an agency addressed in this chapter, does this using various evidence-based models and transdisciplinary practice. Emerging practice areas exist for therapists to address problems such as suicide and the trauma that surrounds active shooters killing peers, teachers, coaches, and others on an all-too-frequent basis. Private practice and community-based programs offer therapists opportunities for addressing the mental health needs of adolescents outside of traditional medical model settings. It may be necessary to advocate for increased services for adolescents with mental health issues and market occupational therapy's unique perspective and training to provide these services. Through this advocacy work, occupational therapists can re-establish, if not establish, a niche in working in this challenging and rewarding area of practice. It is the hope of the authors that the field of occupational therapy continues to research and focus on the adolescent population because this is a critical time of transition that requires support, specifically for adolescents with mental health concerns.

CASE ILLUSTRATION 11-6: FRANK—SUCCESSFUL REWARDING HOME-BASED OCCUPATIONAL THERAPY

Frank was a 13-year-old male at the time he was referred to an occupational therapist in private practice for home-based therapy to address depression and anger management issues. The referring psychiatrist began seeing Frank when he was 12 years old and began exhibiting emotional and behavioral problems following the death of his father, whom he had discovered after he had a massive heart attack. His attendance at outpatient therapy with a counselor had been poor, and he eventually refused to go.

Presenting Problems

Frank's presenting problems included isolating himself in his room at home on his computer, refusing to spend time with his family, school refusal with sporadic attendance, and angry outbursts and aggressive behaviors directed toward his mother and female siblings. He did not have any friends that he saw on a regular basis. He was frequently noncompliant with taking his prescribed antidepressant medications. Occasionally he broke household items, and prior to one of the therapist's initial weekly visits, he had punched a hole in a wall after a fight with his mother. When the occupational therapist suggested that Frank's mother take away his computer privileges, she refused, stating, "I'm too afraid of what he'll do." The occupational therapist interviewed Frank and his mother to establish treatment goals, a therapy schedule, and a fee for services. Frank begrudgingly began therapy, and his mother was supportive of his involvement, as well as her own, in the weekly sessions.

Course of Treatment

Frank was seen for therapy for 4 years. Initial interventions involved working with Frank individually, which was always followed with a wrap-up and review of the session with his mother. To establish trust, the occupational therapist had established with Frank that he would keep the contents of their sessions private that Frank wanted to remain confidential, with the exception of any disclosures that would indicate that he was a threat to himself or others. Initially, some sessions were held with the entire family, using typical board games as well as therapeutic games such as the Ungame to facilitate appropriate communication and interaction among family members. Later, the therapist felt that enough information had been gleaned from assessing family dynamics in these family sessions, and it was determined that the best use of sessions was to meet with Frank individually.

Frank's road to recovery was initially a rocky one. In some early sessions, he would leave for his room in anger and swear at the therapist and his mother or siblings. Interestingly, they would swear back. On one occasion he yelled at the therapist, "And don't think you're coming up here [his room] to talk to me" and slammed the door. On prior occasions, Frank had been amenable to talking, but this was clearly not one of them, and the therapist respected that he was finished with therapy for that day. The volatile nature of this adolescent's mood, as well as his depressive symptoms and behavior, often presented roadblocks to therapy. Occasionally, the occupational therapist would process the session on his way home or on his way to the next appointment and think to himself, *This case is going nowhere*; however, he persevered.

A turning point in Frank's therapy came following what ended up being a necessary change in the therapist's style, which was warm and supportive, to confrontational given the slow, uneven progress seen in the initial 18 months and Frank's resistance to change. The therapist told Frank, "Look, I'm here to help you. You are a depressed kid with a lot of problems that I'm happy to work on with you, but you have to be willing to work with me. If you're not able to do that, I don't see any point in continuing therapy." Frank thought about it for a few minutes and then said, "All right, I'll try."

From that point forward, Frank worked to address issues of attending school, taking medication, responding more appropriately and without aggression or destruction when angry, developing peer relationships, and, ultimately, finding a job that would provide him with opportunities for success in meeting others, getting positive feedback for his work, and moving him in a developmentally appropriate direction as he approached his 17th birthday. Obtaining a driver's license to increase his independence and provide him with opportunities to interact with others outside his home was accomplished as well. All of these goals required a great deal of support, patience, and encouragement but were accomplished in time. Part of the therapist's intervention was realizing and discussing with Frank that his family was a source of annoyance and the more time he spent with peers or in a job would only benefit him. As in all cases, the goals that were worked on also had to be Frank's to provide client-centered and successful care. Concessions necessarily were made over issues that continued to produce power struggles instead of change.

(continued)

CASE ILLUSTRATION 11-6: FRANK—SUCCESSFUL REWARDING HOME-BASED OCCUPATIONAL THERAPY (CONTINUED)

Course of Treatment (continued)

Frank was taking his medication sporadically at best, and although he would tell the occupational therapist that he had been taking his medication, in fact, he had not. His mother had presented his fairly untouched medications, so improvements were being made despite his refusal to take them. The family informed the psychiatrist of this in their scheduled session, and medication compliance was dropped as a goal for treatment.

When he was a senior, he continued to attend school infrequently. Frank's mother wanted him to be home-schooled as a result, but the therapist felt that attending school was a responsibility and part of the role of the adolescent and provided opportunities for social interaction. The family chose to have Frank home-schooled, which was their choice, and school attendance was no longer a treatment issue. By the mutually agreed-upon conclusion of Frank's therapy, he had friends that he hung out with at their homes and places in the community. They would have weekend sleepovers where they brought and played games on their computers. He purchased a car and successfully worked in a restaurant, where he was eventually promoted and offered career opportunities. He began to date. He had successfully resolved his issues and recovered to a remarkable degree, ready to graduate from high school and start considering his future.

A few weeks after their last session, the therapist received an invitation to Frank's graduation party, which he attended. At the party, Frank talked about his plans for the future, and when people walked up to him during their conversation, Frank would stop and say, "This is my counselor," and introduce him by name.

Discussion

The flexibility of home-based therapy allowed for the family and the therapist to practice in an environment that provided an in vivo context for intervention. Client factors and activity demands could easily be worked into sessions as things progressed or regressed. In times of high levels of dysfunction, sessions could be increased to twice a week, and, when considerable progress was being made, reduced to once a week or every other week, which happened frequently as Frank's mental health improved. The therapist, who was paid on a fee-for-service basis and not through a traditional insurance provider, allowed for the length and frequency of therapy to be determined by the client, his family, and the occupational therapist. Because Frank eventually refused to take medication but did agree to continue therapy, Frank's progress and eventual recovery could be directly linked to occupational therapy intervention. Frank's family had been considerably dysfunctional, particularly in their interaction style (e.g., yelling, swearing, and blowing up). Therapeutic use of relationship or self was essential to the successful outcome of this case. Had the occupational therapist not worked for many years in child and adolescent mental health, where behaviors like these were frequently encountered, the foul language and high affect states that the family used as a regular part of their conversations could have been upsetting or appalling. By addressing the issues that led to referral (i.e., symptoms of depression, school refusal, and poor anger management skills) and not the family's longstanding ways of communicating in emotional reactive ways, the therapist was able to focus on the adolescent's recovery in his context, without imposing his own standards or beliefs on civility. In time, the family did interact in a more pleasant manner, and the tone of the home became more placid as well. Oftentimes, therapists and other clinicians do not respond in a therapeutic manner that addresses treatment issues when patients use vulgar or profane language and say, "Now, is that the way we ask for things?" to a swearing client, not taking into account that in that individual's home environment, context, and culture, such interaction and ways of expressing one's self may well be the norm.

The client-centered approach used by the therapist enabled Frank to feel a part of the process, giving Frank positive feedback for his accomplishments and providing the adolescent with choices and avoiding power struggles as mentioned elsewhere in this chapter, which worked effectively as demonstrated in this case. Frank's case also illustrates the qualities needed to practice effectively with adolescents, such as having patience; being genuine, committed, and caring; and being able to empathize and support an individual who is still maturing—not a child but not yet an adult—and looking for guidance as he makes that transition. This is not always easy when dealing with typically developing teenagers, let alone adolescents who are having great difficulty navigating this developmental phase of their lives.

CASE ILLUSTRATION 11-7: ANNA—REACTIVE ATTACHMENT DISORDER AND FAMILY TREATMENT

Anna is a 14-year-old girl referred to an outpatient occupational therapist by a local child and adolescent psychiatrist. She has had traditional outpatient therapy in the recent past, which has proved unsuccessful, and Anna stopped attending. She has a diagnosis of reactive attachment disorder (RAD), and her presenting problems include conflictual family relationships, particularly with her adoptive mother.

Background and History

Anna was born in Russia and adopted at the age of 7 by her current adoptive parents. Prior to her adoption, she grew up in a home where her parents were neglectful due to their active substance abuse. Her biological parents were rarely home, and Anna was cared for by a series of neighbors and relatives who were present on an inconsistent basis. She was often left by herself, and, consequently, she had resorted to stealing food for sustenance. She was removed from the home at 5 years old and placed in an orphanage. Her adoptive parents, Tony and Maria, are financially well off and spent a great deal of money and time arranging for Anna's adoption when they were unable to conceive. Anna was a difficult child with frequent temper tantrums who was cool and distant to her parents and frequently disobedient as she grew older. Her parents have tried numerous interventions, including taking her to a center in a major city that specializes in treating children with RAD when she was 8. Despite their best intentions and attempts at therapeutic interventions to help resolve their problems, things in the household have not changed, but have actually gotten worse as Anna entered adolescence. Additionally, the couple was able to conceive a daughter in the intervening years, who is now 5 years old. Anna has threatened the sister and believes that the parents favor her. The therapist enters the case at this impasse.

The outpatient therapist arrived at the family home and began by interviewing Anna and completing a Kinetic Self-Image Test. Anna draws a picture of herself drawing a picture. Her goal for treatment is "I want to have a happy family." Additionally, he had interviewed her parents and solicited their goals for treatment. Tony would like for Anna to "just get along with her mother. She doesn't really have a problem with me." The therapist will later discover that although she gets along well with her father, whose business keeps him away from home more than 40 hours a week, she has stolen money from his wallet, which he now has to keep locked up.

Because the primary family conflict appears to be with the mother, the therapist arranges a session for them to complete a mother-daughter collage about their family. The therapist notes that they work in a parallel manner, with little to no conversation, although the mother tries to initiate. Later, when processing the session, the mother remarked, "We pretty much worked on our own," and Maria said that she "hadn't really expected anything to be different. This is the way it always is."

Following a subsequent individual session, the mother told the therapist, "I've been able to overhear some of your sessions, and I want you to know she's not telling you the truth about what happens around here. She didn't tell you about how she tried to push me down the stairs when we were arguing about her finishing the vacuuming, and our week was nothing like she described."

At this point, the therapist decides to have family meeting–style sessions where a forum can be created to discuss family events and dynamics. Some progress is made; however, Anna continues to not follow rules, lie, and be disrespectful, especially toward her mother. As her father and mother begin to align to reinforce consequences for negative behavior, Anna begins to be nasty and disrespectful to the father as well. Tony "just can't understand it. We give her all these great things that she could never have had in Russia and she's so ungrateful. Soon as she gets one thing, she wants something else. She's never grateful for anything." The family meetings focused on having the parents present as a united front with regard to limits, expectations, and consequences, although Tony continued to believe that "Maria is too hard on her. I think if we give her more positives, she'll come around" when Maria tried to follow through with limits and consequences.

(continued)

CASE ILLUSTRATION 11-7: ANNA—REACTIVE ATTACHMENT DISORDER AND FAMILY TREATMENT (CONTINUED)

Background and History (continued)

Therapy made progress initially as Tony and Maria assumed more appropriate parental roles. As their position strengthened, Anna became more oppositional, limit testing, and threatening. At home one Friday, the therapist received a call from Tony that "Anna has threatened to kill all of us." Based on her history of threats and the attempt to push her mother down the stairs, the therapist recommended inpatient hospitalization and walked the father through the necessary steps. He asked the father to call him if he had any difficulties. At the next session, it was found that the father did not follow through.

At this point in the therapeutic process, the therapist contacted the referring psychiatrist for guidance. The doctor believed that the therapist was doing the right things in therapy and offered to see the family and possibly start a low dose of medication. The family did not go to the appointment, and in that week's session, Tony stated, "I won't have my daughter turned into a zombie" and not only refused to discuss the matter further, but left the room and the session.

All of the particulars of this case cannot be presented in this case illustration, but eventually, the family and the therapist agreed that "we're just spinning our wheels" and that progress was no longer being made. The therapist reviewed the course of therapy with the parents and provided his interpretation that they were not able to provide consistent limits and consequences; that Anna, who had voiced that she did not want to live with them any longer, continued to pose a threat to them and their younger daughter; and that choices needed to be made regarding Anna remaining in the home or sent to boarding school because she was academically sound, had no desire to work on a relationship with them, posed a threat to the young family, and would be leaving for college in a few short years. He gave them praise for continuing to try to effect change despite what they knew about RAD and how many avenues they had tried, and offered to re-enter the case to assist in Anna's placement if that was what they chose. They thanked the therapist and stated that they had believed this was "their best chance" at improving their situation, but did not call him again.

Discussion

Unlike the previous case illustration of Frank, this case does not have what would appear to be a happy ending. Of course, not all attempts at therapy do. It does, however, illustrate a number of important points and positive outcomes. Therapy based in the home on an outpatient basis increased Anna's involvement in therapy and provided the therapist with a truer picture of family dynamics than might have been had at an outpatient office. Although the parents strengthened their positions and roles to a degree, the fact that they could not agree on how to parent Anna effectively became clear to the therapist as well as to each other. At one point, the therapist suggested marital counseling, and the mother replied, "Many have." As is always the case in providing effective occupational therapy, the patient has to be a willing participant in the therapeutic process, as do the parents when working with adolescents. Therapy clarified relationships and barriers to successfully meeting treatment goals and led the family to the point where they had to be willing to change if change was to occur. When that didn't happen, the therapist used reflection, sought guidance from the referring psychiatrist, presented the parents with options, and knew when to terminate therapy based on the response of the parents and Anna to intervention. It is difficult to come to the decision, based on clinical reasoning, that further intervention will be futile unless the participants are willing to accept what is being presented and make changes accordingly. Perhaps this family was not ready to do that. Perhaps they never will be. Nonetheless, they expressed their gratitude for the therapist's attempts at trying to help them resolve their issues. As is the case with occupational therapy in mental health, and in other settings as well, the therapist often cannot and may never know what the ultimate outcomes of therapy actually were.

ACKNOWLEDGEMENT

The authors would like to acknowledge Kasey Fitzgerald, MS, OTR/L, who contributed significantly to the editing and research for this chapter.

REFERENCES

Achenbach, T. (2001). *Youth self-report for ages 11-18*. Burlington, VT: ASEBA, University of Vermont.

American Occupational Therapy Association. (2014). Occupational therapy practice framework: Domain and process (3rd ed.). *American Journal of Occupational Therapy, 68*(S1), S1-S48.

American Psychiatric Association. (2013). *Diagnostic and statistical manual of mental disorders: DSM-5* (5th ed.). Arlington, VA: Author.

Bates, M. P. (2001). The Child and Adolescent Functional Assessment Scale (CAFAS): Review and current status. *Clinical Child and Family Psychology Review, 4*(1), 63-81.

Brown, C., & Dunn, W. (2002). *Adolescent-Adult Sensory Profile*. San Antonio, TX: Pearson.

Centers for Disease Control and Prevention. (2015). *Understanding youth violence*. Retrieved from https://www.cdc.gov/violenceprevention/pdf/suicide-datasheet-a.pdf

Chaudry, A., & Fortuny, K. (2010). *Children of immigrants: Economic well-being*. Washington DC: Urban Institute.

Costa, D. M. (2009). Eating disorders: Occupational therapy's role. *OT Practice, 14*(11), 13.

DePanfilis, D., & Dubowitz, H. (2005). Family Connections: A program for preventing child neglect. *Child Maltreatment, 10*, 108-123.

Derr, A.S. (2016). Mental health service use among immigrants in the United States: A systematic review. *Psychiatric Services, 67*(3), 265-274.

Gardiner, C., & Brown, N. (2010). Is there a role for occupational therapy within a specialist child and adolescent mental health eating disorder service? *British Journal of Occupational Therapy, 73*(1), 38-43.

Glick, B., & Gibbs, J. C. (2010). *Aggression replacement training: A comprehensive intervention for aggressive youth* (3rd ed.). Champaign, IL: Research Press.

Goertz, H., Benedict, B., Bui, O., Peitz, S., Ryba, R., & Cahill, S. (2008). AOTA's societal statement on youth violence. *American Journal of Occupational Therapy, 62*(6), 709-710.

Guarino, K. K., Soares, P., Konnath, K., Clervil, R., & Bassuk, E. (2009). *Trauma-informed organizational toolkit*. Rockville, MD: Center for Mental Health Services, Substance Abuse and Mental Health Services Administration.

Gutman, S. A. (2005). Understanding suicide: What therapists should know. *Occupational Therapy in Mental Health, 21*, 55-77.

Haworth, C., & Cyrs, G. (2017). Supporting transitions to the workforce for at-risk youth: Developing and using an occupation-based work skills assessment. *OT Practice, 22*(15), 21-24.

Henderson, S.W. & Baily, C.D.R. (2013). Parental deportation, families, and mental health. *Journal of the American Academy of Child & Adolescent Psychiatry, 52*(5), 451-453.

Hoff, D. L., & Mitchell, S. N. (2009). Cyberbullying: causes, effects, and remedies. *Journal of Educational Administration, 47*(5), 652-665.

Ito, M., Horst, H., Bittanti, M., Boyd, D., Herr-Stephenson, B., Lange, P., . . . Robinson, L. (2008). *Living and learning with new media: Summary of findings from the Digital Youth Project*. Building the Field of Digital Media and Learning: MacArthur Foundation. Retrieved from http://digitalyouth.ischool.berkeley.edu/files/report/digitalyouth-TwoPageSummary.pdf

Kaiser, E., Gillette, C., & Spinazzola, J. (2010). Trauma treatment: A controlled pilot-outcome study of sensory integration (SI) in the treatment of complex adaptation to traumatic stress. *Journal of Aggression, Maltreatment, and Trauma, 19*, 699-720.

Kloczko, E., & Ikiugu, M. (2006). The role of occupational therapy in the treatment of adolescents with eating disorders as perceived by mental health therapists. *Occupational Therapy in Mental Health, 22*(1), 63-83.

Law, M., Baptiste, S., Carswell, A., McColl, M. A., Polatajko, H., & Pollock, N. (2015). *Canadian Occupational Performance Measure (COPM)* (5th ed.). Toronto, Canada: Canadian Association of Occupational Therapists.

Lock, J., Le Grange, D., Agras, W., Moye, A., Bryson, S., & Jo, B. (2010). Randomized clinical trial comparing family-based treatment with adolescent-focused individual therapy for adolescents with anorexia nervosa. *Archives of General Psychiatry, 67*(10), 1025.

Masten, A. S. (2001). Ordinary magic: Resilience processes and development. *American Psychologist, 56*, 227-238.

Mayo Clinic. (2017). *Self-injury/cutting*. Retrieved from https://www.mayoclinic.org/diseases-conditions/self-injury/symptoms-causes/syc-20350950

Mental Health America. (n.d.). *Bullying: Tips for parents*. Retrieved from http://www.mentalhealthamerica.net/bullying-tips-parents

Moro, C. (2007). A comprehensive literature review defining self-mutilation and occupational therapy intervention approaches: Dialectical behavior therapy and sensory integration. *Occupational Therapy in Mental Health, 23*(1), 55-67.

Najavits, L. M. (2002). *Seeking safety: A treatment manual for PTSD and substance abuse*. New York, NY: Guilford.

National Institute for Mental Health. (2017). *Suicide prevention*. Retrieved from https://www.nimh.nih.gov/health/topics/suicide-prevention/index.shtml

National Institute for Mental Health. (2018). *Suicide*. Retrieved from https://www.nimh.nih.gov/health/statistics/suicide.shtml

National Research Council, Institute of Medicine. (2009). *Preventing mental, emotional, and behavioral disorders among young people: Progress and possibilities*. Washington, DC: National Academies Press.

New Freedom Commission on Mental Health. (2003). *Achieving the promise: Transforming mental health care in America: Final Report*. Washington DC: U.S. Department of Health & Human Services.

Occupational Therapy Training Program. (2018). *Family programs*. Retrieved from https://www.ottp.org/family-programs

Parent Project. (2018). *Changing destructive adolescent behavior*. Retrieved from https://www.parentproject.com/index.php/about-us/programs-offered/changing-destructive-adolescent-behavior

Petrenchik, T., & Weiss, D. (2015). Childhood trauma. In *American Occupational Therapy Association, School mental health toolkit*. Retrieved from https://www.aota.org/~/media/Corporate/Files/Practice/Children/Childhood-Trauma-Info-Sheet-2015.pdf

Richards, M., Lewis, G., Sanderson, R. C., & Deane, K. (2016). Introduction to special issue: Resilience-based approaches to trauma intervention for children and adolescents. *Journal of Child and Adolescent Trauma, 9*, 1-4.

Schroeder Oxer, S., & Kopp Miller, B. (2001). Effects of choice in an art occupation with adolescents living in residential treatment facilities. *Occupational Therapy in Mental Health, 17*(1), 39-49.

Schurgin O'Keeffe, G., & Clarke-Pearson, K. (2011). The impact of social media on children, adolescents, and families. *American Academy of Pediatrics Clinical Report, 127*(4).

Shearsmith-Farthing, K. (2001). The management of altered body image: a role for occupational therapy. *British Journal of Occupational Therapy, 64*(8), 387-392.

Steinberg, A. M., Brymer, M. J., Decker, K. B., & Pynoos, K. B. (2004). *The University of California at Los Angeles post-traumatic stress disorder reaction index.* New York, NY: Springer.

Substance Abuse Mental Health Service Administration. (2018). *National Registry of Evidence-Based Programs and Practices (NREPP).* Retrieved from https://www.samhsa.gov/nrepp

Weinstein, A., & Lejoyeux, M. (2010). Internet addiction or excessive internet use. *American Journal of Drug and Alcohol Abuse, 5,* 277-283.

Werner E. E. (2005). Resilience research. In: R. D. Peters, B. Leadbeater, & R. J. McMahon (Eds.), *Resilience in children, families, and communities* (pp. 3-11). Boston, MA: Springer.

Williams, K., & Bydalek, K. (2007). Adolescent self-mutilation diagnosis & treatment. *Journal of Psychosocial Nursing and Mental Health Services, 45,* 1219-1225.

Wyman, P. A., Hendricks Brown, C., LoMurray, M., Schmeelk-Cone, K., Petrova, M., Yu, Q., ... Wang, W. (2010). An outcome evaluation of the Sources of Strength suicide prevention program delivered by peer leaders in high schools. *American Journal of Public Health, 100*(9), 1653-1662.

SUGGESTED RESOURCES

American Psychiatric Association: https://www.psychiatry.org

American Psychological Association: Children's Mental Health: http://www.apa.org/pi/families/children-mental-health.aspx

American Academy of Child & Adolescent Psychiatry (AACAP) Resource Centers: http://www.aacap.org/AACAP/Families_and_Youth/Resource_Centers

Mental Health Association: Children's Mental Health: http://www.nmha.org/go/children

National Alliance on Mental Illness: Teens & Young Adults: https://www.nami.org/Find-Support/Teens-Young-Adults

National Center for Children in Poverty: Children's Mental Health: http://nccp.org/publications/pub_687.html

National Federation of Families for Children's Mental Health: http://ffcmh.org

National Library of Medicine Medline Plus: Child Mental Health: https://medlineplus.gov/childmentalhealth.html

National Institute of Mental Health: Child and Adolescent Mental Health: http://nimh.nih.gov/health/topics/child-and-adolescent-mental-health/index.shtml

Substance Abuse and Mental Health Services Administration: https://www.samhsa.gov

SAMHSA's National Registry of Evidence-Based Programs and Practices: https://www.samhsa.gov/nrepp

Western Psychological Services: https://www.wpspublish.com/app/Home.aspx

Mental Health of Emerging Adults

Karen McCarthy, OTD, OTR/L; Anne MacRae, PhD, OTR/L, BCMH, FAOTA;
and Bernadette Hattjar, DrOT, MEd, OTR/L, CWCE

17 + 1 = 18. You're not a teenager; you're a young adult!! —Unknown

This simple quote of unknown origins (probably a birthday card) indicates the beginning age range for the young adult population commercially. In actuality, the exact date and time of graduation to adulthood is astonishingly elusive, and the demarcation points vary in different cultures and have evolved over time as societies change. This chapter reflects the work of Arnett (2016), who argues that the road to adulthood is longer than previous generations and would define this unique stage as "emerging adulthood," instead of "extended adolescence" or "young adulthood."

Occupational therapists need to be skilled in the nuances of lifespan, where there are distinct occupational transitions and challenges. Historically, there has been a lack of focus in occupational therapy on the period of emerging adulthood, collapsing services into either adolescent or adult services. Emerging adults, as a population in their own right, can be hard to isolate due to a variety of health conditions, living environments, and service use. This variety also means that occupational therapists encounter emerging adults across an array of practice areas and must be aware of their unique culture and needs.

DEVELOPMENTAL FRAMEWORK

Young adulthood is a developmental stage that has often been collapsed into adolescence or adulthood, but there are experiences and developmental tasks that are unique to this age group (Bonovitz, 2018). For the first time in their lives, emerging adults are likely to be outside of parental control and the routine of school, living on their own, working, and deciding who they want to be and what future they want to have.

Emerging adulthood is a transition where one experiments with new occupations, roles, and behaviors. With any life transition, there can be a risk of stagnant or damaged transitions, where one "responds passively to adverse life circumstances," or there can also be "repaired and progressive transitions" where one, given the right support, can thrive and succeed (Bynner, 2005, p. 379).

This is a time of life where one's personal identity is drawn, formulated, and executed. Consider individuals in this age group graduating from high school and embarking to college or a career; developing more mature relationships with another individual; possibly riding the wave of autonomy from family and home; and being part of financial, leisure, and general life experiences. Marriage or committed coupling may also occur during this time of life. Additionally, having children, pregnancy, and child rearing may become a part of life. In other words, this time of life

MacRae, A. (Ed.). *Cara and MacRae's Psychosocial Occupational Therapy: An Evolving Practice, Fourth Edition* (pp 201-214).
© 2019 Taylor & Francis Group.

Box 12-1. Social and Emotional Development of Emerging Adults

- **Identity exploration**: A time of deciding who one is and what is wanted or expected out of school, work, and love
- **Instability**: Consider the change of residence for school or college, living with friends, living with a romantic partner
- **Feeling "in between"**: Consider this age where individuals are no longer in the regiment of high school and possibly residing with parents or family. These individuals are no longer children and have additional responsible for societal demands (e.g., voting, driving, college, working) but are not viewed as full-fledged adults. This is a time of determining where one is in this process and where one will fit in.
- **Self-focus**: This life period is marked by young individuals deciding what they want to do, where they want to go, and who they want to be with—before the choices get limited by work, marriage, and children.
- **Possibilities**: This period of life is frequently colored with optimism for the future. Individuals believe that they will have a better life than their parents, find a soulmate, and select a good job or career. This can also be a time when individuals are risk takers and may engage in harmful activities such as drug use, smoking, and alcohol use.

is all about choices. Positive choices will tend to spur the person further in a direction, whereas negative choices can prompt the person to make additional negative or unfulfilling choices for the self, friends and family, and the community and society in general.

This age mismatch further substantiates the problems and issues that surround providing intervention and services to this underserved age group/population. Services and interventions must walk the tightrope between adolescence and young adulthood. Providing these items with the just-right fit for the age and stage of this population can determine the overall effectiveness or lack thereof.

As previously mentioned, this chapter primarily uses the concepts of emerging adulthood, but the term *young adult* is used interchangeably, especially when discussing the higher end of the age range. Emerging adults differ from adolescents because they have to make significant decisions about housing, career, and relationships. They reach adulthood not because of a single event such as marriage or having a child, but as a result of the gradual process of becoming self-sufficient. The endpoint of emerging adulthood and establishment of young adulthood is difficult to bracket into specific age ranges because much of this transition is marked by how much someone feels adult. The heart of emerging adulthood seems to be ages 18 to 25, whereas acknowledging that differences in socioeconomic status, culture, and life events might extend this stage to age 29 (Arnett, 2016). Becoming an adult is a process, and emerging adulthood defines this liminal space between adolescence and adulthood as an arena (or a battleground, on occasion), one that is characterized by trying things out and seeing what works. In other words, this stage is one of transitions, and it is not uncommon for an individual to sometimes feel like a child or youth and other days to feel ready for adulthood.

Physical Development

The young adult period of life is also characterized by males and females adjusting to their new physical sense of self. Females tend to complete this development process earlier than males. Males may not become fully physically mature until about age 21. The young adult time span also is noted to be a time where the individual adjusts to his or her sexually maturing body and feelings associated with his or her sexuality (e.g., finding a partner, intimacy issues, developing a clear sense of sexual identity) and where the individual begins to develop and apply abstract thinking skills (e.g., the ability to put the self into another person's shoes, increased capacity to consider different points of view, the baseline development of philosophical and idealistic attributes). This changes and/or redirects his or her ability to think about him- or herself, others, and the world around him or her.

Social and Emotional Development

This particular range of ages also represents a wide variety of life stages and milestones, including high school graduation, potential college attendance and graduation, securing a full-time job, marriage, and the birth of children. The operative terms frequently used to describe this time of life are *change, the passage into adulthood,* and *a time of not fitting into much of anything,* hence a time of developing relationships outside of the typical family. This may include a group of friends, a Greek organization, a religious or spiritual organization, a volunteer or work group of friends, or many other types of population or group affiliation in order to feel a part of something. The major concepts related to the social and emotional development of emerging adults are synthesized in Box 12-1.

TABLE 12-1. OCCUPATIONS OF EMERGING ADULTS

TYPE OF OCCUPATION	COMMENTS
Leisure occupations	Young adults have choices to make about continuing hobbies or starting new interests as they enter adulthood. Personal and social factors impact leisure, as well as a culture that promotes consumption. Common leisure occupations include active occupations such as structured sports and exercise routines, as well as passive occupations such as watching movies. Some leisure occupations can be compulsive or have a negative impact on well-being, including vandalism, substance misuse, and pornography addiction.
Digital occupations	Young adults today grew up immersed in media and technology, becoming known as *digital natives*. They have always had digital technologies that allow them to communicate instantly with their social world. Young adults use these tools as extensions of their bodies and minds, incorporating them into their daily routines. There is now growing concern about the negative impact of dependence on social media and screen time addiction.
Sexual occupations	The expectation for many young adults today is that they will date multiple people before committing to a life partner, if at all. Dating in young adulthood can range from casual, such as hanging out with friends, to formal, such as going on official dates. Client factors such as their beliefs about sexuality, body functions, and what they value as important in a partner impact their choices. Young adults may be freer than previous generations to search for a partner without the restrictions of archaic dating rules and laws against mixed race or same-sex relationships, but that does not mean that finding the right person has become any easier.
Spiritual occupations	Part of forming one's identity is developing an ideology or worldview. Many young adults are still in the process of forming their beliefs, and they are less likely to identify with the belief system of their parents. This group might be more skeptical of formal religious institutions and more inclined to create their own beliefs based on various traditions and philosophies.

OCCUPATIONS OF EMERGING ADULTS

We emerge as adults through our engagement in occupation. Our occupational choices reflect who we are, our values, and who we want to become. Emerging adults tend to have more choice in occupations, with increased autonomy and diminishing parental influence, possessing more of a "self-focus" in their decision making (Arnett, 2015). What will I eat today? When will I go home tonight? Whom will I meet up with? For the most part, they decide. Some individuals may experience a limitation of autonomy that is so critical at this age due to financial constraints or continued ties to parental influences. For example, some may need to work in a low-paying job with the inability to afford college tuition or to pay rent to move out of their parents' home. When young adults are not engaged in occupations of value, they can experience occupational alienation, and life can seem meaningless (Townsend & Wilcock, 2004). Without choice and opportunity to engage in personally meaningful occupations, feelings of isolation, powerlessness, loss of control, and frustration may follow. Table 12-1 describes some of the primary occupations of emerging adults. However, the most complex and formative are work and education occupations; therefore, expanded discussion of these occupations is warranted.

Work and Education Occupations

Most Americans have a part-time job, often only lasting a few months, while in high school. These are primarily low-skill service jobs with the intention of earning extra money for leisure, not as preparation for their career (Arnett, 2004). For some youth, both in America and in other parts of the world, early work experience is often to help the family meet basic needs or assist in the family business. However, it is becoming less common for people to stay in the family business, and eventually the focus shifts to preparation for a future career and exploring educational opportunities that will help propel them along their chosen career path. As they experiment with different jobs or educational paths, they discover more about themselves and what they want to do. Changes in society, including increased gender diversity in the workplace and delaying of marriage, have opened up new opportunities for work and educational choices for women. Disability legislation such as the Americans with

CASE ILLUSTRATION 12-1: KEVIN'S EDUCATIONAL AND VOCATIONAL CHALLENGES

Kevin is a 19-year-old man who was recently released from a juvenile detention facility where he was serving a 6-month drug-related charge, which occurred before his 18th birthday. His only legal job was in a fast food restaurant, and he hated it. So, after he left home, he sold weed to get by. School records show that Kevin was diagnosed with attention deficit disorder but did not respond to medication. There were also repeated reports of fights in school resulting in suspensions, but there was evidence that these fights were primarily defensive responses to bullying. At age 16, Kevin quit high school, stating he "had enough."

Kevin uses both marijuana and alcohol in excess, trying to "feel better" about himself and fit in. He acknowledges a long history of depression, but he only occasionally took medication and refused therapy. He also reports high anxiety bordering on "panic" at the thought of heading back to jail, but he has no idea what he can do for legal work. He feels that he has already "screwed up" his life, and he doesn't see much hope for the future.

Discussion

An occupational therapy work readiness assessment could help Kevin identify potential vocational opportunities that not only match his interests, but also his real and potential skills. (See Chapter 5 for a detailed description of a work readiness program.) For example, many young people with attention deficit disorder have no interest in and perhaps minimal ability for tolerating a typical desk job. However, outdoor and/or very active jobs, such as construction and gardening, might be a good match. Jobs with the greatest potential for career development and advancement typically do require some form of advanced training. However, this does not necessarily mean degree programs. Many skilled labor jobs have apprentice programs and licensure requirements that use a series of short course work and experiential education.

Disabilities Act, which was passed in 1990, has also opened some doors for those with a psychiatric disability to pursue employment and higher education, receiving reasonable accommodations. The form and function of work have also changed for the millennial generation, with many young adults choosing to have jobs outside of their main source of income, aka the *side hustle*. The side hustle is a necessity for many young adults to make the rent/mortgage or pay back student loans. For others, it can be a way to diversify work experience; pursue other passions; and avoid that feeling of being stuck, dull, or cheated by life. Young adults can use app-based employment such as Uber or Task Rabbit, which promote freelance or contract work. This type of work can make the 9-to-5 job seem obsolete, but they are lacking the benefits that often come with full-time work, such as retirement matching or health insurance. Participating in the work environment is one of the catalysts to reaching adulthood. Threats to successfully managing this transition include high unemployment, stigma, and discrimination.

Postsecondary Education

Postsecondary education has become almost essential in recent times to obtain a good job in American society, and many other countries are following this pattern. The rising costs of higher education in America and other exclusionary policies in education can present insurmountable challenges, preventing young adults from experiencing key developmental passages that could be of benefit (Côté, Skinkle, & Motte, 2008). Many adolescents who experienced mental health issues have not completed their high

school education for a variety of reasons. According to the Learning Disabilities Association of America (n.d.), children with learning disabilities are at higher risk of developing a mental illness or emotional disturbance as they age. Resulting anxiety and depression are particularly common, but the social alienation and bullying that too often occurs to young people with learning disabilities can also lead to addiction issues or a wide variety of other high-risk behaviors. Case Illustration 12-1 highlights a young man's struggles with these multiple challenges.

Postsecondary education can involve 4-year universities, 2-year colleges (including junior college, community college, technical college, or city college), as well as shorter-duration programs in vocational/trade schools with more hands-on experience. Each setting provides a unique environment and culture, where students will engage in diverse experiences, requirements, and occupations. In a 4-year university, students might try out different majors or courses and experiment with different social groups or clubs. These explorations are part of their identity formation. They are trying to find out what type of career would fit them or what type of future they would like to have, in pursuit of an elusive moment where it all clicks and they know their path. Some find it and some do not, but a 4-year university might give them the breathing space and the opportunity to explore. Vocational and trade schools are more focused on specific skill attainment and job training, so exploration and experimentation with different job paths might not be as applicable in this context.

CASE ILLUSTRATION 12-2: MAUREEN'S EXACERBATION OF SCHIZOPHRENIA

Maureen is a 23-year-old college student who was preparing for midterm examinations, which she described to her roommates as being "hella stressful." The voices apparently worsened over the past several days to the point where she was unable to sleep at all or concentrate on any activities. Her behavior became increasingly erratic and prompted her roommate to take her to the emergency psychiatric services at the county hospital. She arrived in a wildly agitated state, shouting, "Let me die." During an initial interview, Maureen admitted that she had been hearing voices commanding her to kill herself. It was decided that Maureen was a danger to herself, and she was admitted to the acute inpatient locked unit. Further interviews revealed that Maureen had a history of repeated psychotic episodes starting in high school. Six years prior, she had been diagnosed with schizophrenia. When she took her medication, her symptoms remained under control and she was able to function relatively well. However, she often stopped her medications because she felt they made her drowsy so she couldn't study. She does acknowledge that each time she stopped her medication, an acute exacerbation of her symptoms occurred.

Discussion

Although stress does not cause schizophrenia, it can adversely affect one's function by increasing both the severity and frequency of symptoms. Therefore, helping Maureen develop a number of skills, including stress and time management, would be beneficial. In addition, psychotropic medication, although not a cure, clearly helped Maureen maintain her functional abilities and decrease episodes of psychosis. She may benefit from a change in medications to decrease drowsiness, but she could also benefit from strategies to manage the side effects of medication. (See Chapter 1 for further discussion.)

Those students that can attend postsecondary education, whether it be certificate courses, junior college, or a 4-year university, will experience a unique transition. Postsecondary education differs from high school because it relies more on a student's self-discipline and motivation to attend. Attendance might be optional, with most of the coursework happening outside the classroom, requiring strong organization and executive functioning skills.

Pursuing postsecondary education, whether part-time or full-time, will bring with it changes in habits, routines, and occupations. In a traditional 4-year university setting, besides a few scheduled courses, students have far more control over their daily time use. Occupations around coursework, including studying, writing, and group projects, will become a prominent part of their routine, with the potential for procrastination to emerge as a dominant habit.

All of these new occupational opportunities can present challenges for some students. Students with social anxiety might tend to isolate from others or miss class. Those who struggle with focus and executive functioning skills might feel overwhelmed with deadlines and settle into a routine of immersing in distracting activities to reduce anxiety.

MENTAL HEALTH
ISSUES AND DIAGNOSES

When identity and fitting in are in question, such as during emerging adulthood, the potential for mental health problems increases. This young adult age group tends to normally experience angst, moodiness, or grumpiness; social inconsistencies, including social withdrawal or social engagement; anger; irritability; weight loss or weight gain; and symptoms consistent with mild depression (Foundations Recovery Network, n.d.). When any or all of these symptoms endure longer than a few days or a few weeks, a mental health problem may be presenting. It is estimated that approximately one in five adolescents or young adults experience a diagnosable mental health disorder. The most common disorders found in this age group are anxiety, depression, substance abuse, eating disorders, and autistic spectrum disorder. Schizophrenia, although not the most common disorder of this age group, is the one that has the potential for causing the greatest level of dysfunction. It is important to note that at least part of the dysfunction associated with schizophrenia is triggered by stigma rather than symptoms. (See further discussion on stigma in Chapter 5.) Symptoms of schizophrenia typically begin to emerge between ages 16 and 25 in men and a few years later in women (Schizophrenia.com, n.d.). As shown in Case Illustration 12-2, the stress commonly experienced by young adults does play a part in acute exacerbations of the illness; however, for many people, the condition can be medically managed. (See Chapter 1 for more information on psychopharmacology.)

It is interesting to note that about 50% of all substance abuse and mental health disorders have roots or can be identified before the age of 14 years. This number is based on behavioral issues; social, school, and family roles; and

CASE ILLUSTRATION 12-3: THE STORY OF CARLOS—UNDERSTANDING THE EMERGING ADULT

Carlos, age 28, completed two 365-day deployments in the Middle East in an active combat role before receiving an honorable discharge to civilian status. He is currently considering work and college options using his GI Bill benefits. Carlos is accustomed to having his routines, which provided structure and a strong connection with his fellow service members. His mind was drawn to the past, with memories from active duty coming up and feeling so real that he sometimes came-to from a flashback in a deep sweat. He reached out to the Veterans Administration and began using psychiatry, receiving a diagnosis of posttraumatic stress disorder and a referral to occupational therapy.

Together, the occupational therapist and Carlos set goals around job acquisition, social connection, and finding a meaningful hobby. Carlos craves active leisure and the thrill of physical occupations. The occupational therapist invites Carlos to join their weekly veteran surfing group. Carlos finds the challenge of surfing combined with the beauty of the ocean to be a healing force in his life. Surfing group ends each week with a campfire social; he enjoys the banter with other veterans. He mentions to the occupational therapist that in the future, he would like to mentor other veterans returning to civilian life.

Discussion

The transition out of active duty and into civilian life involves a physical move as well as a transition to different roles, identity, occupations, and time use. Occupational therapy is part of a comprehensive team approach, which also includes the support of his family, friends, and peers. His engagement with his peers at the Veterans Administration is helping him to recreate his valued identity as a service member. Carlos is on a journey to becoming his future self, which might include mentoring other veterans. The journey to recovery is often nonlinear and unique to each person. Through engaging in surfing, he used one tool in his recovery toolkit: occupation.

---

performance patterns. However, by the age of 24 years, this number rises to 75% within this population as a whole (Foundations Recovery Network, n.d.). Any life disruption or distinct change can be associated with increased stress levels related to the changes as well. This situation is documented throughout the world.

Suvisaari et al. (2009) conducted a study of 1,863 Finnish young adults (ages 19 to 34) and found that mental health issues that were apparent were depression or depressive disorders (17.7%), substance abuse or dependence (14.2%), and anxiety disorders (12.6%) during the young adult time of life. Patel, Fisher, Hetrick, and McGarry (2007) report that mental illnesses account for "a large proportion of the disease burden in young people in all societies [and] is strongly related to other health and development concerns in young people, notably lower educational achievements, substance abuse, violence, and poor reproductive and sexual health" (p. 1302).

THE ROLE OF THE OCCUPATIONAL THERAPIST WITH EMERGING ADULTS

Occupational therapists draw on theoretical perspectives to enhance their understanding of the lived experience of others. Occupational science, in addition to psychology, provides additional lenses through which to view development and occupational engagement. This section will highlight the significant concepts of transition, identity, time, and occupational balance. Case Illustration 12-3 illustrates how these concepts are relevant for understanding the individual and providing occupational therapy.

Transition

A transition is "a passage, evolution, development or abrupt change that leads to movement from one life state, stage or place to another" (Orentlicher, Schefkind, & Gibson, 2015, p. 20). In this transition, there are natural social and cultural guidelines that direct our behaviors and influence our expectations. A helpful way to view transitions is to consider the separate phases of each transition, including preparation, actual transition, and consolidation. Young adulthood can encompass all three of these phases, which can be viewed as dynamic and cyclical rather than a linear process (Figure 12-1).

Identity

The transition into adulthood involves the process of questioning, experimenting, and embracing an adult identity. Am I an adult? Do I feel like an adult? These are questions related to one's embodiment of an adult identity. In occupational science literature, there is an underlying belief that identity is created by and expressed through our engagement in occupations (Alsaker & Kroger, 2006). Christiansen (1999) proposed the following four central concepts of occupation and identity:

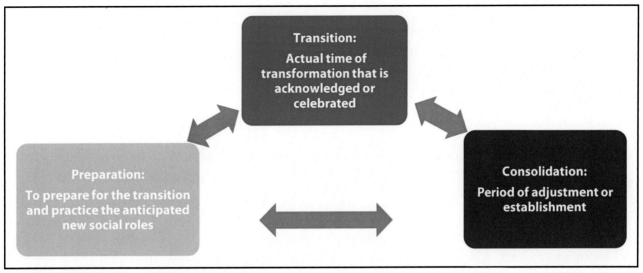

Figure 12-1. The dynamic and cyclical process of transitions.

1. Identity is an overarching concept that shapes and is shaped by our relationships with others.

2. Identities are closely tied to what we do and our interpretations of those actions in the context of our relationships with others.

3. Identities provide an important central figure in a self-narrative or life story that provides coherence and meaning for everyday events and life itself.

4. Because life meaning is derived in the context of identity, it is an essential element in promoting well-being and life satisfaction.

It is important to acknowledge that identity is not just an individual quest for a sense of self, but it is also social and cultural. (See Chapters 7 and 8 for further discussion.) Our interactions with others and our culture influence our expectations and actions in relation to occupation and our identity. Identity is also not just in the present tense, or *being*, but incorporates who we would like to be in the future, or *becoming* (Wilcock, 1999). The occupational therapy role can include helping clients to build their identity.

Time

Another dimension to examine in young adulthood is the concept of time and how one develops a sense of self over time (Bonovitz, 2018). Children and adolescents might experience time as unlimited, recalling summers as a child that seemed to last forever, whereas in young adulthood, adulthood, and middle age, time might seem to pass quicker. In occupational science literature, this concept of *tempo*, or *pace of life*, can relate to a stage in your life and is impacted by our occupational choices (Farnworth, 2003). In young adulthood, the meaning of time changes, and the focus is on what time is left, an awareness of aging, and projecting yourself into the future (Colarusso, 1991). This future focus relates to Farnworth's concept of temporality, which she defines as "one's sense of past, present, and future" (2003, p. 119). As occupational therapists, it is important to consider our clients' senses of tempo and temporality as they contribute to their identity, occupational choices, and life narrative.

Occupational Balance

The process of becoming adult brings with it many new occupations, roles, and responsibilities, making striking the right balance difficult to attain. Making choices about what occupations to pursue and what to abandon is part of becoming an adult. Occupational balance is defined as getting the "right mix of occupations" (Wagman, Hakansson, & Bjorklund, 2012, p. 325). This balance of occupations is subjective and determined by the individual. The perfect balance isn't so much about equal time spent doing different categories of occupations, such as self-care, productivity, and leisure, but more about linking your occupations with your values. Having a life of *occupational integrity* (Pentland & McColl, 2008) can be defined as the "extent to which an individual can design an occupational life that is consistent with his or her values … the extent to which he or she feels a sense of balance and well-being" (p. 6). As occupational therapists, we can help our clients to explore their values and make strong connections between their ideals and their choices in occupations. How people spend their time becomes more important than how much time is spent. As a young adult, time use, which focuses on what one does with one's time and why (Farnworth, 2003), reflects values and choices and can lead to a sense of balance.

Box 12-2. Occupational Self-Analysis Questions

- **History**: What were your childhood occupations? How did your occupations change over time? How did your past occupations influence who you are today?
- **Culture**: What cultural occupations were (are) important to you? How do you express your culture through what you do?
- **Context**: Where do you engage in occupations (physical, virtual, social)? Who do you engage in occupations with?
- **Temporal aspects**: How do you spend your time? How do weekends differ from weekdays? Is there a time in the week/day where time seems to pass slowly or quickly? What occupations are you doing at this time?
- **Wellness**: What occupations have a positive impact on your health and well-being? What occupations have a negative impact on your health and well-being? What occupations are calming, challenging, fatiguing, uplifting, (insert other relevant emotion or quality)?
- **Meaning**: What occupations help you to feel that you are living a full and meaningful life? When do you feel a sense of purpose? What occupations help you to feel productive?
- **Barriers and strengths**: What are the physical, cognitive, emotional, cultural, or spiritual barriers or supports to occupational engagement?
- **Goals**: What would you do if you were not afraid? What would you like to change about your lifestyle? What would you like to accomplish in the next 5 years? What supports or resources will help you to accomplish your goals?

Assessment With Emerging Adults

Occupational therapists can help emerging adults to be occupationally enlightened through the process of occupational self-analysis, which includes the exploration of routines and occupational patterns. The occupational therapist can then help service users modify their lifestyles to improve quality of life (Clark et al., 2015). Box 12-2 provides sample questions that can be used for occupational self-analysis. Occupational therapists can facilitate a discussion or activities around past, present, and future occupations, exploring occupational history, environments, routines, rituals, meaning, identity, challenges, and opportunities. The process of assessment is described in Chapter 4; therefore, Table 12-2 focuses on assessments that are of particular use with emerging adults.

Intervention With Emerging Adults

Where possible, interventions should actively engage service users in their occupations within their lived environment. Replicating the context in which the occupation takes place helps to increase transferability of skills and future performance of that occupation.

As previously discussed, young adults are digital natives and will use technology to complete their occupations. Therefore, it is helpful to incorporate technology into intervention where appropriate. For example, looking up social groups online, tracking nutrition using fitness apps, or creating a dating profile could all be included in an intervention plan. Another example of technology in intervention is telehealth, which the American Occupational Therapy Association (2013) defines as "the application of evaluative, consultative, preventative, and therapeutic services delivered through telecommunication and information technologies" (p. S69). Also, because this generation is accustomed to immediate communication, texting is a very effective method for checking in on goal progress and providing reminders.

The use of humor during assessment and intervention can be crucial in forming a strong therapeutic alliance as well as having potential health benefits for service users. Literature has supported the use of humor in occupational therapy practice (Vergeer & MacRae, 1993). Being humorous with clients in a compassionate way promotes relaxation, hope, and openness (Wooten, 1996). Humor can also be used as a motivator to empower clients to take control of their situation (Leber & Vanoli, 2001). Although there are many benefits to using humor, it should only be used when it is meaningful and purposeful to the service user. Certain forms of humor, such as sarcasm, can be difficult to translate cross-culturally or could be perceived as offensive. In general, occupational therapists should use their observation skills to determine when humor is a strength, value, and mode of being for the service user.

TITLE	SOURCE	COMMENTS
TABLE 12-2. OCCUPATIONAL THERAPY ASSESSMENTS FOR USE WITH EMERGING ADULTS		
Canadian Occupational Performance Measure	Law et al. (1998)	Uses a semi-structured interview to set client-centered goals, where the client can rate his or her sense of importance, performance, and satisfaction. The Canadian Occupational Performance Measure can be used as an outcome measure to track changes in perceived performance and satisfaction with occupations.
Assessment of Communication and Interaction Skills	Forsyth, Salamy, Simon, & Kielhofner (1998)	A Model of Human Occupation observational assessment that measures a client's social performance while engaged in occupations
Social Interaction Scale	Williams & Bloomer (1987)	An observational assessment of seven verbal and nonverbal behaviors in five contexts: one-on-one interview, over a meal, an unstructured group, a structured activity group, and a structured verbal group
Picture Card Sort Interview: The New Client-Centered Assessment for Young Adults	Authentic Occupational Therapy (www.authenticot.com/services-opportunities/products)	Contains 50 photo cards of occupations and allows older teen and adult clients to communicate nonverbally and reflect on their desires for leading full occupational lives
Transition to Work Inventory (3rd ed.)	Liptak (2012)	Designed for people with little to no work experience or limited education, it provides a list of 96 nonwork activities and asks individuals to rate how much they like each one. Simple self-scoring allows them to connect their answers to the 16 career clusters, which then lead to a list of related jobs, self-employment options, and paths for education and training.
Careerscope V10: Comprehensive Career Assessment	Lustig, Brown, & Lott, (1998)	Helps clients to identify their attraction to careers and gives comprehensive reports that link to career recommendations that align with the client's interests and aptitudes
Test of Grocery Shopping Skills	Brown, Rempfer, & Hamera (2009)	A performance-based assessment to determine a person's ability to locate items in a grocery store in an accurate and efficient way
Worker Role Interview Version 10.0	Braveman et al. (2005)	A semi-structured interview developed to address psychosocial and environmental factors that impact return to work. This tool is useful for someone who took a leave of absence from work and is hoping to return to employment.
Work Environment Impact Scale	Moore-Corner & Kielhofner (1995)	A semi-structured interview and rating scale influenced by the Model of Human Occupation, the Work Environment Impact Scale focuses on how the work environment impacts occupational performance. The tool uses the client's perspective of his or her current work environment and has him or her rate how it positively or negatively impacts work performance and satisfaction.
Weekly Calendar Planning Activity	Weiner, Toglia, & Berg (2012)	Useful for clients who have difficulties in executive functioning or higher-level cognitive independent activities of daily living. The Weekly Calendar Planning Activity involves following and organizing a list of appointments or errands into a weekly schedule while keeping track of rules, avoiding conflicts, monitoring passage of time, and inhibiting distractions, giving the occupational therapist an opportunity to observe how the client manages a cognitively challenging task.

TABLE 12-3. INDIVIDUAL INTERVENTIONS FOR EMERGING ADULTS

OCCUPATION	INTERVENTION
Leisure (exploration and participation)	• Explore leisure interests online. • Participate in leisure together. • Ask the service user to teach his or her favorite hobby (to therapist and/or peers).
Health management and maintenance: exercise, nutrition, healthy lifestyle	• Track exercise and diet using smartphone app or weekly diary. • Prepare meals or healthy snacks together. • Visit a farmer's market, plan menus, and shop. • Visit the gym, go on walks, or participate in active sports.
Sleep (preparation and participation)	• Create a healthy sleep routine guide; set reminders on phone. • Engage in relaxation training such as using mindfulness techniques and guided meditation. • Practice assertive communication with sleep partners/roommates.
Social participation	• Join online social groups or clubs/organizations. • Role play initiating conversation. • Explore dating apps.
Education	• Input semester assignments and exam dates on the calendar. • Break down assignments into small chunks of activity. • Explore strategies for decreasing procrastination.
Work	• Advise on work accommodations. • Role play an interview. • Practice work readiness soft skills (e.g., communication with coworkers and supervisors, conflict resolution).

Depending on intervention context, emerging adults may engage in a variety of occupational therapy groups, many of which are described throughout this text. The primary benefit of groups, especially for this population, is the support of peers. However, there is also great benefit in one-on-one practitioner–service user sessions that can be specifically tailored to the unique needs of the individual in the emerging adult stage. Table 12-3 lists examples of individual occupational therapy interventions for emerging adults.

NONTRADITIONAL SETTINGS AND PROGRAMS FOR YOUNG ADULTS

Although this text does address nontraditional and emerging practice areas in several different chapters, the majority of examples of practice remain in the clinical realm, either by diagnostic groupings or behavioral health settings. This text provides various examples of intervention settings and programs. Although most occupational therapists work in clinical or hospital settings, these environments often neglect the preventative approach to mental health.

Where are your adults in the context of their occupations, as they are first starting to struggle with their mental health and well-being? Community programs can also benefit from using alternative funding streams outside health insurance, such as education funds, local grants, and social services. As occupational therapists, we are called to be innovative and creative in our approaches. Therefore, in this section, the focus is on occupations therapy for young adults in nonclinical settings.

Homeless Youth

Housing instability and homeless youth is largely a hidden problem in the United States, with many young adults altering between shelters, couch surfing with family or friends, temporarily living in their cars, or various camping out scenarios. This housing instability can expose youth to risks and can be warning signs of future long-lasting or permanent homelessness. According to the report by Chapin Hall, titled *Missed Opportunities: Youth Homelessness in America*, 1 in 10 young adults between the ages of 18 and

25 years experiences some level of homelessness (Morton, Dworsky, & Samuels, 2017). Homeless youth have complex issues facing them, with 29% of youth reporting substance use problems and 69% reporting mental health difficulties. The study also points to unique challenges for rural youth with little access to support services. Other risk factors include those with less than a high school diploma or General Equivalency Diploma, those with a household income less than $24,000 per year, and those who are Hispanic; African American; lesbian, gay, bisexual, transgender, and queer/questioning (LGBTQ); or unmarried and parenting (Morton et al., 2017).

Homeless youth often experience a lack of structure and changing environment that might prevent them from attaining life skills, including activities of daily living (e.g., bathing, dressing, grooming, eating), instrumental activities of daily living (e.g., meal preparation, cleaning, household maintenance, money management), and community skills (e.g., accessing transportation, time management, social interaction). Shelters for youth might provide them with meals without providing training on how to shop for groceries on a budget and prepare a healthy meal. Occupational therapists can start with life skills assessments, including the Ansell-Casey Life Skill Assessment and the Occupational Self-Assessment specifically recommended for homeless youth (Aviles & Helfrich, 2004).

It is important when creating a therapeutic alliance with homeless youth to maintain a caring and respectful relationship. Many of these youth did not grow up in supportive environments and will need a safe, family-like environment to succeed in therapy (Aviles & Helfrich, 2004). These young adults might also benefit from creating healthy routines and health-promoting habits with the help of an occupational therapist. The occupational therapist can build on their strengths and interests to embed new occupations into their routines.

In addition to interventions with young adults who are already experiencing housing instability, it is also important to take a preventative approach when working with youth who might be at risk of becoming homeless or preventing long-term homelessness. Occupational therapists can identify early risk factors that might contribute to future homelessness and help link clients with resources in the community.

Lesbian, Gay, Bisexual, Transgender, and Queer/Questioning Youth

The gap between when a person realizes his or her sexual orientation and decides to disclose or come out averages about 8 years. Twelve years old is the median age when LGBTQ youth first felt they might be something other than straight, 17 years is the median age for knowing for sure they were LGBTQ, and 20 years is the median age when they first come out to someone close to them (Pew Research Center, 2013). The process of coming out is not a one-time event, but rather can happen throughout one's lifetime as a person encounters different social contexts and work environments. Sexual orientation and gender identity involve myriad occupations, including dress, self-care, leisure, and social occupations. Through the process of coming out or transitioning gender, one's occupations are also in transition. An occupational therapist might work with a client on experimenting with and embracing new occupations that reflect his or her identity. Minority stress can also affect the mental health and well-being of LGBTQ young adults, with peer and family being positive support factors (Shilo & Savaya, 2011). An occupational therapist might also link service users with resources such as LGBTQ support groups or create a peer mentoring program.

Occupational Therapy in Higher Education

Young adulthood is characterized by identity explorations, and attending college allows young people to explore various possible educational directions that would lead to different occupational futures (Arnett, 2004, p. 121). College students with mental health concerns are at risk of losing this opportunity. Young adults with mental health concerns experience longer delays in entering college (Newman et al., 2011) and exhibit high dropout rates (Salzer, Wick, & Rogers, 2008). Meanwhile, institutions of higher education are seeing a dramatic increase in the number of students with psychiatric diagnoses (Sharpe & Bruininks, 2003; Sharpe, Bruininks, Blacklock, Benson, & Johnson, 2004).

This uptick in the number of students in the United States who are known to have psychiatric disabilities might be due to increased services under the Individuals with Disabilities Education Act (2004), as well as several other federal laws, which have protected the rights of students with disabilities to attend postsecondary education. Title II of the Americans with Disabilities Act of 1990 requires persons with disabilities to have equal access to public programs and services. Section 504 of the Rehabilitation Act (1973) safeguards that programs receiving federal assistance do not discriminate on the basis of disability and that students are provided with reasonable accommodations.

The Higher Education Opportunity Act of 2008 expanded opportunities for students with disabilities to access higher education by providing grants and loans. Despite this federal legislation, supportive services for people with physical and learning disabilities are more commonly offered in postsecondary education than services for people with psychiatric disabilities (Hutchinson, Anthony, Massaro, & Rogers, 2007). Even in colleges that provide supportive mental health services, students often do not access these services or are not aware of them.

CASE ILLUSTRATION 12-4: THE STORY OF PETER—COMPLEX OCCUPATIONAL ISSUES

Peter, an international student from Hungary, studied abroad for 1 year at a large U.S. university. He registered with Disability Services with anxiety and Crohn's disease, receiving accommodations for extra time on exams and a referral to the on-campus occupational therapist. In occupational therapy, he reported challenges with time management/procrastination and feeling stressed by assignment deadlines. Peter has been engaged in limited occupations outside college, often choosing to stay home because he feared a flare-up of Crohn's disease or getting a flat tire and being stranded on a busy freeway. Peter completed the Canadian Occupational Performance Measure and identified his main goals areas: improving time management and stress management and trying new leisure occupations. Peter addressed time management as he broke down college assignments into smaller, more achievable tasks. Peter learned new strategies such as deep breathing exercises to improve stress management. To overcome his safety concerns, he created detailed plans for his excursions, including an emergency services contact list. He produced a bucket list of activities he would like to engage in before he returned to Hungary, and after two semesters, he checked off country line dancing, rock climbing, beach volleyball, and even a solo road trip to Las Vegas. On discharge, he stated, "I feel that I am moving from talking to doing."

Discussion

Some of Peter's occupations were due to his disability, whereas others were due to moving to the United States and transitioning to a new culture. Peter had received accommodations for his disability but needed extra support provided by an occupational therapy on-site supported education model. Through exploring strategies, planning, and preparation with the occupational therapist, Peter moved through the stages of change model from contemplation and preparation into an action phase.

Supported education services were established to help students succeed in higher education. These supported education interventions include supports "to assist people with psychiatric disabilities to take advantage of skill, career, educational and inter-personal development opportunities within postsecondary educational environments" (Collins, Bybee, & Mowbray, 1998, p. 597). Supported education programs exist in a variety of settings and tend to fall into three distinct models: onsite, mobile support, and self-contained classroom.

Despite the increase of supported education for young adults with psychiatric disabilities, occupational therapists have not commonly become involved in this critically needed service area. Occupational therapists have a unique lens and can have a strong contribution to supported education services. The American Occupational Therapy Association has outlined the role of occupational therapy in working with students with disabilities in higher education (Jirikowic, Campbell, DiAmico, Frauwith, & Mahoney, 2013).

In contrast to secondary education, college students must self-disclose their disabilities and are required to register for disability services in order to receive accommodations (National Alliance on Mental Illness, n.d.). This need for student initiation requires students to self-advocate. Occupational therapists can help students to enhance their self-advocacy skills and communicate with support staff and professors.

It is important to add that not all occupational therapists working in postsecondary education settings are working with students with disabilities. Occupational therapists can use a preventative/wellness approach and work with all college students who have occupational needs. Case Illustration 12-4 highlights a college student who has complex occupational issues related to both symptoms and context.

SUMMARY

Throughout this chapter, the challenges of the emerging adult time of life have been highlighted. If we look back to this time in our own lives, the age and stage, occupational role progression, level of independence or autonomy, and development of our own life progression is of paramount importance. When these issues are layered over mental health problems, the frequently overlooked life stage can become unbearable, an impediment, or a cause for symptoms increasing or presenting for the first time. This is, however, a time when life-appropriate health care services may not be accessed due to lack of insurance, embarrassment, or the denial of symptoms.

Occupational therapy's placement in traditional or nontraditional settings might promote an easier transition during this time of life through evaluation and interventions designed to address issues and problems; identify needs, limitations, and strengths; and promote meaningful health and wellness options in this underserved group.

References

Alsaker, F. D., & Kroger, J. (2006). Self-concept, self-esteem and identity. In S. Jackson & L. Goossens (Eds.), *Handbook of adolescent development* (pp. 90-117). Oxfordshire, England: Taylor & Francis.

American Occupational Therapy Association. (2013). Telehealth [Position paper]. *American Journal of Occupational Therapy, 67*(Suppl), S69-S90. doi:10.5014/ajot.2013.67S69

Americans with Disabilities Act of 1990, 42 U.S.C. §§ 12101-12213 (1990).

Arnett, J. J. (2004). *Emerging adulthood: The winding road from the late teens through the twenties.* New York, NY: Oxford University Press.

Arnett, J. J. (2015). *Emerging adulthood: The winding road from the late teens through the twenties* (2nd ed.). New York, NY: Oxford University Press.

Arnett, J. J. (2016). Does emerging adulthood theory apply across social classes? National data on a persistent question. *Emerging Adulthood, 4*(4), 227-235.

Aviles, A., & Helfrich, C. (2004). Life skill service needs: Perspectives of homeless youth. *Journal of Youth and Adolescence, 33*(4), 331-338.

Bonovitz, C. (2018). All but dissertation (ABD), all but parricide (ABP): Young adulthood as a developmental period and the crisis of separation. *Psychoanalytic Psychology, 35*(1), 142-148. doi:10.1037/pap0000128

Braveman, B., Robson, M., Velozo, C., Kielhofner, G., Fisher, G., Forsyth, K., & Kerschbaum, J. (2005). *Worker Role Interview (WRI)* (Version 10.0). Chicago, IL: Model of Human Occupation Clearinghouse, Department of Occupational Therapy, College of Applied Health Sciences, University of Illinois at Chicago.

Brown, C., Rempfer, M., & Hamera (2009). *Test of Grocery Shopping Skills.* Bethesda, MD: American Occupational Therapy Association.

Bynner, J. (2005). Rethinking the youth phase of the life-course: The case for emerging adulthood? *Journal of Youth Studies, 8*(4), 367-384. doi:10.1080/13676260500431628

Christiansen, C. H. (1999). Defining lives: Occupation as identity: An essay on competence, coherence and the creation of meaning. *American Journal of Occupational Therapy, 53,* 547-558.

Clark, F. A., Blanchard, J., Sleight, A., Cogan, A., Florindez, L., Gleason, S., ... Vigen, C. (2015). *Lifestyle Redesign®: The intervention tested in the USC well elderly studies* (2nd ed.). Bethesda, MD: AOTA Press.

Colarusso, C. A. (1991). The development of time sense in young adulthood. *The Psychoanalytic Study of the Child, 46,* 125-144.

Collins, M. E., Bybee, D., & Mowbray, C. T. (1998). Effectiveness of supported education for individuals with psychiatric disabilities: Results from an experimental study. *Community Mental Health Journal, 34*(6), 595-613.

Côté, J., Skinkle, R., & Motte, A. (2008). Do perceptions of costs and benefits of post-secondary education influence participation? *Canadian Journal of Higher Education, 38*(2), 73-93.

Farnworth, L. (2003). Time use, tempo and temporality: Occupational therapy's core business or someone else's business. *Australian Occupational Therapy Journal, 50,* 116-126.

Forsyth, K., Salamy, M., Simon, S., & Kielhofner, G. (1998). *The Assessment of Communication and Interaction Skills* (Version 4.0). Chicago, IL: Department of Occupational Therapy, University of Illinois at Chicago.

Foundations Recovery Network. (n.d.). *Common mental health disorders in young adults.* Retrieved from https://www.dualdiagnosis.org/mental-health-and-addiction/common-young-adults

Higher Education Opportunity Act, Pub. L. No. 110-315 (2008).

Hutchinson, D., Anthony, W., Massaro, J., & Rogers, E. S. (2007). Evaluation of a comorbid supported computer education and employment training program for persons with psychiatric disabilities. *Psychiatric Rehabilitation Journal, 30,* 189-197.

Individuals With Disabilities Education Act, 20 U.S.C. § 1400 (2004).

Jirikowic, T., Campbell, J., DiAmico, M., Frauwith, S., & Mahoney, W. (2013). *Students with disabilities in postsecondary education settings: How occupational therapy can help.* Retrieved from https://www.aota.org/About-Occupational-Therapy/Professionals/CY/Postsecondary-Education.aspx

Law, M. M., Baptiste, S., Carswell, A., McColl, M. A., Polatajko, H., & Pollock, N. (1998). *Canadian Occupational Performance Measure* (3rd ed.). Ottawa, Canada: CAOT Publications ACE.

Learning Disabilities Association of America. (n.d.). *Mental health and learning disabilities: Why a higher risk?* Retrieved from https://ldaamerica.org/mental-health-and-learning-disabilities-why-a-higher-risk/

Leber, D. A, & Vanoli, E. G. (2001). Therapeutic use of humor: Occupational therapy clinicians' perceptions and practices. *American Journal of Occupational Therapy, 55,* 221-226. doi:10.5014/ajot.55.2.221

Liptak, J. L. (2012). *Transition to Work Inventory* (3rd ed.). St. Paul, MN: JIST Publishing.

Lustig, D. C., Brown, C. D., & Lott, A. C. (1998). Reliability of the CareerScope career assessment and reporting system. *Vocational Evaluation and Work Adjustment Bulletin, 31,* 19-21.

Moore-Corner, R. A., & Kielhofner, G. (1995). *Work Environment Impact Scale.* Chicago, IL: Department of Occupational Therapy, University of Illinois at Chicago.

Morton, M. H., Dworsky, A., & Samuels, G. M. (2017). Missed opportunities: Youth homelessness in America. *National estimates.* Chicago, IL: Chapin Hall at the University of Chicago. Retrieved from https://voicesofyouthcount.org/wp-content/uploads/2017/11/ChapinHall_VoYC_NationalReport_Final.pdf

National Alliance on Mental Illness. (n.d.). *Managing a mental health condition in college.* Retrieved from https://www.nami.org/Find-Support/Teens-Young-Adults/Managing-a-Mental-Health-Condition-in-College

Newman, L., Wagner, M., Knokey, A., Marder, C., Nagle, K., Shaver, D., & Wei, X. (2011). *The post-high school outcomes of young adults with disabilities up to 8 years after high school: A report from the national longitudinal transition study-2 (NLTS2).* National Center for Special Education Research, Institute of Education Sciences. Retrieved from https://ies.ed.gov/ncser/pubs/20113005/pdf/20113005.pdf

Orentlicher, M. L., Schefkind, S., & Gibson, R. W. (Eds.). (2015). *Transitions across the lifespan: An occupational therapy approach.* Bethesda, MD: AOTA Press.

Patel, V., Fisher, A. J., Hetrick, S., & McGarry, P. (2007). Mental health of young people: A global public-health challenge. *Lancet, 369,* 1302-1313.

Pentland, W., & McColl, M. A. (2008). Living a life of occupational integrity: Another perspective on life balance. *Canadian Journal of Occupational Therapy, 75*(3), 135-138.

Pew Research Center. (2013). *A survey of LGBT Americans.* Retrieved from http://www.pewsocialtrends.org/2013/06/13/a-survey-of-lgbt-americans

Rehabilitation Act of 1973, 29 U.S.C. § 701 et seq. (1973).

Salzer, M. S., Wick, L. C., & Rogers, J. A. (2008). Familiarity with and use of accommodations and supports among postsecondary students with mental illnesses. *Psychiatric Services, 59,* 370-375.

Schizophrenia.com (n.d.). *Schizophrenia facts and statistics.* Retrieved from http://www.schizophrenia.com/szfacts.htm

Sharpe, M. N., & Bruininks, B. D. (2003). *Services for students with psychiatric disabilities in the big ten schools* [Unpublished manuscript]. Minneapolis, MN: University of Minnesota.

Sharpe, M. N., Bruininks, B. D., Blacklock, B. A., Benson, B., & Johnson, D. M. (2004). The emergence of psychiatric disabilities in postsecondary education (Issue Brief No. 1). *National Center on Secondary Education and Transition (NCSET).* Minneapolis, MN: University of Minnesota.

Shilo, G., & Savaya, R. (2011). Effects of family and friend support on LGB youths' mental health and sexual orientation milestones. *Family Relations, 60*(3), 318-330. doi:10.1111/j.1741-3729.2011.00648.x

Suvisaari, J., Aalto-Setala, T., Tuulio-Hendriksson, A., Harkanen, T., Saarni, S., Perala, J., & Lonnqvist, J. (2009). Mental disorders in young adulthood. *Psychological Medicine, 39*(2), 287-299. doi:10.1017/S0033291708003632

Townsend, E., & Wilcock, A. A. (2004). Occupational justice and client centred practice: A dialogue in progress. *Canadian Journal of Occupational Therapy, 71*, 75-87.

Vergeer, G., & MacRae, A. (1993). Therapeutic use of humor in occupational therapy. *American Journal of Occupational Therapy, 47*(8), 678-683.

Wagman, P., Hakansson, C., & Bjorklund, A. (2012). Occupational balance as used in occupational therapy: A concept analysis. *Scandinavian Journal of Occupational Therapy, 19*(4), 322-327.

Weiner, N. W., Toglia, J., & Berg, C. (2012). Weekly Calendar Planning Activity (WCPA): A performance-based assessment of executive function piloted with at-risk adolescents. *American Journal of Occupational Therapy, 66*(6), 699-708.

Wilcock, A. A. (1999). Reflections on doing, being and becoming. *Australian Occupational Therapy Journal, 46*, 1-11.

Williams, S., & Bloomer, J. (1987). *The Bay Area Functional Performance Evaluation* (2nd ed.). Palo Alto, CA: Consulting Psychologists Press.

Wooten, P. (1996). Humor: An antidote for stress. *Holistic Nursing Practice, 10*(2), 49-55.

SUGGESTED RESOURCES

Active Minds: A nonprofit organization that aims to raise mental health awareness among college students, utilizing peer support and campus chapters. http://www.activeminds.org

Association on Higher Education and Disability (AHEAD): An association that disseminates knowledge and advocates for full participation by students with disabilities in postsecondary education. https://www.ahead.org

Job Accommodation Network (JAN): This network provides guidance and practical strategies for workplace accommodations and disability employment issues. https://askjan.org

Trevor Project: A national 24-hour, toll-free confidential suicide hotline for LGBTQ youth. https://www.thetrevorproject.org/#sm.oooh bn1zwxpzdtu11ku2hao6w4ez8

Mental Health of Mid-Life Adults

Anne MacRae, PhD, OTR/L, BCMH, FAOTA

As with all of the chapters in this text that address lifespan issues, readers are cautioned to avoid thinking of these age groups in terms of chronology alone because there are many factors that influence one's development. Although there is much overlap between the age groups, this chapter generally focuses on ages 30 to 35 years through 55 to 60 years.

Mid-life adults experience some unique psychosocial stressors that not only affect their current quality of life, but also may be precursors to serious physical and mental illness in later life. Furthermore, although this age group is not typically associated with a high risk of mental health issues, the incidence of some forms of mental illness and addiction are actually quite significant. This chapter addresses the age-stage identity of mid-life and developmental theory in order to understand psychosocial stressors. In addition, a review of common diagnoses and health concerns of this age group is provided.

It is particularly important for occupational therapists to understand that people in this age group may be secondary recipients of services or clients (Vergis & Brintell, 2018). For example, the primary client could be a child or an elder, but often the expectation for needed caregiving is on the mid-life adult relative. The therapist therefore must attempt to understand the life worldviews of all individuals affected by services rendered.

AGE-STAGE IDENTITY

Please don't retouch my wrinkles. It took me so long to earn them. —Anna Magnani

This quote by Italian actress Anna Magnani perfectly summarizes the dilemma of mid-life. On one hand, the contemporary view of this age bracket is that striving for perennial youth is the ideal goal, and it is one that is reinforced daily by the media. An exorbitant amount of money and time is dedicated to advertisements of products aimed to achieve a youthful appearance or perceived virility. In these advertisements, youth is linked to beauty, and women are especially targeted. As Scherker (2017) states, "Every year, women spend billions of dollars in exchange for beautiful hair, luxurious eyelashes and smooth, silky skin. Still, many of our culture's most common beauty procedures were virtually nonexistent a century ago." What effect does this elusive quest for eternal youth have on the self-esteem and mental health of mid-life adults? Conclusive scholarly evidence is scarce but certainly worthy of further exploration.

On the other hand, the historical view of mid-life is that it is a time of our greatest stability, productivity, and accomplishments. Therefore, mid-life and older adults should be respected for their experience and wisdom. Although this is still somewhat true in many cultures, it is not evident

MacRae, A. (Ed.). *Cara and MacRae's Psychosocial Occupational Therapy:*
An Evolving Practice, Fourth Edition (pp 215-224).
© 2019 Taylor & Francis Group.

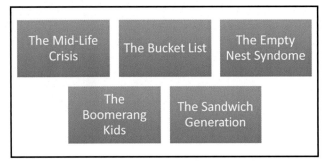

Figure 13-1. Mid-life markers and clichés.

in countries with a heavy media presence, especially the United States. Once again, if respect for one's life experiences is decreased, what is the effect on the mental health of mid-life adults? What can or should societies in general and mental health providers in particular do to reclaim respect and reinforce self-esteem of mid-life adults?

DEVELOPMENTAL THEORY

The scholarly literature has paid far more attention to the age-stage development of children, adolescents, and older adults than to developmental markers of mid-life adults. Furthermore, the majority of developmental theories seem to be somewhat dated and out of step with the everyday lived experiences of this age group. The best explanations for this phenomenon are found in popular literature rather than the scholarly literature. For example, Gail Sheehy authored a series of self-help books about "passages" starting in 1976. However, less than 20 years after her original publication, Sheehy stated in a revision that there have been some dramatic societal changes in the life experiences of adults and, subsequently, how we define the mid-life age stage. Long accepted markers of age-stage development have shifted and now occur 10 years later or earlier than the accepted norm. For example, it is not uncommon for 30-year-old men to still live with their parents, 40-year-old women to have a first pregnancy, and 50-year-old men to be forced into early retirement (Sheehy, 1995).

One developmental psychologist whose work seems to have survived the test of time, at least for this age group, is Erik Erickson. Since the original publication of his theory of psychosocial development in 1950, there have been numerous reprints, and the material continues to be taught today. The age span of 40 to 65 years is the seventh of Erikson's eight stages of development and is dubbed *generativity versus stagnation*. Generativity refers to accomplishments for self and society. For those who do not achieve this milestone, there is a sense of stagnation or failure that may lead to isolation and despair. The potential occupational disruptions or dysfunctions related to stagnation may include decreased interest in personal self-care, poor job performance, and strained relationships. Cherry

(2018) elaborates on the concept of generativity vs. stagnation stage by identifying further conflicts within this stage:

- Inclusivity vs. exclusivity
- Pride vs. embarrassment
- Responsibility vs. ambivalence
- Productivity vs. inadequacy
- Parenthood vs. self-absorption
- Honesty vs. denial

Markers, Myths, and Clichés

It is important to recognize that not everyone experiences the same developmental events, and they certainly do not experience them in the same way. Nevertheless, common markers are helpful to frame our understanding of any life stage. Mid-life markers are primarily focused on family and career, but what is somewhat unique to the mid-life stage are markers that basically have become clichés. The most common ones are highlighted in Figure 13-1 and discussed in the subsequent subsections. These are well-known phrases in the general public that are very entrenched in our thinking as truisms but sometimes do not accurately represent the real experiences of the mid-life adult.

Mid-life crisis is probably the most overused of the clichés for this age group and is generally associated with unhappiness with one's current situation followed by dramatic alterations in one's lifestyle. However, research has not shown this to be a widespread phenomenon (Clay, 2003). On the other hand, some research suggests that, not only is the mid-life crisis real, it is happening more frequently and at an earlier age. Bentley (2010) reports that people aged 35 to 44 years are the unhappiest in society because of increasing work hassles, money worries, and loneliness. These different interpretations are partly because there are many different ways of defining a mid-life crisis. Perhaps a more accurate and helpful way to frame the discussion is to think of mid-life as a crossroad. For some, the choices to be made may represent a crisis and could signify the onset of depression. For others, the time can be a mid-life epiphany rather than a crisis, and healthy changes can be made. The occupational therapy perspective on resiliency, adaptation, and coping are valuable for people struggling with this crossroad.

Bucket list is a term that became popular after the 2007 release of a film of the same name. The storyline involved two men with terminal illnesses who set out to accomplish certain goals or fulfill wishes before they *kicked the bucket* (died). The euphuism is now widely used to denote a list of things that an individual would want to accomplish before the end of life. However, unlike in the movie, common usage now does not imply that death is imminent. Rather, it represents an awareness that one's time is finite and is therefore related to the previously discussed mid-life crisis or epiphany. It is in mid-life that individuals are most likely to acknowledge their own mortality, but this does not necessarily show regret or fear. Rather, it is a time to re-evaluate one's activities, redirect energy, plan for near-future adventures, and, in general, make the most out of life. Although it is typical to include some rather grandiose, and perhaps unrealistic, items on one's bucket list (such as traveling around the world), most lists include achievable goals. These may include personal relationships such as reconnecting with family members, making amends, or dating again. Personal bucket lists also often include new learning or new hobbies that are especially important to those who have gone through major life changes such as divorce or early retirement.

Empty nest syndrome denotes the experience of having one's children leave home to pursue their independence. It has been widely assumed to be a cause of grief, loneliness, and depression for a mid-life parent and is most likely to occur in parents who had a significant amount of their own identity intertwined with the accomplishments and activities of their children. For years this has been an accepted phenomenon or norm, especially thought to be experienced by mothers. However, the entire notion is controversial, and some suggest that the concept is rooted in ageist and sexist constructs. Recent research does suggest that, although feelings of loss and depression can and do occur in some parents whose children have left home, for many others, this is a time of positive action and healthy transitions (Mount & Moas, 2015). For example, an empty nest often means that there is more time available to pursue new activities and reconnect with partners and friends. For the occupational therapist working with a mid-life adult, our unique skills in facilitating transitions can be invaluable.

Boomerang kids is a relatively new term that recognizes a significant number of emerging adults who had previously left home but have returned to live with their parents. Sometimes this is a temporary situation while the young adult is searching for employment, considering relocating, returning to school, or ending a relationship. However, in times of economic downturn or in locations where the cost of housing is extremely high, the length of time staying at the mid-life parents' home is uncertain. Although some parents apparently delight in having their children back in the nest, many others find that having one's children return to the home can be a source of conflict. A study conducted in Europe found that parents of boomerang kids experienced a decline in their quality of life and well-being (Sellgren, 2018). Furthermore, it must be acknowledged that some boomerang kids simply were not able to thrive independently. This may be due to poor skill development, physical or mental illness, or, in some situations, substance use disorders. Case Illustration 13-1 describes the conflicts and range of emotions experienced by the parents of a boomerang kid who has returned to their home. The previous chapter provided multiple examples of strategies and interventions for helping the emerging adult, but too little attention is given to the people who love and house them. Coping with the reality of one's adult child's failure to thrive can cause a parent to experience a whole range of emotions, including anxiety, guilt, and anger. Occupational therapists who encounter the mid-life parents of boomerang children, whether as primary or secondary clients, can offer invaluable support by encouraging these parents to attend to their own well-being and self-care. Box 13-1 highlights suggestions for mid-life self-care that not only apply to living with boomerang kids, but also to coping with many different roles and responsibilities. Although some of these suggestions may seem obvious, mid-life adults typically do for others before themselves and benefit from reminders and implicit permission to take care of themselves first.

The *sandwich generation* are "middle age adults (between the ages of 30 and 60) who manage the responsibility of caring for elderly parent(s) or parent(s) in law and young and or adult child(ren)/grandchild(ren)" (Vergis & Brintell, 2018). In the United States, approximately 15% of middle-age adults are sandwiched financially, and in Canada, 8% of caregivers are considered sandwiched (Boyczuk & Fletcher, 2016). "Typically, middle-aged adults are at the peak of their careers and face extensive demands in the workplace" (Riley and Bowen, 2005, p. 52). Therefore, the stress of balancing the needs of both the older and younger generations with their own needs can be both stressful and complicated. There are many reasons for the emergence of the sandwich generation, including the previously mentioned boomerang kids. However, the most prominent reasons are the trend of women having children later in life and the demographics of people generally living longer (DeRigne & Ferrante, 2012). A scoping review conducted by Vergis and Brintell (2018) determined that sandwiching can negatively affect occupational performance in the area of productivity-paid work, including increased absenteeism, reduced hours, and decreased work performance. People in the sandwich generation also had decreased time for leisure and self-care, as well as additional strain on social and marital relationships. However, they also report that, for some people, caregiving is a rewarding experience that can bring comfort and closeness to family relationships.

Whether caring for multiple generations or a single generation, caregiving has become a primary occupation of mid-life adults. Providing care for a family member, partner, or friend with a chronic, disabling, or serious health condition—known as *family caregiving*—is nearly universal today. It affects most people at some point in their lives. The need to support family caregivers will grow as our population ages, more people of all ages live with disabilities, and the complexity of care tasks increases (Reinhard, Friss Feinberg, Choula, & Houser, 2015). Occupational therapists working in all areas of practice have a major role in training and supporting caregivers. Case Illustration 13-2 describes the stressors of a mid-life couple unexpectedly in the position of raising their granddaughter. Because mid-life is the primary time to be assuming the caregiver role, it is essential that occupational therapists take into account the mid-life experiences and developmental stages described in this chapter.

CASE ILLUSTRATION 13-1: JASON RETURNS HOME

Jennifer is a 46-year-old women currently being seen in occupational therapy for an exacerbation of her rheumatoid arthritis symptoms. She reports an increase in pain and difficulty in performing activities of daily living. During the initial assessment, Jennifer mentions that her 25-year-old son, Jason, has recently moved back to the home that she shares with Toby, Jason's stepfather. The occupational therapist realizes that the changes in the family dynamics may be negatively impacting Jennifer's ability to successfully engage in her occupations. As the occupational profile is developed and a trusting therapeutic relationship is formed, several significant psychosocial stressors are identified:

- Jason, Jennifer's son, has a long history of polysubstance abuse with several failed attempts at rehabilitation. The current move back home was precipitated by the loss of his job and eviction from his apartment. Jennifer states, "He always finds a way to blame other people for things that go wrong."
- Toby, Jennifer's husband, has a strained relationship with his stepson and does not approve of his move back into his home. Toby retreats into his work world, logging many overtime hours and volunteering for additional business trips.
- Jennifer reports that she has run out of pain medication and confides that she is sure that Jason has been stealing her prescriptions. She said that she tried to hide the medication but "Jason keeps finding them." Jennifer is hesitant to refill her prescription for fear that it will enable Jason's drug habit.
- Jason denies continued drug use but also does not contribute to the household in any way. Jennifer states that she understands that he is not in a position to financially help, but she wishes he would "at least help with chores around the house."
- Jennifer tolerates her son's behavior because she feels responsible for "the way he turned out." She shares that Jason's biological father was verbally abusive and she was "too weak" to protect her son. When she finally filed for divorce from her first husband, it was a long, drawn-out, contentious proceeding, and Jennifer feels that Jason was "caught in the middle." She feels guilty for not seeing "the signs" of his distress and not doing more to help him when he was young.

Discussion

The occupational therapist was able to recognize and elicit detailed information regarding the psychosocial stressors exacerbating Jennifer's physical symptoms. However, the pressure for productivity and insurance restrictions often inhibits occupational therapists from adequately addressing psychosocial issues in physical medicine settings. The strategies, therefore, should be twofold. First, the link between psychosocial stressors and exacerbation of physical symptoms is indisputable. Therefore, helping Jennifer develop assertive communication techniques and set boundaries is a critical part of her needed work simplification regime. In addition, Jennifer could benefit from stress management techniques and adapting her activities of daily living, including negotiating shared household responsibilities with all family members. The second strategy acknowledges that, even though psychosocial issues can and should be addressed in conjunction with physical rehabilitation, the time and reimbursement constraints are sometimes substantial. Therefore, it is up to the occupational therapist to go beyond the direct service role and provide referrals to additional resources, including behavioral health services for further assessment as well as counseling and support groups. Also, because of the unique set of circumstances, Jennifer could benefit from specialized and interdisciplinary pain management services.

DIAGNOSES AND HEALTH ISSUES IN MID-LIFE

Health issues in mid-life can generally be divided into three categories:

1. *Substance use disorders*, which include alcohol abuse/addiction and drug abuse/addiction. These conditions may have predated the mid-life stage or be of new onset and are further discussed in the subsequent section.

2. *Pre-existing conditions*, which include serious and persistent mental illnesses such as schizophrenia and bipolar disorder, and also many insidious but long-lasting, or at least intermittent, mental illnesses, including eating disorders (Micali et al., 2017) and attention deficit hyperactivity disorder (Stuart-Smith, Thapar, Maughan, Thapar, & Collishaw, 2017). It is important to recognize that some people who have managed their serious mental illness for decades may experience a decompensation in mid-life due to age-related stressors or changes in physiology that alter the effectiveness

Box 13-1. Suggestions for Mid-Life Self-Care

- Set limits with family members and define roles and responsibilities.
- Remind yourself and your family that you need to stay healthy to be available for others.
- Ask for and accept help in difficult situations.
- Spend time doing activities you enjoy with people you like.
- Eat well-balanced meals.
- Exercise regularly.
- Get enough quality sleep.
- Join a support group.
- Cut down on unnecessary or burdensome tasks.
- Practice relaxation skills.

CASE ILLUSTRATION 13-2: RAISING ABBY

Child Protective Services has been following the case of a 5-year-old girl named Abigail based on a series of complaints registered by neighbors. The investigation concluded that the child was often left alone while her mother was "out partying," and there was also concern that the child was undernourished and generally neglected. Abby was subsequently removed from the home, and her grandparents petitioned for and were granted custody of the child.

Immediately upon being placed in her new home, the grandparents noticed that Abby appeared to be unusually hyperactive, easily upset, aggressive, and combative on a regular basis. At first, the grandparents assumed that the behaviors were due to being in a new environment and not having a healthy routine early in life. However, Abby's new kindergarten teacher not only concurred with the grandparents' observations, she also reported evidence of both cognitive and motoric developmental delays. Upon a complete medical and psychological assessment, it was determined that Abigail has fetal alcohol syndrome. The pediatric team, including an occupational therapist, was tasked with developing a comprehensive treatment plan for Abby.

The occupational therapist initially assigned to Abby's case provided extensive written instructions to the grandparents as part of a comprehensive home program. However, on subsequent visits, it became obvious that the grandparents were unable or unwilling to follow through with recommendations but appeared to be increasingly anxious and reported feeling exhausted. The director of occupational therapy suggested reassigning Abby's case to another occupational therapist with an extensive background in mental health and also approved home visits.

Although the grandparents are relatively young (52 years old), they both have some health challenges as well as financial limitations. The grandparents want to protect Abby and feel an obligation to do so, but they were not prepared for the depth of her issues. The occupational therapist visiting at home realized that the grandparents were overwhelmed with their new responsibilities and decided to provide a low-stress home program to simplify the daily routine for everyone. Referrals were also initiated for in-home respite and additional social support for the family.

Discussion

This case exemplifies the need for all occupational therapists to be consistently aware of psychosocial stressors involving not only primary clients but also their caregivers. As stated in the *Occupational Therapy Practice Framework*, "Occupational therapy practitioners understand and focus intervention to include the issues and concerns surrounding the complex dynamics among the client, caregiver, and family" (American Occupational Therapy Association, 2014, p. S11). Effective instruction for caregivers must include an awareness of the developmental issues, environmental limitations, and psychosocial stressors of all those responsible for providing care. However, organizational protocols and payment schemas often limit intervention for caregivers to those actions that can be shown to directly address the goals of the primary client, in this case 5-year-old Abigail. If additional support and services are warranted for the caregivers, the occupational therapist can be a conduit for referrals and collaborative interventions.

Box 13-2. Long-Term Consequences of Psychiatric Medication in Mid-Life Adults

- Sedation and orthostatic hypotension: May incur an increased risk of falls
- Anticholinergic effects: Possible gastrointestinal disturbances, dehydration, and confusion
- Weight gain and high cholesterol levels: May lead to diabetes and cardiac disorders
- Potential kidney and liver damage
- Extrapyramidal symptoms, late onset: Tardive dyskinesia

of medication. As a result, the coping mechanisms that worked in the past become less effective. Because these individuals have a more difficult time "pulling it together," they are at risk for further decompensation and more pronounced symptoms.

3. *New-onset mental illnesses*, which may include post-traumatic stress disorder, sleep-related disorders or symptoms, and mood disorders. Trauma is discussed throughout this book but is mentioned here as a reminder that traumatic events can happen anytime throughout the lifespan and must always be considered as a possible root cause of decreased function and increased symptoms.

Changes in sleep patterns are very common in mid-life and, although they may or may not reach the threshold of being considered disordered, too much or too little sleep or poor-quality sleep can have a significant impact on functional ability and is often a precursor for myriad health problems in later life. There has been much recent interest regarding the role of occupational therapists in addressing problems with adequate and restorative sleep (American Occupational Therapy Association, 2014; Gentry & Loveland, 2013; Marger Picard, 2017). The focus of the occupational therapy literature is either nonspecific to age or stage or solely addresses issues with children or older adults. However, occupational therapists should also be aware that there is evidence that sleep disturbances in mid-life are common (Polo-Kantola, 2011) and therefore should be assessed in services provided to mid-life adults. Sleep disturbances in mid-life are often associated with physiological changes, such as menopause in women, but can also occur with other disorders, such as chronic pain, or be caused by the multiple stressors of mid-life.

Comorbidities with mid-life conditions are especially prevalent. Physiological changes may be the cause or the effect of psychosocial issues, or they can simply coexist without an obvious relationship. Kanesarajah, Waller, Whitty, and Mishra (2018) conducted a review of research studies and concluded that there is substantial comorbidity in mid-life, with clusters of mental health conditions and cardiovascular disease. Furthermore, mid-life comorbidity is consistent with poor health-related quality of life.

It is not possible in this chapter to adequately cover the full range of potential health problems found in mid-life. The remainder of this chapter focuses on areas of health and illness that are especially important in providing intervention because of prevalence and unique presentation in this age group.

Pharmacology and Substance Use in Mid-Life

Mid-life adults with serious and persistent mental illnesses, such as schizophrenia, often have been on powerful medications for years. It is important to understand that, although many pharmaceuticals have serious side effects and long-term consequences, the benefit:risk ratio is taken into consideration, and in general, the risks to people with schizophrenia stopping medication outweighs the benefits. This is, of course, assuming that the medication was properly prescribed, adjusted, and monitored. (See Chapter 1 for further discussion.) Nevertheless, it is important to acknowledge the potential health risks of long-term use of psychiatric medicine, especially as they often do not surface until mid-life and/or after decades of use, and changes in medication regimes can often minimize the deleterious effects. Box 13-2 lists the common long-term consequences of psychiatric medication in mid-life adults.

Alcohol abuse among young people tends to be the most noticeable because of concurrent legal issues, high risk-taking behaviors, and a high incidence of binge drinking. Alcohol abuse among mid-life people is still quite prevalent, even if it is sometimes subtle in presentation. Mid-life alcohol abusers may have developed strategies to hide drinking behavior and are more likely to have family members and coworkers enabling their continued drinking. However, it is in mid-life that the physical consequences of long-term alcohol abuse are most likely to emerge, including kidney, heart, liver, and gastrointestinal damage, as well as cognitive decline.

The most recent and tragic substance use issue for mid-life adults is opioid dependence. In 2017, the U.S. Department of Health and Human Services (2018) declared the opioid crisis to be a public health emergency. This declaration is designed to provide support and foster solutions for combating the epidemic. However, at the time of this writing, there are few clear or consistent policies in effect. Although there are many causes for the catastrophic increase in opioid use, it is generally agreed that the primary cause was intensive marketing by pharmaceutical companies and misinformation regarding the safety and addictive properties of many of these drugs. Therefore, although opioid addiction happens at all ages, because of legal overprescribing by physicians, mid-life adults are especially affected. Because opioid use by mid-life adults is most often related to chronic pain, the occupational therapy approach to this issue is discussed in the subsequent section.

Chronic Pain

People with chronic pain disorders experience high rates of depression, anxiety, and other forms of psychiatric comorbidity and psychosocial distress (Taylor, 2006). In addition to facing multiple losses in functioning and quality of life, otherwise nondisabled individuals with intractable pain are often stigmatized in health care settings (Taylor, 2006). For example, some physicians who could not find a physical cause for a client's pain simply suggested that it was imaginary. Research pointed out that clients tended to attribute most of their medical symptoms to being rooted in pain rather than depression (Sharp & Keefe, 2006). Therefore, pain among clients with depression or other psychiatric disorders is often dismissed or misdiagnosed as somatization disorder (Dewar, 2007).

Thus, it is essential that occupational therapists understand how to assess and respond to pain in the most optimal way; that is, a way that not only supports occupational engagement, but also protects the psychological well-being and self-esteem of our clients. Chronic pain syndromes can occur during any life stage, and it is sometimes difficult to find the underlying cause. However, there are several known physical conditions common in mid-life that are strongly associated with chronic pain. Among them are the following:

- Arthritis (rheumatoid, osteoarthritis)
- Cancer
- Peripheral neuropathy
- Fibromyalgia
- Lower back pain
- Chronic headaches

As previously mentioned, the current opioid crisis especially affects people in mid-life who have or had some form of long-lasting pain. For people with terminal illness in palliative care, the goal is comfort, and the addiction potential is not a primary consideration. However, many people who are using opioids to control or mask chronic pain experience rapid addiction requiring increased doses to achieve the same effect, loss of quality of life, and loss of function. Although occupational therapists do not prescribe medication, we are in a position to observe clients and hear their stories and can therefore report back to the team to develop appropriate pain management and coping strategies. Some possible signs for the risk of opioid addiction are clients repeatedly running out of medication early, complaints

about the need for additional prescriptions, unapproved use of prescribed medication to self-medicate other problems, and multiple episodes of "stolen" prescriptions (Breivik, 2005). Practitioners should be aware of clients' histories of personal problems, such as alcohol or drug abuse. They should document medication doses and monitor clients closely for any symptoms of abuse.

The challenge now is to find nonpharmacological methods to effectively address chronic pain to either eliminate or decrease the use of opioids. Clients who receive occupation-focused, client-centered interventions may be more likely to experience positive outcomes in rehabilitation that include fewer somatic symptoms, lower perceived risk for pain, and shorter duration of pain (Jellema et al., 2006; Kielhofner, 2008). Through the application of assessments and interventions from the Model of Human Occupation and from the Intentional Relationship Model (Taylor, 2008), therapists may achieve a more detailed clinical understanding of how to manage both the somatic and psychosocial issues faced by clients with pain disorders. As therapists learn more about clients' experience of their symptoms and the meaning of their daily activities and behaviors, they may be able to develop increased empathy and intentionality, leading to improved therapeutic reasoning and well-planned intervention.

Mood Disorders

Mood disorders can range from very subtle disturbances (often undiagnosed) to extremely debilitating illness that may include episodes of psychosis and often present as a complex configuration of symptoms and dysfunctions. Many people living in the 21st century can identify with the term *depression* because they have some idea of what it feels like to be sad, blue, or under the weather or to temporarily lose a sense of meaning in their lives. Many people can also identify with the term *mania* because, due to today's fast-moving society, they have some idea of what it is like to feel pressured, pressed, speedy, or hyper. Perhaps because of our general ability to experience a range of emotions, depression and mania (to a lesser extent) have become household words. Because these terms have become familiar and people can generally identify the emotions associated with each term, novice therapists are often not prepared for the depth of the symptoms in the clients seen in psychiatric practice.

Bipolar disorder, marked by episodes of both mania and depression, is generally thought to have its onset in young adulthood or adolescents. However, recent evidence shows that, whereas the average age of onset for men is 25 years, onset for women tends to be later, sometimes even into the fifth decade of life (Parial, 2015).

Although by definition mania and depression are polar opposites, there is a wide range of presentation with this illness, especially in mid-life. Thus, it is possible to have some symptoms found in either or both mania and depression. Table 13-1 lists the common symptoms of mania and

TABLE 13-1. MOOD DISORDER SYMPTOMS AND BEHAVIORS

MANIA	DEPRESSION	EITHER/BOTH
High energy	Low energy	Poor concentration and attention
Euphoria	Hopelessness	Poor attention to detail
Grandiosity	Hypohedonia	Sleep disturbance
Impulsivity	Worthlessness	Agitation
Risk taking	Guilt	Low frustration tolerance
Pressured speech	Negative thinking	Loss of appetite
Hypersexuality	Low libido	Poor boundaries with sexual behavior

depression, as well as the symptoms that can be found at both ends of the mood spectrum.

Major depression affects people of all ages but has its peak incidence between 30 to 40 years of age. This may be due to the previously discussed psychosocial stressors of the stage or because of the comorbidity with the onset of many physical illnesses. According to the World Health Organization (WHO, 2018), depression is the leading cause of disability worldwide, affecting more than 300 million people.

Because major depression is extremely common, occupational therapists can expect to encounter people with this condition in all treatment settings. Table 13-2 lists the common problems found with depression as well as interventions used by occupational therapists.

SUMMARY

This chapter attempts to fill a void in the psychological and occupational therapy discourse on what it means to be a middle-aged adult. Although there are tremendous variables of norms and behaviors, there are some important event markers. These milestones or occurrences are important for occupational therapists to know, even when the mid-life person is not the primary client, but instead a family member or caregiver.

Although the mid-life age group is not typically associated with a high incidence of mental illness, there are significant issues of comorbidity, chronic pain, and addiction. Moreover, people with persistent mental illness who are in the mid-life stage may experience exacerbations of illness that requires developmentally sensitive occupational therapy interventions. It is critical that occupational therapists be very aware of the high incidence of mood disorders, especially depression, in this age group and be prepared to address this for both primary and secondary clients.

ACKNOWLEDGEMENTS

Elizabeth Cara, PhD, OTR/L, MFT, contributed Table 13-2 on interventions for depression and to the discussion of mood disorders. Renee R. Taylor, MA, PhD, and Chia-Wei Fan, MS, OTC, contributed to the section on chronic pain.

REFERENCES

American Occupational Therapy Association. (2014). Occupational therapy practice framework: Domain and process (3rd ed.). *American Journal of Occupational Therapy, 68*, S1-S51.

Bentley, P. (2010, September 30). Mid-life crisis arriving earlier as loneliness, work and money troubles take their toll from mid 30s. *Daily Mail*. Retrieved from http://www.dailymail.co.uk/news/article-1316109/Mid-life-crisis-arriving-earlier-loneliness-work-money-troubles-toll.html#ixzz5GWyIs4If

Boyczuk, A. M., & Fletcher, P. C. (2016). The ebbs and flows: Stresses of sandwich generation caregivers. *Journal of Adult Development, 23*, 51-61.

Breivik, H. (2005). Opioids in chronic noncancer pain, indications and controversies. *European Journal of Pain, 9*(2), 127-130.

Cherry, K. (2018, October 1). *Generativity vs. stagnation: The seventh stage of psychosocial development*. Retrieved from https://www.verywellmind.com/generativity-versus-stagnation

Clay, R. (2003). Researchers replace midlife myths with facts. *Monitor on Psychology, 34*(4). Retrieved from http://www.apa.org/monitor/apr03/researchers.aspx

DeRigne, L. & Ferrante, S. (2012). The sandwich generation: A review of the literature. *Florida Public Health Review, 9*, 95-104.

Dewar, A. (2007). Chronic pain and mental illness: A double dilemma for all. *Journal of Psychosocial Nursing, 45*(7), 8-9.

Erikson, E. H. (1950). *Childhood and society*. New York, NY: Norton.

Gentry, T., & Loveland, J. (2013). Sleep: Essential to living life to the fullest. *OT Practice, 18*(1), 9-14. doi:10.7138/otp.2013.181f1

Jellema, P., van der Horst, H. E., Vlaeyen, J. W., Stalman, W., Bouter, L., & van der Windt, D. (2006). Predictors of outcome in patients with (sub)acute low back pain differ across treatment groups. *Spine, 31*, 1699-1705.

Kanesarajah, J., Waller, M., Whitty, J., & Mishra, G. (2018). Multimorbidity and quality of life at mid-life: A systematic review of general population studies. *Maturitas, 109*, 53-62.

TABLE 13-2. INTERVENTIONS FOR DEPRESSION

SYMPTOMS	PROBLEMS	INTERVENTIONS
Emotional	• Loss of interest in formerly valued activities or pursuit of narrow or single interests exclusively and in a compulsive manner • Tendency to isolate oneself and withdraw from others	• Engage in valued activities; expand opportunities to engage in more than one activity • Monitor value and pleasure while doing or completing activities and engage in values clarification activities
Cognitive and motivational	• Indecision and ambivalence • Inability to concentrate and attend to usual daily activities • Negative attitudes that predominate in all usual activities • Inability to initiate or sustain activity • Tendency to isolate	• Engage in group activities; initially provide occupations and do not require too many choices • Provide opportunities to successfully accomplish short-term, simple, concrete activities; engage in movement activities and mindfulness-based activities • Set realistic, step-by-step goals and behavioral to-do lists, grading activities and environment for successful completion • Re-establish normal routines: structured planning of daily occupations, simple behavioral lists • Engage in cognitive therapy (i.e., recognizing, monitoring, and changing thoughts) • Perform reality testing and question unrealistic beliefs • Engage in psychoeducational groups concerning symptoms and behavior, such as recognizing precursors to mood changes and managing medicines
Self-concept	• Worthlessness and guilt	• Provide opportunities to successfully accomplish short-term, simple, concrete activities • Set realistic, step-by-step goals and behavioral to-do lists, grading activities and environment for successful completion • Perform cognitive therapy; challenge distorted ideas • Engage in activities that focus on self-exploration, such as recognizing and dealing with emotions, self-expression, and self-exploration through creative media and expanding coping styles
Vegetative	• Failure to sustain basic needs for food, rest, etc.	• Provide external structure

Kielhofner, G. (2008). *Model of human occupation: Theory and application* (4th ed.). Philadelphia, PA: Lippincott Williams & Wilkins.

Marger Picard, M. (2017). *Occupational therapy's role in sleep.* Retrieved from https://www.aota.org/About-Occupational-Therapy/Professionals/HW/Sleep.aspx

Micali, N., Martini, M., Thomas, J., Eddy, K., Kothari, R., Russell, E., … Treasure, J. (2017). Lifetime and 12-month prevalence of eating disorders amongst women in midlife: A population-based study of diagnoses and risk factors. *BMC Medical, 15*(12), 1-10. doi:10.1186/s12916-016-0766-4

Mount, S., & Moas, S. (2015). Re-purposing the "empty nest." *Journal of Family Psychotherapy, 26,* 247-252. doi:10.1080/08975353.2015.1067536

Parial, S. (2015). Bipolar disorder in women. *Indian Journal of Psychiatry, 57*(2), S252-S263. doi:10.4103/0019-5545.161488

Polo-Kantola, P. (2011). Sleep problems in midlife and beyond. *Maturitas, 68*(3), 224-232.

Reinhard, S. C., Friss Feinberg, L., Choula, R., & Houser, A. (2015). Valuing the invaluable: 2015 update: Undeniable progress, but big gaps remain. *AARP Public Policy Institute*. Retrieved from https://www.aarp.org/content/dam/aarp/ppi/2015/valuing-the-invaluable-2015-update-new.pdf

Riley, L., & Bowen, C. (2005). The sandwich generation: Challenges and coping strategies of multigenerational families. *The Family Journal: Counseling and Therapy for Couples and Families, 13*(1), 52-58. doi:10.1177/1066480704270099

Scherker, A. (2017, July 12). 7 ways the beauty industry convinced women that they weren't good enough. *Huffington Post*. Retrieved from https://www.huffingtonpost.co.za/entry/beauty-industry-women_n_5127078

Sellgren, K. (2018, March 8). Empty-nesters 'resent boomerang kids.' *BBC News*. Retrieved from http://www.bbc.com/news/education-43321512

Sharp, J., & Keefe, B. (2006). Psychiatry in chronic pain: A review and update. *Journal of Lifelong Learning in Psychiatry, 4*(4), 573-580.

Sheehy, G. (1995). *New passages: Mapping your life across time*. New York, NY: Ballentine Books.

Stuart-Smith, J., Thapar, A., Maughan, B., Thapar, A., & Collishaw, S. (2017). Childhood hyperactivity and mood problems at mid-life: Evidence from a prospective birth cohort. *Social Psychiatry and Psychiatric Epidemiology, 5*, 87-94.

Taylor, R. R. (2006). *Cognitive behavioral therapy for chronic illness and disability*. New York, NY: Springer.

Taylor, R. R. (2008). *The intentional relationship: Occupational therapy and use of self*. Philadelphia, PA: F. A. Davis.

U.S. Department of Health and Human Services. (2018). *What is the U.S. opioid epidemic?* Retrieved from https://www.hhs.gov/opioids/about-the-epidemic/index.html

Vergis, P., & Brintnell, S. (2018). *Occupational performance of the sandwich generation: World issue*. Paper presented at the 17th World Federation of Occupational Therapists (WFOT) Congress, Cape Town, South Africa.

World Health Organization. (2018). *Depression*. Retrieved from http://www.who.int/en/news-room/fact-sheets/detail/depression

Mental Health of
Older Adults

Jerilyn (Gigi) Smith, PhD, OTR/L, FAOTA
and Anne MacRae, PhD, OTR/L, BCMH, FAOTA

This chapter, while focusing on mental health issues that affect aging individuals, also addresses the health of the older adult from a broader perspective. The interdependence of context with physical and mental health is even more pronounced in the elderly population than in the general population. Furthermore, as discussed throughout this chapter, there are several external factors that confound the ability to address psychiatric or psychological problems of this age group. Many occupational therapists have long held the belief that the medical model is insufficient to meet all of the health-related needs of the world's population. Nowhere is that more evident than in meeting the needs of the older adult. The health conditions of this population are more likely to be of a chronic nature. Many individuals have multiple medical problems that, when combined with changes that occur in the normal aging process and further superimposed with mental health issues, present a complicated case for assessment and intervention. As will be shown in this chapter, the mental and physical health of the older population is explicitly contingent on physical, social, and personal contexts. The medical profession has attempted to address the specific issues of aging with the development of specialties in geriatric medicine and psychiatry. The American Psychological Association (2014) has published a document, "Guidelines for Psychological Practice with Older Adults," that addresses attitudes, general knowledge about adult development, aging and older adults, clinical issues related to aging and psychopathology, assessment and intervention, and the need for ongoing education with respect to working with older adults with mental health issues. The guidelines stress that an interdisciplinary, coordinated-care approach is essential in the treatment of this older population to ensure the most effective care.

THE DEMOGRAPHICS OF AGING

According to the Administration on Aging (AoA, 2016), the population of older adults (aged 65 years) in the United States in the year 2015 totaled 47.8 million people. This represents 14.9% of the U.S. population, or more than one in every seven individuals. By the year 2060, this population is expected to more than double to 98 million. Minority populations are projected to increase from 10.6 million (22% of the elderly population) in 2015 to 21.1 million (28% of the elderly population) in 2030. The worldwide demographic changes are even more dramatic.

The number of persons aged 60 years or older was estimated to be 901 million in 2015 and is projected to grow to almost 2 billion by 2050, at which time there will be more people over 60 years of age than adolescents and youth aged 1 to 24 years (United Nations, Department of Economic and Social Affairs, Population Division, 2015).

This rise in the numbers of older adults will have significant effects on all areas of human and societal function, particularly economics and family dynamics. To provide effective care for this population, all health professionals

MacRae, A. (Ed.). *Cara and MacRae's Psychosocial Occupational Therapy: An Evolving Practice, Fourth Edition* (pp 225-241).

will need to expand their focus beyond a medical model and become advocates for change in social, economic, and health care policies and systems.

In 2015, 17% of individuals in the United States aged 64 to 75 years assessed their health as fair or poor, with this number rising to 43% in those aged 85 and above (AoA, 2016). Most older adults have at least one chronic condition, and many have multiple chronic conditions. Self-report of health has repeatedly been shown in the literature to have a high correlation to disability and function. Clearly, the health care needs of this population are significant. However, these data also show that the majority of older people are healthy, active, and productive members of their communities. In 2015, 54% of community-dwelling older persons aged 64 to 75 years rated their overall health as excellent or very good (AoA, 2016). This group is commonly referred to as the *well-elderly*. Some of the factors that help the older adult stay healthy are obvious and are tied to known healthy living factors of the general population (e.g., no smoking, good diet, management of pre-existing health conditions). Interestingly, however, many of the factors identified in the promotion of elder health are related to the psychological and social well-being of the individual, which is discussed in this chapter.

PSYCHIATRIC DIAGNOSES

There has been much debate in the literature regarding the prevalence of mental health issues and psychiatric disorders in older adults and whether these rates increase or decrease in later life. In general, it has been reported that older adults have a lower incidence of all psychiatric diagnoses, excluding cognitive disorders, than other age groups. However, more recent studies show that previously reported incidence rates underestimated the burden of late-life psychiatric disorders (Gum, King-Kallimanis, & Kohn, 2009). Statistics reporting low incidence of mental health issues among older adults must be viewed with caution for several reasons:

- Most older adults receive their health care through a primary physician or a general medicine clinic or institution. There is a serious lack of training in geriatric mental health and administrative support for identifying symptoms of mental illness and making appropriate referrals, as well as a significant gap in the overall number of geriatric practitioners and the number of older adults requiring mental health care (Popeo, Blazek, & Lehmann, 2017).

- There is generally a greater concern in the older population than in the general population about the stigma of mental illness; therefore, treatment specified as *psychiatric* or *psychological* is often avoided (Tzouvara, Papadopoulos, & Randhawa, 2018).

- Almost all (93%) older adults in the United States are at least partially dependent on Medicare, a government-sponsored health care payment program, primarily for those over age 65 years (AoA, 2016), which is woefully inadequate in reimbursement for mental health. The consequence of this is twofold: The individual avoids such treatment and the health care providers are often unwilling to diagnose and treat conditions that may not be reimbursable.

- Presentation of mental illness in the elderly compared with older adults is often symptomatically different and more chronic in nature and, therefore, difficult to diagnose and treat. Most notably is the tendency of the elderly to emphasize and describe somatic (physical) concerns rather than emotional concerns (Hegeman, de Waal, Comijs, Kok, & van der Mast, 2014). This often leads to both underrecognized psychiatric illness and unnecessary medical treatment. Additionally, validated diagnostic tools that are used with adults are often less suitable for diagnosing mental disorders in elderly people due to the length and complexity of testing material. Differentiation between older age groups—young-old (55 to 64 years), middle-old (65 to 74 years), old-old (75 to 84 years), and oldest (85+ years)—has not been the focus in studies reporting the incidence of psychiatric disorders in late life. A comprehensive study of the prevalence of psychiatric disorders across older adult age groups showed that, although there was a leveling off of prevalence rates in the oldest population (85+), there were relatively high rates of psychiatric disorders in the other adult age groups (Reynolds, Pietrzak, El-Gabalawy, Mackenzie & Sareen, 2015).

As the demographics change, there is a need for health care professionals to increase their understanding of geriatric mental health conditions and the unique mental health needs of an aging population. Although there is the demand for psychologists who are trained in the cultural and clinical needs of an aging population is rising, relatively few have received formal training in the psychology of aging. This has considerable implications for addressing the mental health needs of elderly adults.

It is estimated that there are approximately 2.8 million older adults in the United States with serious mental illness (National Institute of Mental Health, 2015) Older adults with serious mental illness have complicated issues due to their psychiatric condition, ineffective or lack of available treatment interventions, and additional complications brought on by the aging process. The consequences of psychiatric disorders in the elderly population are dire and include social deprivation, decreased quality of life, cognitive decline, disability, suicide, increased risk for somatic illness, and nonsuicidal mortality (Skoog, 2011).

Even in cases where the individual may not meet the full criteria for a psychiatric disorder, many psychiatric symptoms may be found in the elderly population due to general medical conditions, side effects of medications, or life stressors and daily life demands that can lead to psychosocial distress. Many of these symptoms (described in Table 14-1) are treatable if recognized. Although these

TABLE 14-1. PRESENTATION OF PSYCHIATRIC SYMPTOMS IN OLDER ADULTS

PSYCHIATRIC CONDITION	DIAGNOSTIC ISSUES
Anxiety	Until a few years ago, anxiety disorders were believed to decline with age. However, experts now say that anxiety is as common among the old as among the young and is commonly experienced by community-dwelling older adults (Koychev & Ebmeier, 2016). Anxiety is a common symptom that is associated with other medical and psychiatric conditions as well as changes in environment and other life stressors associated with aging. Anxiety and depression are often seen as comorbidities. Both are associated with a depletion of resources for coping with challenges, which can make the individual more susceptible to negative health conditions (Zisberg, 2017). Generalized anxiety disorder is the most common anxiety disorder in late life. Generalized anxiety disorder is a chronic disorder that is unlikely to resolve without treatment. It is three times as prevalent in order adults with chronic obstructive pulmonary disease (Fuller-Thompson & Lacombe-Duncan, 2016).
	New onset of anxiety in older adults may also be associated with medication side effects, bereavement, chronic grief, alcohol use, or other stresses and changes that often accompany aging. Fears about changes in health and aging in general can lead to anxiety. The anxiety is accompanied by physical symptoms, such as agitation, fatigue, and sleep disturbances. Other signs of anxiety disorder include excessive worry or fear, refusal to do routine activities or an excessive preoccupation with routine, overconcern about safety, complaints of racing heartbeat, shallow breathing, trembling, nausea, sweating, muscles tension, feeling weak and shaky, hoarding, and self-medicating with alcohol or other central nervous system depressants (Geriatric Mental Health Foundation, n.d.). Anxiety disorders cause a great deal of distress for elderly individuals and have a significant negative impact on their ability to fully participate in life, often resulting in isolation and depression. Anxiety symptoms are associated with greater disability, significant impairment in health-related quality of life, greater health care usage among older adults, and increased mortality. Phobias (including social phobias), obsessive compulsive disorders, panic disorders, and posttraumatic stress disorders are also types of anxiety disorders. The Geriatric Anxiety Inventory, Anxiety Disorder Scale, and Fear questionnaire are tools that have been developed to screen for anxiety in the older adult population (Koychev & Ebmeier, 2016).
Depression	Depression in later life frequently coexists with other medical illnesses and disabilities. Late-life depression is common in older individuals who have chronic or disabling medical disorders such as diabetes, cardiovascular disease, lung disease, thyroid disease, arthritis, oncological diseases, intestinal disorders, and stroke (Hegeman et al., 2014) and often leads to increasing negative health outcomes, a worsening of self-rated health and self-perceived disability, increased somatization, higher rates of hospital and nursing home admissions, and premature mortality.
	Social isolation is a significant contributor to the development of geriatric depression. There are many factors that contribute to social isolation, including mobility limitations, medical illnesses, financial constraints, loss of a spouse, significant others, and social networks. Social isolation results in impaired social engagement and decreased participation in social activities. Although living alone does not necessarily lead to social isolation, it is a risk factor. Regardless of where a person lives, seniors who feel lonely and isolated are more likely to report also having poor physical and/or mental health. Many studies have shown that feelings of loneliness are associated with more depressive symptoms in older adults (Liu, Gou, & Zou, 2016).
	Depression is not a normal part of aging; however, many believe this to be true, which contributes to it being underrecognized, underdiagnosed, and undertreated. Like most other psychiatric disorders, depression in the older population presents itself differently than it does in younger individuals, which leads to frequent misdiagnosis or underdiagnosis by physicians.

(continued)

TABLE 14-1 (CONTINUED). PRESENTATION OF PSYCHIATRIC SYMPTOMS IN OLDER ADULTS

PSYCHIATRIC CONDITION	DIAGNOSTIC ISSUES
Depression (continued)	A depressed or sad mood may not be reported by the individual. More commonly reported symptoms include anergy (lack of energy), anhedonia (absence of pleasure), loss of appetite, sleeplessness, somatic complaints (e.g., unexplained pain, headaches, chronic fatigue, anorexia, gastrointestinal complaints, weight loss), anxiety, apathy, withdrawal, and cognitive impairment (Hegeman et al., 2014).
	Geriatric depression is a serious medical condition that can lead to a significantly compromised quality of life. Depression among the elderly can lead to suicide. Older white males have the highest rate of suicide among all age groups. Over 70% of older suicide victims visited their primary physician during the month prior to their attempt, and many had depressive illness that went undetected during this visit. The majority of older adults with depression improve when they receive treatment with antidepressant medication, psychotherapy, cognitive behavioral therapy, or a combination of these treatments (Blackburn, Wilkins-Ho & Wiese, 2017).
Bipolar disorder	Diagnosis of bipolar disorder in the older adult is typically designated as early onset (individuals who developed their illness during early adulthood) and late onset (those who experienced their first mood episode at an older age; Depp & Jeste, 2004). Research shows that older individuals with bipolar disorder have substantially compromised cognitive functioning, which negatively affects daily functioning and compliance with treatment (Cullen et al., 2016). Deficits in executive functions and verbal memory are prevalent, and when added to the changes that accompany aging in general, they present a considerable challenge for the individual. This has important clinical implications in terms of determining effective intervention strategies that take into account the often-significant cognitive deficits that accompany this disorder.
	Mania may also be a symptom of cognitive disorders or confused with the irritability and lability found in dementia and delirium.
Psychosis	Psychotic symptoms are associated with myriad different psychiatric and medical disorders, including delirium, major depression, affective illness, Alzheimer's-type dementia, schizophrenia or other primary psychotic disorders, general medical conditions, and substance abuse or dependence (Reinhardt & Cohen, 2015). Psychotic features, including hallucinations, thought disturbances, poverty of thinking, irrationality, delusions, and behavioral disturbance, vary depending on the etiology of the psychosis. Management of psychosis in the elderly is complicated and involves careful, multidisciplinary assessment of the individual.
Substance abuse	Alcohol and substance abuse are underrecognized in the elderly population, and warning signs (e.g., falls, relationship conflicts, and memory impairment) may be misattributed to the aging process. The negative effects of use and abuse of and addiction to alcohol and other substances are intensified in the older adult as a result of the aging changes, chronic disease processes, and dangerous interactions with over-the-counter and prescribed medications (Clay, 2010). Alcohol or other substance abuse is also commonly found in elders with depression and may be used as a maladaptive coping strategy. Alcohol abuse impairs memory and information processing and may go unrecognized in the early stages of dementia despite causing significant functional deterioration. Toxicity from over-the-counter medications and combinations of prescribed medications can cause both serious medical consequences and cognitive impairments that may erroneously lead to a diagnosis of early dementia (Hall, 2002). Risk factors for the initiation or exacerbation of substance abuse or addiction in elders include female sex, polypharmacy, chronic physical illness, poor health, and concurrent or a history of psychiatric or other substance use disorder (Simoni-Wastila & Yang, 2006).

CASE ILLUSTRATION 14-1: MR. SORENSEN—DIFFERENTIAL DIAGNOSIS: DEPRESSION AND DEMENTIA

Mr. Sorensen is a widower who lives in an elder assisted living facility. His wife of 42 years, who visited him every day, suddenly passed away, and the family had to put their aging dog to sleep because no one was able to care for him. The staff noted that Mr. Sorensen was not eating well and was spending more time alone. He was generally noncommunicative and often appeared confused. He needed prompting to get out of bed in the morning and supervision to complete personal care.

Discussion

Grief and multiple losses are common in the elderly and can lead to depression if not addressed. The staff at the facility may not realize the magnitude of Mr. Sorensen's personal losses and dismiss his current behavior as to be expected given the recent losses in his life. Mr. Sorensen may indeed have a progressive dementia, but the life stressors he is enduring certainly warrant intervention, including counseling and/or medication, for what may be a treatable depression.

CASE ILLUSTRATION 14-2: MRS. DEVAUGHN—DIFFERENTIAL DIAGNOSIS: TOXICITY AND DEMENTIA

Mrs. DeVaughn has been displaying increased confusion, memory loss, and irritability. Her daughter, Edna, arranged for a home health care team to evaluate her safety in the home. She fully expected that a recommendation would be made for Mrs. DeVaughn to move to a supervised living situation because of what Edna sees as deteriorating dementia. Mrs. DeVaughn refused to let the visiting nurse go over her medications with her but agreed to let the occupational therapist help her organize her bathroom and kitchen cabinets "just to make things easier." The occupational therapist found 14 prescription medications prescribed by five different medical specialists as well as her primary care physician. She also found a plethora of over-the-counter medications as well as herbal supplements. The occupational therapist contacted the case manager nurse, who arranged with the physician to have Mrs. DeVaughn hospitalized so her medicines could either be discontinued, reduced, or changed. Within 3 days, Mrs. De Vaughn's mental status markedly improved and, much to her daughter's surprise, she was able to return to independent living.

Discussion

Although physicians and pharmacists have increased their awareness of drug interactions and symptoms, and although methods for tracking medical prescriptions are much improved, the problems associated with using multiple health care providers still exist. The older adult tends to trust health care providers and is unlikely to question a prescription or offer information about other medications unless specifically asked. The occupational therapist is in an ideal position to evaluate actual medication regimens in the home by addressing daily living habits and routines and can then coordinate with the team for treatment recommendations. In any case of suspected dementia, it is vital that all other, often treatable, causes are ruled out. In the case of Mrs. DeVaughn, there may have also been a metabolic or general medical condition, such as decreased kidney function, that would increase the likelihood of toxicity (i.e., increased concentration of substances because of decreased elimination resulting in a change in mental status).

symptoms are seen in various age groups, they present differently in the older population. These psychiatric symptoms are sometimes seen in dementia but may also be indicative of a separate and distinct disorder that too often goes undiagnosed and therefore untreated. Two such situations are highlighted in Case Illustrations 14-1 and 14-2.

One disorder that is unique to the elderly population (at least in terms of high incidence) is dementia, an emotionally, socially, and physically devastating condition that warrants further discussion.

Dementia

Dementia is a syndrome identified by the presence of multiple cognitive deficits. Dementia has an insidious onset, characterized by the slow onset of short-term memory loss. It is a chronic, progressive, and irreversible condition in which the individual retains normal levels of alertness. Attention and concentration are globally affected, and language impairment and confabulation are common. In addition to memory impairment and other cognitive deficits, a person with dementia demonstrates a significant decline in overall function. In most progressive dementia, there is no cure or treatment that actually stops the progression (Alzheimer's Association, n.d.). An estimated 5.2 million people in the United States suffer from severe dementia, and another 1 to 5 million people experience mild to moderate dementia. Five to eight percent of people over the age of 65 have some form of dementia, and the number doubles every 5 years over age 65 (HealthCommunities.com, 2015). As the U.S. population aged 65 years and older continues to increase, the number of individuals with dementia is expected to rapidly increase. Worldwide, it is estimated that 50 million people are living with dementia, and this number is projected to increase to 82 million in 2030 and 152 million in 2050 (World Health Organization [WHO], 2017).

Dementia may be caused by a wide variety of conditions, including degenerative disorders of the central nervous system such as Parkinson's disease or Huntington's disease; cardiac disorders, which may result in vascular dementia; metabolic disorders such as diabetes that may result in vascular dementia or uncontrolled thyroid conditions; nutritional, especially vitamin, deficiencies; toxicity or drug related, such as substance-induced dementia; brain tumors; trauma; and infections, most notably Creutzfeldt-Jakob disease and HIV. From a medical viewpoint, it is critical to determine the underlying reason for the dementia because many of the aforementioned conditions can be medically treated or at least controlled. However, more than half of all diagnosed dementia is caused by Alzheimer's disease, a progressive condition for which there is no known cure.

Vascular dementia and Alzheimer's disease are both strongly age related. The percentage of individuals with Alzheimer's dementia increases with age: 3% of people aged 65 to 74 years, 1% aged 75 to 84 years, and 32% aged 85 years and older have been diagnosed with Alzheimer's dementia (Alzheimer's Association, 2018). The World Alzheimer Report 2016 (Alzheimer's Disease International [ADI], 2016) estimates that in 2015, there were 46.8 million people living with dementia worldwide and projects that this number will increase 131.5 million by 2050. This is a dramatic increase from the estimated 18 million people who were identified with dementia in 2000. The implications of societal costs of dementia and the impact of these on families, health, and social care services are staggering.

Alzheimer's disease is progressive and often difficult to diagnose in its early stages; therefore, the diagnosis may be made retrospectively or when all other causes of the dementia have been ruled out. The relatively minor memory problems consistent with early stages of the disease may be found in any older adult and are not necessarily indicative of the relentless pending decline in function and cognition seen in Alzheimer's disease.

Table 14-2 outlines the stages of the disease as described by Reisberg, Ferris, and Crook (1983) in the Global Deterioration Scale. The staging is helpful in anticipating common reactions and behaviors and adjusting intervention to address them.

People who exhibit symptoms of dementia may have potentially treatable conditions, such as nutritional deficits, side effects from medications, or depression, and this should be taken into careful consideration by the individual's physician.

Delirium is sometimes confused for dementia in the elderly. Delirium is an acute confusional state accompanied by agitation. It has an abrupt onset, fluctuating levels of alertness, and variable states of orientation. These changes in mental functions are well beyond the typical forgetfulness that often occurs in aging. Delirium affects elders primarily in acute care settings. Older adults with dementia are at an even higher risk for delirium because the aging neurologic system is more vulnerable to insults caused by underlying systemic conditions (Fong, Tulebaev, & Inouye, 2009). Delirium is one of the most common complications of medical illness, prolonged hospital stays, or recovery from surgery among elderly individuals. Approximately one-third of individuals over the age of 70 who are admitted to an acute hospital experience delirium, and about two-thirds of elderly patients experience delirium after major surgery (Health in Aging, 2017). Delirium is typically considered to be a temporary problem of short duration, but it may persist for months if the underlying cause is not determined and treated. Reversible causes of delirium include drugs (especially narcotics, other pain relievers, sedatives, corticosteroids, and drugs that affect acetylcholine levels in the brain), electrolyte disturbances (dehydration and thyroid problems), lack of drugs (stopping use of long-term sedatives), infection, reduced sensory input (e.g., poor vision or hearing), urinary problems, myocardial problems, chronic obstructive lung disease, and alcohol abuse (Mayo Clinic, 2018). Delirium is considered a serious medical situation that requires medical attention. The primary goal for treatment of delirium is to identify and treat the underlying cause or causes. This includes looking at medical and environmental factors. Potentially modifiable risk factors include sensory issues such as hearing and vision, impact of immobilization such as catheters or restraints, contextual factors (environmental overstimulation or deprivation), emotional distress from hospitalization, and disturbance to sleep patterns. Evidence suggests that an early goal-directed, multidisciplinary, multi-intervention approach to working with elders with delirium may help reduce the duration of delirium. The relationship between quality of sleep and circadian rhythms, as well as their contribution to delirium, has been widely discussed in the literature (Rains & Chee, 2017). Poor quality of sleep and disruptions in circadian rhythms are common problems experienced by those in a hospital setting. Occupational therapy has a key role in addressing the areas of cognition, memory, sleep hygiene, and function. Occupational therapists work with individuals in the area of rest, sleep preparation and participation,

TABLE 14-2. CLINICAL COURSE OF ALZHEIMER'S DISEASE

STAGE	DESCRIPTION	EXAMPLES OF PERFORMANCE AND BEHAVIORS
Stage 1	No cognitive decline	Normal functioning; occasional lapses of memory
Stage 2	Very mild cognitive decline	No deficits noted in occupational or social roles; however, the individual may express concern over "forgetfulness." Often forgets names or misplaces objects
Stage 3	Mild cognitive decline	Immediate recall is impaired and agnosia may be present. Because of decreased performance in demanding employment and social situations, it is in this stage that family, friends, and coworkers may recognize a problem. Anxiety overperformance is common at this stage, but there is usually significant denial as well.
Stage 4	Moderate cognitive decline	Deficits are now obvious, including poor concentration, decreased knowledge of recent and current events, and difficulties traveling alone (especially to unfamiliar places) and in handling personal finances. The individual usually remains orientated to time and familiar places and persons. There is often a withdrawal from new or challenging situations, and the person will generally still be in denial of the seriousness of his or her condition.
Stage 5	Moderately severe cognitive decline	Individuals at stage 5 generally need assistance to live safely. They are likely to forget important phone numbers or emergency procedures and are frequently disoriented to time or place but will usually remember their own name and names of close friends and family. They begin to have problems with multistep activities of daily living (ADL), such as dressing, but do not need assistance with many personal care tasks such as eating or toileting.
Stage 6	Severe cognitive decline	The individual occasionally forgets spouse's name or the names of other significant people in his or her life. Retains some sketchy knowledge of past life but is largely unaware of recent events and experiences. Disoriented to time and place. Sleep patterns are frequently disturbed. There is often marked personality/emotional changes in this stage that may include delusions, obsessiveness, anxiety, agitation, apathy, and, occasionally, violent behavior.
Stage 7	Very severe cognitive decline	Profound physical symptoms such as incontinence and limited mobility (may be unable to walk). Communication is severely impaired and may be limited to grunting. Needs assistance with all personal care.

Adapted from Reisberg, B., Ferris, S. H., & Crook, T. (1983). Global Deterioration Scale. In B. Reisberg (Ed.), *A guide to Alzheimer's disease*. New York, NY: Free Press.

and activities related to obtaining restorative rest and sleep (American Occupational Therapy Association [AOTA], 2014).

MENTAL HEALTH ASSESSMENT

All health care providers should be cognizant of the presence of psychiatric disorders in their elderly clients, particularly ones that are too often overlooked, such as depression and substance abuse. Simple screening tools may identify treatable conditions. The most commonly used depression screen for older adults is the Geriatric Depression Scale (GDS), originally designed by Yesavage et al. (1983) and now available in the public domain. The GDS is a 30-item self-report assessment consisting of questions related to seven common characteristics of depression in later life (somatic concern, lowered affect, cognitive impairment, feelings of discrimination, impaired motivation, lack of future orientation, and lack of self-esteem).

The questions are answered with yes/no responses. The short version containing 15 questions (Shiekh & Yesavage, 1986) probably has the most widespread usage. The GDS has been shown to be a reliable and cost-effective screening tool, especially when used in conjunction with other tests (Midden & Mast, 2018). The Geriatric Anxiety Inventory has been shown to be a valid tool in detecting anxiety in the elderly, especially in those with depression (Johnco, Knight, Tadic & Wuthrich, 2015). There are several screening tools used to identify geriatric alcohol abuse. One of the most popular is the Short Michigan Alcoholism Screening Test-Geriatric Version (University of Michigan Alcohol Research Center, 1991). Many self-screening tools are available on the internet and offer recommendations to individuals and their families on how to access help for the specific problem.

Given the global effects of dementia on individuals and their families, it is important to arrive at a working diagnosis as early as possible. There are several specific assessments to screen, diagnose, and classify the stages of Alzheimer's disease as well as other dementias. Examples are the Memory Impairment Screen, the General Practitioner Assessment of Cognition, and the mini-Cog (Cordell et al., 2013). These brief cognitive assessments require 5 minutes or less to administer, are validated for use in a primary care or community setting, have excellent psychometric properties, and are easily administered by health professionals who are not physicians.

Occupational Therapy Assessment

Assessment of the overall mental health of older adults is often conducted as an interdisciplinary effort. The focus of the interdisciplinary assessment corresponds with many of the traditional domains of occupational therapy; therefore, occupational therapy assessments, especially those that focus on cognition, occupation, environment, and social relations, are valuable for this population. Many assessments are described throughout this book that can be used with the older adult population, and readers are encouraged to explore a wide variety of assessments to fit the individual needs of particular clients. A crucial contribution of occupational therapy in the assessment of the elderly individual with psychiatric illness lies in the occupational therapist's unique skill in performing functional evaluations, either through formal assessment or task analysis, in vivo, or in the client's natural environment. A study by Hoppes, Davis, and Thompson (2003) on the environmental effects on the assessment of people with dementia concluded that "while it may be time consuming to assess clients in specific settings of interest, this may be the only valid way to determine abilities to function in those settings" (p. 401).

In Chapter 3 of this text, Case Illustration 3-1 (Uyen—Performance in the Community) described an in-clinic assessment that overestimated the client's functional capabilities. Case Illustration 14-3 demonstrates the opposite situation.

Quality-of-Life Assessment

Life satisfaction or quality-of-life assessment is now an important part of an interdisciplinary assessment and is recognized as a desired outcome of treatment by both the World Health Organization (2013) and AOTA (2014), as well as many other occupational therapy and health care organizations around the world. Despite this recent focus, there is little agreement in the literature on a definition of quality of life. The definition of "quality of life" is deeply personal and is different for each individual. Some key elements needing assessment are as follows:

- The ability to think, make decisions and have control in one's daily life
- Physical and mental health
- Living arrangements
- Social relationships
- Religious beliefs and spirituality
- Cultural values
- A sense of community
- Financial and economic circumstances.

The important point in a quality-of-life assessment is to recognize the unique and subjective nature of the client's responses, as shown in Case Illustration 14-4. Clients will have interests and priorities in life that may be quite different from what the therapist thinks is important. A truly client-centered approach using active listening is essential for a meaningful quality-of-life assessment. This information is then used to establish goals and formulate an individualized intervention plan.

Quality of life should be addressed in all occupational therapy assessments, but it has particular significance for the older adult because the more conventional outcomes of restoration, rehabilitation, or improvement of function may not always be realistic goals for many older individuals, depending on the nature of their disability and other complicating factors. This presents one of the many challenges for occupational therapists working with the older adult because functional progress is often the basis for reimbursement, and conventional rehabilitation may be viewed by employers as the only occupational therapy services that should be offered. Occupational therapists need to advocate for a broadening of their role in many settings and engage in research that demonstrates the long-term cost-effectiveness of quality-of-life intervention.

OCCUPATIONAL THERAPY INTERVENTION

Intervention for the older adult, as with assessment, is best provided with a holistic and coordinated approach that includes professionals, family members, caregivers, and other significant individuals. However, for the purposes

CASE ILLUSTRATION 14-3: MRS. AYALA—IN VIVO ASSESSMENT

Mrs. Ayala is a 76-year-old woman with a history of vascular disease who was recently hospitalized for a transient ischemic attack. The hospital interdisciplinary team determined that she had a moderate level of dementia, most likely of the vascular type. The hospital-based occupational therapist performed a kitchen assessment in the occupational therapy clinic to determine Mrs. Ayala's safety and functional abilities in ADL. During the assessment, it was noted that Mrs. Ayala became quite agitated and confused. She did remember to turn off the electric range top, but then placed a plastic bowl on the burner. The occupational therapist needed to intervene to prevent the bowl from melting and then provided moderate assistance to complete the task safely.

The hospital-based team recommended that Mrs. Ayala not be allowed to stay at home alone after discharge. She lives with her daughter's family, but all family members are either at work or school during the day. The family refused to consider placement for her outside the home but did agree to home health care services.

The home health occupational therapist received the discharge notes from the hospital-based therapist. Therefore, she was quite surprised when arriving at Mrs. Ayala's home to find her in the kitchen alone successfully making pancit (a traditional Filipino meal made of rice stick noodles, vegetables, and shrimp or meat) as well as homemade lumpia (egg rolls) for her family's dinner. When the occupational therapist expressed her concern, Mrs. Ayala laughingly replied, "I've been doing this all of my life!"

Discussion

In her own home, Mrs. Ayala demonstrated a much higher functional ability than previously seen in the hospital. She was able to perform cooking tasks that were actually much more complicated than what was asked of her during the hospital evaluation. The familiarity of the tools (such as a gas range instead of an electric one) and the layout of the kitchen often help people with memory or other cognitive deficits perform tasks automatically. The cultural familiarity with the items being prepared is also an important factor. A third critical factor is the motivation and satisfaction of being able to preserve an important and meaningful role as a contributing member of the family.

CASE ILLUSTRATION 14-4: PROFESSOR FUJIYAMA'S QUALITY OF LIFE

Dr. Fujiyama is an emeritus professor of neurobiology at a prestigious university. He is in the early-to-moderate stage of Alzheimer's disease. All of his adult life, he took immense pride in his intellectual ability and is having great difficulty in adjusting to his memory lapses and generally decreased function. He became withdrawn and was often irritable. The home health occupational therapist wanted to engage him in self-care activities but was met with great resistance. The occupational therapist decided to change her approach and offered to work with him on cognitive activities. She showed the doctor some interactive computer programs on biology and engaged him in several pencil-and-paper tasks using memory strategies. Eventually, he started asking questions about cognitive rehabilitation and the theories behind her choice of activities for him. He developed an interest in using the computer and researching websites about Alzheimer's disease.

The occupational therapist would leave worksheets and suggested activities for the professor after every visit, and upon her return, he would confidently show the occupational therapist his completed "homework." Although Dr. Fujiyama continued to avoid most ADL and depended on his wife or an aide to perform such tasks, his affect was brighter, he had fewer angry outbursts, and he appeared more engaged and interested in life.

Discussion

Although the occupational therapist was unable to engage Dr. Fujiyama in many of the traditional activities used by home health therapists, she was able to adjust her intervention to include tasks that were personally meaningful and appropriately challenging to the professor. This provided a quality of life to this client that could not be found in more conventional therapy.

CASE ILLUSTRATION 14-5: THE OCCUPATIONS OF MR. HATFIELD

Mr. Hatfield is a retired factory worker who is currently being evaluated for depression and dementia. He reported to the occupational therapist that the only thing that he ever liked doing was fishing, but he can't drive his truck to the pier anymore. Through further conversation, the occupational therapist learned that Mr. Hatfield always tied his own flies for fly fishing, and she asked him to teach her the craft. He wrote a shopping list of all the supplies that he needed, and together they shopped for supplies and continued to tie fancy fishing flies for several sessions. Mr. Hatfield seemed to enjoy the sessions and reminisced about past great fishing trips. However, he clearly still missed his prime occupation of actually going fishing. The occupational therapist helped Mr. Hatfield contact a local volunteer organization to find a fishing companion willing and able to accompany and transport Mr. Hatfield to local fishing spots. A successful match was made, and a trip was planned for the following week. His volunteer companion also told Mr. Hatfield that there was a fly-tying club over in the next town and he would be glad to take him to a meeting. Although Mr. Hatfield remained somewhat forgetful and he needed guidance to perform many tasks, his affect greatly improved.

Discussion

Although Mr. Hatfield's interests seem limited, his passion for fishing opened up possibilities for new leisure and social pursuits and provided the motivation to engage in cognitively challenging activities such as constructing a craft and shopping for supplies. The need to teach an activity (to the occupational therapist) also provided a sense of purpose and an opportunity to demonstrate mastery and competence.

---

of this chapter, the discussion is limited to those interventions most frequently used by occupational therapists specifically for older adults. Depending on the condition being addressed, expected outcomes may include restoration of function and rehabilitation, but goals addressing quality of life, prevention, and adaptation are also crucial for the older adult population.

Occupation

The overarching purpose of occupational therapy is to promote "participation in life through engagement in occupation" (AOTA, 2014, p. S4); this is illustrated in Case Illustration 14-5. A study conducted by Aubin, Hachey, and Mercier (1999) suggested that:

> perceived competence in daily tasks and rest, and pleasure in work and rest activities are positively correlated with subjective quality of life. The influence of occupation and its meaning on quality of life, an occupational therapy assumption, is supported by these results. (p. 53)

A critical review of 23 other studies concurred:

> Occupation has an important influence on health and well-being. Ranging from physiological to functional outcomes, it is clear that the performance of everyday occupations is an important part of everyday life. Withdrawal or changes in occupation for a person have a significant impact on a person's self-perceived health and well-being. (Law, Steinwender, & Leclair, 1998, pp. 89-90)

Evidence from a review of the literature from diverse sources supports the efficacy of occupational therapy intervention focusing on engagement in occupation for individuals with dementia and their caregivers (Walker, Allen, Koch, Sprehe & Webber, 2017). The positive effects of occupation were seen both in the clients and in their caregivers. Pimouguet, Le Goff, Wittwer, Dartigues, and Helmer (2017) found that participation in everyday occupation contributed to the well-being of both the caregiver and the older individual with dementia, reduced the caregiver's burden, and facilitated continuity of relationships for the caregiver. Successful engagement in everyday occupations by the care receiver was an important source of satisfaction for the caregiver as well. In a seminal study conducted by Baum (1995), it was found that "individuals who remained active in occupation demonstrated fewer disturbing behaviors, required less help with basic self-care, and their carers experienced less stress" (p. 59).

Although considerable research is being conducted on the effects of occupation, it is difficult to draw generalizations. In order for occupation to be effective as an intervention, it must be personally meaningful and present an appropriate level of challenge. A task that is overly simple may be seen as demeaning, yet an overly complex task may promote feelings of failure. In order for occupation to be used as a therapeutic modality (rather than a simple diversion), it must address the goals established in the occupational therapy assessment. The occupational therapist chooses the activity or occupation in collaboration with the client. Adaptations or gradations to the activity may be necessary to meet specific goals and provide the just-right challenge for the client. Interventions used by occupational therapists often use occupations or activities that are commonplace in daily life, which may lead to an erroneous conclusion by some that occupation-based interventions may be competently and less expensively conducted by para- or nonprofessionals. Although some purely diversional activities groups are helpful and welcomed by the older adult, a groundbreaking 3-year well elderly study conducted by Clark et al. (1997) concluded that "superior outcomes can be expected when an activity-centered intervention is administered by professional therapists as opposed to being conducted by nonprofessionals" (p. 1325). Pimouguet et al. (2017) studied 421 individuals with dementia who received occupational therapy services and found that functional performance remained stable at 3 months during occupational therapy intervention, behavioral symptoms decreased significantly, and reported quality-of-life scores improved during intervention. Caregiver burden scores and time spent providing care also significantly decreased during intervention. The occupational therapist is trained to continually assess and modify the intervention based on the client's performance to elicit outcomes that are geared toward established goal attainment. An individual untrained in occupation-based theory will not have the knowledge to make these modifications.

Environmental Support and Adaptation

Understanding the context in which treatment is provided is critical to the occupational therapy process. Environment plays a vital role in both the overall functioning and the quality of life of the older adult. In the United States and in other parts of the world, the preference of older adults is to remain in their homes or communities for as long as possible. A phenomenological study conducted in Scandinavia "showed that moving to sheltered housing meant for a majority of participants that their self-image changed from being self-reliant and independent to becoming dependent and perceiving themselves and their care to be a burden" (Sviden, Wikstrom, & Hjortsjo-Norberg, 2002, p. 10). To meet the needs of the older population and honor their choices, facilitating aging in place has "benefits that extend beyond cost savings to include social and emotional benefits to both seniors and the broader community" (Office of Policy Development and Research, U.S. Department of Housing and Urban Development, 2013).

As discussed in Chapter 6 of this text, occupational therapists are specifically trained in environmental adaptation that addresses the physical, social, emotional, spiritual, and cognitive contexts. Given the often-complex needs of the older adult, this holistic view of the environment is essential for successful intervention. Aging in place can be facilitated through a variety of environmental interventions, including home modifications. There are many design principles, environmental interventions, and technology

tools designed to facilitate successful engagement in ADL; however, further research is needed to examine the efficacy of these interventions for individuals with mental health issues such as dementia.

Although much attention is paid to the physical environment for successful aging in place, the role of the social environment on mental health and well-being must also be considered. This concept is demonstrated in Case Illustration 14-6. Social capital is a concept in which social networks and relationships are a central component of the environment. Social capital—specifically, participation in groups, having neighbors willing to help, and having a sense of belonging and trust in neighbors—has been found to play a significant role in self-rated physical and mental health of older adults (Norstrand, Glicksman, Lubben, & Kleban, 2012). Occupational therapy intervention can include providing the older adult with tools to develop social capital.

The social context of the environment includes the roles of caregivers, family, and the community as well as the individual client, and it is often appropriate for the occupational therapist to include all or some of these others in the client's intervention program. Additionally, education, training, and support should be considered for those who make up the social context of the client. Research indicates that friends of both the older adult and the caregivers provide valuable emotional and social support (Donnellan, Bennett, & Soulsby, 2017) and should be included in assessment and treatment as needed. Evaluating the needs of the caregiver, facilitating coping and caregiving strategies, and empowering caregivers are vital roles of the occupational therapist. As an older adult declines in function, the role of the caregiver increases, thereby increasing his or her stress. If supported by outside services, including receiving necessary education to facilitate the caregiver role, the caregiver may be more effective and may be able to successfully continue in this role for a longer period of time. The cost-effectiveness of a family approach to treatment results in the older adult being able to remain in the home rather than being moved to an institutional placement. Case Illustration 14-7 continues the story of Mrs. Christie's life path that was originally discussed in Case Illustration 14-6.

Social isolation has been associated with adverse health effects, including dementia (Seegert, 2017). The occupational therapist, along with the social worker, plays a critical role in reconnecting an isolated individual with his or her community by making appropriate referrals to community and social groups and by facilitating the ability to access social support systems. These community referrals may also benefit the caregiver by providing support and respite.

Although aging in place is preferred by many older adults and has many advantages, care must be taken not to assume that one's home always provides the ideal living situation. For many people, the responsibility of home management is not possible or is overly stressful. According to the AoA (2016), 73% of older men lived with their spouse,

CASE ILLUSTRATION 14-6: MRS. CHRISTIE—THE MEANING OF HOME

Mrs. Christie lives in a large Victorian home in the city where she raised her four children. After her husband passed away, her grown children, all with families of their own, wanted her to move to a smaller home or apartment out in the suburbs, closer to them. Two of the four children also offered to have her move in with them. Although Mrs. Christie freely admits that she has slowed down "quite a bit," she still feels quite able to care for herself. Her biggest functional change has been to give up driving. She has groceries delivered or walks to the corner store and either takes a taxi or has a friend drive her to appointments. Mrs. Christie's children all agree that the house is too much work for her, and they think she would be safer out of the city. Also, if she were in the suburbs, they could check up on her more frequently. She steadfastly resists, stating that she would miss her friends and her garden.

Discussion

Many older adults freely choose to move to a low-maintenance residence or move in with family; however, many others wish to stay in a familiar place. Although the concerns expressed by Mrs. Christie's children could be realistic, they fail to take into account the personal meaning of home. In some cultures, such as the Anglo-American culture of Mrs. Christie, independence is highly prized, and moving in with one's children may be seen as an imposition or failure (even if invited).

A familiar home often provides a sense of community. It is likely that Mrs. Christie knows her neighbors, grocer, church minister, and pharmacist. She has also shown the ability to be adaptive, maintaining her mobility in the community without driving. Her home is a place full of memories and favorite occupations such as gardening. Intervention geared toward helping Mrs. Christie stay as independent as possible in her own home and doing the things she likes to do, rather than encouraging her to abandon her home, would be preferable.

whereas fewer than one-half (47%) of older women did. Additionally, older women were more than twice as likely as older men to live alone (35% and 20%, respectively). In the case of Mrs. Christie (see Case Illustration 14-6), living alone was clearly her choice, and she was still actively involved in her community and had a social support network. However, for many older adults, living alone can be a frightening and lonely experience. A move to a socially active senior residence or to a family member's home may ease the loneliness as well as provide necessary support to maintain maximal well-being.

Another aspect of the environmental conditions that must be evaluated is the potential for elder abuse, which can occur in any setting and affects elders across all socioeconomic groups, cultures, and races. Women and older elders are more likely to be victimized, as are seniors with dementia or other mental health and substance abuse issues.

Elder abuse can take many different forms. Physical abuse, sexual abuse, emotional or psychological abuse, neglect, abandonment, financial or material exploitation, and self-neglect (a refusal or failure to provide him- or herself with adequate food, water, clothing, shelter, personal hygiene, medication, or safety) are examples of elder abuse (U.S. Department of Health and Human Services, n.d.). According to the best available estimates, between 1 and 2 million Americans over the age of 65 have been injured, exploited, or otherwise mistreated by someone on whom they depended for care or protection. This may be an underestimation because victims of elder abuse rarely

report such incidences, and they are not likely to be seen in public where others may report their concerns. The older person may fear being abandoned by the very person responsible for the abuse or may be afraid of further abuse. Cognitive impairment may impede the individual's ability to report abuse. Case Illustration 14-8 describes a tragic but all-too-common tale of elder abuse.

Behavioral Techniques and Humanistic Philosophy

Behavioral techniques used by both professionals and caregivers can greatly increase the comfort and safety of not only the older adult, but also those around him or her. Box 14-1 outlines helpful strategies for dealing with people with dementia. However, conflict can occur between a behavioral approach, which emphasizes safety of the older adult, and a humanistic philosophy, which emphasizes choice and respect for the older adult. The *Global Alzheimer's Disease Charter* (ADI, 2008) emphasizes the importance of a humanistic, client-centered approach with the following statements:

- "I have a voice and should have a say in the care that I am given, for as long as I can."
- "People looking after me should know about my life, family, and history so they can provide personalized care that's right for me. My care should be shaped around my personality, preferences and lifestyle." (p. 1)

CASE ILLUSTRATION 14-7: MRS. CHRISTIE—1 YEAR LATER

The family arguments about Mrs. Christie living alone have escalated. In the past year, she has fallen off a step stool while reaching for something in a high cabinet; gotten lost while shopping, although she was able to call a neighbor for help; and was hospitalized once for dehydration. She said the doctors told her to stop drinking so much tea and start drinking more water, which she says she now does.

Mrs. Christie's oldest daughter is especially upset by what she sees as her mother's stubbornness and takes the drastic move to apply to the courts to be named her conservator. After a comprehensive psychiatric and physical evaluation, the courts turn down the daughter's request, stating that Mrs. Christie is aware of the consequences of her actions and is competent to make her own decisions. The psychiatric team recommends family counseling for the mother and daughter to be able to make compromises regarding Mrs. Christie's activities and minimize the family stress.

Discussion

Mrs. Christie is asserting her right of free choice, and her daughter's well-meaning, but misguided, attempts to control her mother's actions have created considerable distress. Family intervention, including psychological counseling and occupational therapy, can help this family understand the mother's needs and develop adaptive strategies in daily activities to ease the daughter's worry and increase Mrs. Christie's safety in the home and community.

CASE ILLUSTRATION 14-8: THE ABUSE OF MR. DEMPSEY

Mr. Dempsey is an 82-year-old former prizefighter with Parkinson's disease and dementia. His once-strong physique is now quite frail. Mr. Dempsey is unable to walk, eat, or use the toilet without assistance, and he is sometimes incontinent. Mr. Dempsey lives with his son, Charlie, in a small, run-down flat. Charlie greatly resents having to "clean up Dad's messes and put up with his babbling." However, Charlie is out of work and depends on his father's Social Security check for income. Charlie's resentment often turns to rage, especially when he has been drinking. On several occasions, he has punched his father, but more often, Charlie ignores his father's physical needs, sometimes forgetting to feed him or change his clothes and bed sheets.

Discussion

Elder abuse can take many forms, and it is not uncommon for the abuser to financially benefit from the relationship. Victims are usually either incapable of reporting the crime or are too frightened to do so. There is also a high incidence of denial from both the abuser and the victim. Assessment of potential elder abuse requires strong observation skills and an understanding of the physiology of age-related diseases. The level of force needed to injure a frail person is minimal, and the consequences of improper care can lead to myriad serious health consequences. In the United States, it is required that all health professionals report suspected abuse to Adult Protective Services.

Prevention and Health Maintenance

A phenomenological study with elderly Swedish women (Hedelin & Strandmark, 2001) found that "the essence of mental health is the experience of confirmation, trust and confidence in the future, as well as a zest for life, development, and involvement in one's relationship to oneself and to others" (p. 9). This finding concurs with the criteria for quality of life and eloquently gives us important guidelines for prevention and health maintenance interventions for the older adult.

Although occupation is the cornerstone of occupational therapy intervention, the well elderly study by Clark et al. (1997) suggests that activity, or "keeping busy," alone is insufficient for health maintenance or promotion. Rather, a systematic application of occupational therapy principles is needed, which includes highly individualized programs (even when conducted in a group setting), instruction in life management skills, and choice of occupations that are viewed as meaningful and health promoting. This study showed significant results of preventative occupational therapy in many areas, including improvement in general mental health and physical functioning as well as increased social functioning and activity, vitality, and life satisfaction. A subsequent study (Clark et al., 2012) supported the beneficial effects of a lifestyle-oriented occupational therapy intervention for improving vitality, social functioning, mental health, composite mental functioning, life

Box 14-1. Approaches to Dealing With Challenging Behaviors

Dealing with troubling behaviors can be very frustrating for both the individual with dementia and the family or caregiver. Creativity, flexibility, patience, and compassion will help the caregiver to successfully interact with and manage challenging behaviors. Although we cannot change the person, we can try to accommodate the behavior rather than try to control the behavior. For example, it the person insists on sleeping on the floor, place a mattress on the floor to make him or her more comfortable. Changing our behavior (or the physical environment) will often result in a positive change in behavior of the individual.

AGGRESSION AND ANGER

- Assure the individual who behaves aggressively that he or she is okay, that you understand that he or she cannot help him- or herself.
- Approach the individual slowly, in full view.
- Speak in a soothing, reassuring voice. Explain in short, simple statements what you are going to do, such as, "I'm going to help you sit down."
- Distract the person with a snack or an activity.
- Sit or stand a little to the side rather than face the person directly. You are less intimidating this way. Do not confront the individual with his or her behavior, and do not try to restrain the person during a period of agitation.
- Be prepared to accept some insults and verbal abuse.
- Ask yourself if too much is being expected of the individual.
- Maintain structure by keeping the same routines. Keep furniture in the same place.
- Try soothing music or reading, or provide familiar, comforting smells (e.g., bread baking, potpourri).

CONFUSION

- Provide a nightlight to help the person see and locate familiar things and prevent falls in the dark; protect against wandering.
- Consider the side effects of some sedatives and cold remedies as well as prescribed drugs.
- Encourage reminiscence. Gently assist with keeping facts reasonably accurate and related to the past.
- Use communication rich in reminders, cues, gestures, and physical guiding (if appropriate) to increase personal awareness. Keep explanations simple.
- Avoid unrealistic promises.
- Keep your mood and responses consistent; provide frequent reassurance.
- Provide special personal space filled with familiar things where the confused person can go, rest, and feel safe and secure.
- Ask permission if something must be moved or changed. This helps to establish feelings of trust and control.
- Overprotection leads to feelings of helplessness and boredom. Provide reminders, directions, adequate time, and praise for self-care efforts on an adult level.
- Schedule respite care regularly in the caregiving routine so it becomes accepted and predictable.

DEPRESSION

- Respond to the impaired person with kind firmness.
- Try to rebuild self-esteem through reminiscence, participation in activities, and decisions. Notice pictures and mementos. Ask about them and listen.
- Alert the person's doctor; medications may help.
- Spend time with the person. Do not ignore quiet, uncomplaining individuals.
- Encourage him or her to talk freely.
- Be familiar with the factors that predispose people to depression. They include problems with health, living situation, losses, and family history of depressive illness.
- A gentle touch with a reassuring smile projects a caring attitude.

(continued)

Box 14-1 (continued). Approaches to Dealing With Challenging Behaviors

HOARDING, RUMMAGING BEHAVIOR

Because of memory loss, people with dementia frequently look for something that is "missing" (e.g., rooms, clothes, personal items). These things may not look familiar, so they are constantly looking for familiar things.

- Do not scold or try to rationalize with the person.
- Distract the impaired person when he or she is somewhere he or she is not supposed to be.
- Learn the impaired person's hiding places.

INCONTINENCE

- Establish a routine for using the toilet.
- Schedule fluid intake. Limit intake in the evening before bedtime.
- Use signs to show which door leads to the bathroom.
- Use easy-to-remove clothing.

REPETITIVE QUESTIONING

Distraction often helps to redirect the individual to another topic.

SLEEPLESSNESS/SUNDOWNER'S SYNDROME

This occurs when impaired people become confused, restless, and insecure late in the afternoon and after dark.

- Set up a daily routine. It will reduce anxiety about decision making and what happens next.
- Increase daytime activities, especially physical exercise.
- Alternate activity with programmed rest.
- Reduce all stimuli during rest periods.
- Strive to keep daily activities within the person's coping ability.
- Plan for afternoon and evening hours to be quiet and calm; provide structured, quiet activity such as a walk outdoors and listening to soothing music.
- Turn on lights well before sunset and close the curtains at dusk. This may help reduce confusion. Keep a nightlight in the person's room, hallway, and bathroom.
- Make sure the living environment is safe: block off stairs with gates, lock doors, put away dangerous items.

SUSPICIOUSNESS, DISTRUST

This occurs most often with people with dementia when they cannot make sense of what is happening.

- Avoid grand gestures and promises that cannot be carried out.
- Do not argue about or rationally explain disappearances of the person's possessions.
- Offer to look for an item if the person says that it is missing, then distract him or her to another activity.
- Try nonverbal reassurances such as a gentle touch. Reassure the person that you understand his or her feelings.
- Learn the person's favorite hiding places.
- Explain to family members and other helpers that suspicious accusations are a part of progressive dementia.

WANDERING

- Does the person need to burn off some energy by going for a walk? If so, escort him or her on the walk. Involve him or her in an exercise group. Make time for regular exercise to minimize restlessness.
- Consider the reasons that the person is walking and try to accommodate that need. Although walking may appear aimless, it most certainly has a purpose behind it, even if the person with dementia cannot explain it.
- Minimize risks; create a safe area for him or her to walk.
- Set up simple alarms so that the individual cannot leave the area without your knowledge.

(continued)

BOX 14-1 (CONTINUED). APPROACHES TO DEALING WITH CHALLENGING BEHAVIORS

WANDERING (CONTINUED)

- Use a barrier like a curtain or colored streamer to mask the door. A stop sign or "do not enter" sign often helps.
- Put away essential items such as coats, purses, glasses, keys. The individual may not consider going out without them.
- Divert the person from wanting to walk by giving him or her a clear task to perform.
- Make sure that the person has a contact phone number on him or her at all times.
- Tell neighbors and other people in advance that the person may get confused or lost.
- Always have a recent photograph of the person with dementia on hand in case he or she does wander off.

satisfaction, and reducing depressive symptoms for ethnically diverse elders. Based on this study, a plethora of programs have been developed addressing lifestyle redesign.

Although substantial evidence that shows the effectiveness of occupational therapy in prevention and health maintenance now exists, the conventional, medically oriented model often does not allow occupational therapists to use their full repertoire of skills. Occupational therapists must be proactive in advocating for change in health care systems and in increasing professional recognition in order to provide necessary and meaningful intervention for the large older adult population.

SUMMARY

Although the majority of older adults are well elderly, the devastating and global effects of chronic and mental illness in the older population have significant consequences for the individual, family, and society as a whole. Given the demographic data provided in this chapter, it is clear that there is very high demand for occupational therapists to work with older adults.

Occupational therapists have a unique role in preserving and fostering the mental and physical health of the older adult. The emphasis on meaningful occupation in a context that is focused on quality-of-life issues and prevention as well as restoration of function is a critical component of health care for the older adult.

REFERENCES

Administration on Aging. (2016). *A profile of older Americans: 2016.* Washington, DC: U.S. Department of Health and Human Services. Retrieved from https://www.acl.gov/sites/default/files/Aging%20and%20Disability%20in%20America/2016-Profile.pdf

Alzheimer's Association. (n.d.). *What is dementia?* Retrieved from https://www.alz.org/what-is-dementia.asp

Alzheimer's Association. (2018). *2018 Alzheimer's disease facts and figures.* Retrieved from https://www.alz.org/media/HomeOffice/Facts%20and%20Figures/facts-and-figures.pdf

Alzheimer's Disease International. (2008). *Global Alzheimer's Disease Charter.* Retrieved from https://www.alz.co.uk/global-charter

Alzheimer's Disease International. (2016). *World Alzheimer's Report 2016.* Retrieved from https://www.alz.co.uk/research/world-report-2016

American Occupational Therapy Association. (2014). Occupational therapy practice framework: Domain and process (3rd ed.). *American Journal of Occupational Therapy, 68,* S1-S40.

American Psychological Association. (2014). Guidelines for psychological practice with older adults. *American Psychologist, 69*(1), 34-65.

Aubin, G., Hachey, R., & Mercier, C. (1999). Meaning of daily activities and subjective quality of life in people with severe mental illness. *Scandinavian Journal of Occupational Therapy, 6,* 53-62.

Baum, C. M. (1995). The contribution of occupation to function in persons with Alzheimer's disease. *Journal of Occupational Science, 2,* 59-67.

Blackburn, P., Wilkins-Ho, M., & Wiese, B. (2017). Depression in older adults: Diagnosis and management. *British Columbia Medical Journal, 59*(3), 171-177.

Clark, F., Azen, S. P., Zemke, R., Jackson, J., Carlson, M., Mandel, D., ... Lipson, L. (1997). Occupational therapy for independent-living older adults: A randomized controlled study. *Journal of the American Medical Association, 278,* 1321-1326.

Clark, F., Jackson, J., Carlson, M., Chou, C. P., Cherry, B. J., Jordan-Marsh, M., ... Azen, S. P. (2012). Effectiveness of a lifestyle intervention in promoting the well-being of independently living older people: Results of the Well Elderly 2 Randomised Controlled Trial. *Journal of Epidemiology and Community Health, 66,* 782-790.

Clay, S. W. (2010). Treatment of addiction in the elderly. *Aging Health, 6*(2), 177-189.

Cordell, C. B., Borson, S., Boustani, M., Chodosh, J., Reuben, D., Verghese, J., ... Fried, L. B. (2013). Alzheimer's Association recommendations for operationalizing the detection of cognitive impairment during the Medicare Annual Wellness Visit in a primary care setting. *Alzheimer's & Dementia, 9,* 141-150.

Cullen, B., Ward, J., Graham, N. A., Deary, I. J., Pell, J. P., Smith, D. J., & Evans, J. J. (2016). Prevalences and correlates of cognitive impairment in euthymic adults with bipolar disorder: A systematic review. *Journal of Affective Disorders, 205,* 165-181.

Depp, C. A., & Jeste, D. V. (2004). Bipolar disorder in older adults: A critical review. *Bipolar Disorders, 6,* 343-367.

Donnellan, W. J., Bennett, K. M., & Soulsby, L. K. (2017). Family close but friends closer: Exploring social support and resilience in older spousal carers. *Aging and Mental Health, 21*(11), 1222-1228.

Fong, T. G., Tulebaev, S. R., & Inouye, S. K. (2009). Delirium in elderly adults: Diagnosis, prevention and treatment. *Nature Reviews Neurology, 5*(4), 210-220.

Fuller-Thompson, E., & Lacombe-Duncan, A. (2016). Understanding the association between chronic obstructive pulmonary disease and current anxiety: A population-based study. *COPD: Journal of Chronic Pulmonary Disease, 13*(5), 622-631.

Geriatric Mental Health Foundation. (n.d.). *Anxiety and older Americans: Overcoming worry and fear.* Retrieved from http://www.aagponline.org/index.php?src=gendocs&ref=anxiety

Gum, A. M., King-Kallimanis, B., & Kohn, R. (2009). Prevalence of mood, anxiety and substance-abuse disorders for older Americans in the national comorbidity survey-replication. *American Journal of Geriatric Psychiatry, 17*(9), 769-781.

Hall, C. (2002). Special considerations for the geriatric population. *Critical Care Nursing Clinics of North America, 14*(4), 427-434.

HealthCommunities.com (2015). *Dementia.* Retrieved from http://www.healthcommunities.com/dementia/dementia-overview-types.shtml

Health in Aging. (2017). *Aging & Health A to Z: Delirium.* Retrieved from http://www.healthinaging.org/aging-and-health-a-to-z/topic:delirium

Hedelin, B., & Strandmark, M. (2001). The meaning of mental health from elderly women's perspectives: A basis for health promotion. *Perspectives in Psychiatric Care, 37*(1), 7-14.

Hegeman, J. M., de Waal, M. W., Comijs, H. C., Kok, R. M., & van der Mast, R. C. (2014). Depression in later life: A more somatic presentation? *Journal of Affective Disorders, 170,* 196-202.

Hoppes, S., Davis, L. A., & Thompson, D. (2003). Environmental effects on the assessment of people with dementia: A pilot study. *American Journal of Occupational Therapy, 57*(4), 396-402.

Johnco, C., Knight, A., Tadic, D., & Wuthrich, V. M. (2015). Psychometric properties of the Geriatric Anxiety Inventory (GAI) and its short-form (GAI-SF) in a clinical and non-clinical sample of older adults. *International Psychogeriatrics, 27*(7), 1089-1097.

Koychev, I., & Ebmeier, K. P. (2016). Anxiety in older adults often goes undiagnosed. *Practitioner, 260*(1789), 17-20.

Law, M., Steinwender, S., & Leclair, L. (1998). Occupation, health and well-being. *Canadian Journal of Occupational Therapy, 65*(2), 81-91.

Liu, L., Gou, Z., & Zuo, J. (2016). Social support mediates loneliness and depression in elderly people. *Journal of Health Psychology, 21*(5), 750-758.

Mayo Clinic. (2018). *Delirium.* Retrieved from https://www.mayoclinic.org/diseases-conditions/delirium/symptons-causes/syc-20371386

Midden, A. J., & Mast, B. T. (2018). Differential item functioning analysis of items on the Geriatric Depression Scale-15 based on the presence or absence of cognitive impairment. *Aging and Mental Health, 22*(9), 1136-1142. doi: 10.1080/13607863.2017.1337716.

National Institute of Mental Health. (2017). *Transforming the understanding and treatment of mental illness.* Retrieved from https://www.nimh.nih.gov/health/statistics/mental-illness.shtml.

Norstrand, J. A., Glicksman, A., Lubben, J., & Kleban, M. (2012). The role of the social environment on physical and mental health of older adults. *Journal of Housing for the Elderly, 26,* 290-307.

Office of Policy Development and Research, U.S. Department of Housing and Urban Development. (2013). *Aging in place: Facilitating choice and independence.* Retrieved from https://www.huduser.gov/portal/periodicals/em/fall13/highlight1.html#title

Pimouguet, C., Le Goff, M., Wittwer, J., Dartigues, J. F., & Helmer, C. (2017). Benefits of occupational therapy in dementia patients: Findings from a real-world occupational study. *Journal of Alzheimer's Disease, 56*(2), 509-517.

Popeo, D., Blazek, M., & Lehmann, S. (2017). Revisiting the 2012 IOM Report: A renewed call for action. *American Journal of Geriatric Psychiatry, 25*(3), S21-S22.

Rains, J., & Chee, N. (2017). The role of occupational and physiotherapy in multi-model approach to tackling delirium in the intensive care. *Journal of the Intensive Care Society, 18*(4), 318-322.

Reinhardt, M., & Cohen, C. (2015). Late-life psychosis: Diagnosis and treatment. *Current Psychiatry Report, 17*(1), 1-13.

Reisberg, B., Ferris, S. H., & Crook, T. (1983). Global Deterioration Scale. In B. Reisberg (Ed.), *A guide to Alzheimer's disease.* New York, NY: Free Press.

Reynolds, K., Pietrzak, R. H., El-Gabalawy, R., Mackenzie, C. S., & Sareen, J. (2015). Prevalence of psychiatric disorders in U.S. older adults: Findings from a nationally representative survey. *World Psychiatry, 14*(1), 74-81.

Seegert, L. (2017). Social isolation, loneliness negatively affect health for seniors. *Association of Health Care Journalists.* Retrieved from https://healthjournalism.org/blog/2017/03/social-isolation-loneliness-negatively-affect-health-for-seniors/.

Sheikh, J. I., & Yesavage, J. A. (1986). Geriatric Depression Scale (GDS): Recent evidence and development of a shorter version. *Clinical Gerontologist: The Journal of Aging and Mental Health, 5*(1-2), 165-173. http://dx.doi.org/10.1300/J018v05n01_09

Simoni-Wastila, L., & Yang, H. K. (2006). Psychoactive drug abuse in older adults. *American Journal of Geriatric Pharmacotherap, 4*(4), 380-394.

Skoog, I. (2011). Psychiatric disorders in the elderly. *Canadian Journal of Psychiatry, 56*(7), 387-397.

Sviden, G., Wikstrom, B. M., & Hjortsjo-Norberg, M. (2002). Elderly person's reflections on relocating to living at sheltered housing. *Scandinavian Journal of Occupational Therapy, 9,* 10-16.

Tzouvara, V., Papdopoulos, C., & Randhawa, G. (2018). Self-stigma experiences among older adults with mental health problems residing in long-term care facilities: A qualitative study. *Issues in Mental Health Nursing, 39*(5), 403-410.

United Nations, Department of Economic and Social Affairs, Population Division. (2015). *World Population Ageing 2015.* Retrieved from http://www.un.org/en/development/desa/population/publications/pdf/ageing/WPA2015_Report.pdf

University of Michigan Alcohol Research Center. (1991). *Short Michigan Alcohol Screening Test—Geriatric Version (Short MAST-G).* Ann Arbor, MI: University of Michigan.

U.S. Department of Health and Human Services. (n.d.). *Elder abuse.* Retrieved from https://eldercare.acl.gov/Public/Resources/Factsheets/Elder_Abuse.aspx

Walker, B. A., Allen, J., Koch, M., Sprehe, C., & Webber, K. T. (2017). Identifying effective strategies in occupational therapy to support persons with Alzheimer's disease and their caregivers. *American Journal of Occupational Therapy, 71*(4 Suppl 1).

World Health Organization. (2013). *International classification of functioning, disability and health (ICF).* Geneva, Switzerland: Author.

World Health Organization. (2017). *Mental health of older adults.* Retrieved from http://www.who.int/mediacentre/factsheets/fs381/en/

Yesavage, J. A., Brink, T. L., Rose, T. L., Lum, O., Huang, V., Adey, M., & Leirer, V. O. (1983). Development and validation of a geriatric depression screening scale: A preliminary report. *Journal of Psychiatric Research, 17,* 37-49.

Zisberg, A. (2017). Anxiety and depression in older patients: The role of culture and acculturation. *International Journal for Equity in Health, 16*(177), 1-10.

SUGGESTED RESOURCES

Alzheimer's Association: http://www.alz.org/index.asp

National Council for Aging Care: Aging in Place Initiative: http://www.aginginplaceinitiative.org/

U.S. National Library of Medicine MedlinePlus: Seniors' Health: https://medlineplus.gov/seniorshealth.html

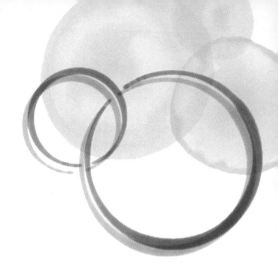

Financial Disclosures

Tiffany (Debra) Boggis has no financial or proprietary interest in the materials presented herein.

Dr. Elizabeth Cara has no financial or proprietary interest in the materials presented herein.

Dr. Elizabeth Carley has no financial or proprietary interest in the materials presented herein.

Dr. Bernadette Hattjar has no financial or proprietary interest in the materials presented herein.

William L. Lambert has no financial or proprietary interest in the materials presented herein.

Dr. Anne MacRae has no financial or proprietary interest in the materials presented herein.

Dr. Karen McCarthy has no financial or proprietary interest in the materials presented herein.

Dr. Jerilyn (Gigi) Smith has no financial or proprietary interest in the materials presented herein.

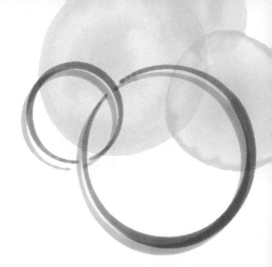

Index